HEALTH PROGRAM
MANAGEMENT

For Carolyn
Praiseworthy

HEALTH PROGRAM MANAGEMENT

FROM DEVELOPMENT THROUGH EVALUATION

Second Edition

Beaufort B. Longest, Jr.

JB JOSSEY-BASS™

A Wiley Brand

Published by Jossey-Bass
A Wiley Brand
One Montgomery Street, Suite 1200, San Francisco, CA 94104-4594—www.josseybass.com

Jossey-Bass books and products are available through most bookstores. To contact Jossey-Bass directly call our Customer Care Department within the U.S. at 800-956-7739, outside the U.S. at 317-572-3986, or fax 317-572-4002.

Wiley publishes in a variety of print and electronic formats and by print-on-demand. Some material included with standard print versions of this book may not be included in e-books or in print-on-demand. If this book refers to media such as a CD or DVD that is not included in the version you purchased, you may download this material at http://booksupport.wiley.com. For more information about Wiley products, visit www.wiley.com.

Library of Congress Cataloging-in-Publication Data

Longest, Beaufort B., Jr., author.
 [Managing health programs and projects]
 Health program management: from development through evaluation/Beaufort B. Longest, Jr. – Second edition.
     p.; cm.
 Preceded by Managing health programs and projects/Beaufort B. Longest Jr. 1st ed. c2004.
 Includes bibliographical references and index.
   ISBN 978-1-118-83470-1 (pbk.) – ISBN 978-1-118-83463-3 (pdf) –
ISBN 978-1-118-83476-3 (epub)
 I. Title.
 [DNLM: 1. Health Planning–methods. 2. Health Services Administration. 3. Organizational Innovation. 4. Program Evaluation. 5. Total Quality Management. W 84.1]
 RA427
 610.68′5–dc23
                                                                                            2014015932

Printed in the United States of America

SECOND EDITION

PB Printing
10   9   8   7   6   5   4   3   2   1

CONTENTS

LIST OF FIGURES, TABLES, AND EXHIBITS

Figures

Tables

Exhibits

This book is about managing health programs. Effective management of programs is important because these are mechanisms through which a great many health services are organized and provided in both the public health and health care sectors. I provide information drawn from management research to assist you in developing a comprehensive approach to the practice of management in health programs. A focused reader will take away a solid overview of the current best practices in management that apply to managing health programs.

Health programs target any of the determinants of health. They can focus on some aspect of the physical environments in which people live and work, on human behavior, on biology, on the social factors that affect people, or on the health services offered to them. There is therefore a broad array of health programs. For example, at the prevention end of the health services spectrum, people receive information about safe sex practices or how to eat healthier in the context of health education programs. At the advanced acute care end of the spectrum of services, people receive kidney transplants within the context of transplant programs.

A persistent, decades-long trend has created ever larger and more elaborate structures that organize, deliver, and finance health services throughout the industrialized world. Current manifestations of this phenomenon can be seen in major public health agencies, such as the California Department of Public Health (www.cdph.ca.gov), or large health services organizations, such as the Massachusetts General Hospital (www.massgeneral.org). Within these large and complex structures, however, health services are provided directly through relatively small units called programs.

A substantial literature exists pertaining to the management of large and complex public- and private-sector health agencies, organizations, and systems. I have contributed to this literature myself. Nevertheless, there is a relative paucity of literature about managing at the level of health programs, where so much of the direct delivery of health services occurs. With this book, I seek to partially address this imbalance.

The intended audience for this book includes students in public health, in health services management, and in a wide variety of health professions who want to prepare themselves for the challenges of managing health programs. Even those who aspire to leadership positions in large agencies, organizations, and systems may begin their management career at the level of programs. The book will also be useful for those who already occupy a program management position, because it comprehensively and systematically presents current information about management.

Programs are defined in this book as organizational units intended to accomplish one or more objectives through a plan of action that describes what work is to be done, by whom, when, and how, as well as what resources will be used. Programs are embedded in organizations and should be of benefit to the larger host organization. Program management is defined as the activities through which the mission and objectives of a program are established and pursued by means of various processes using human and other resources.

As a way of organizing the discussion of program management, and to give a sense of the structure of the book itself, I present in Chapter 1 a model of the activities managers engage in as they manage programs. These activities are divided into two sets: core activities and facilitative activities. All health program managers engage in three core activities as they perform management work: developing/strategizing, designing, and leading. In addition, managers also engage in other activities that facilitate and support the accomplishment of a program's mission and objectives. Program managers engage extensively in such facilitative activities as decision making and communicating as they carry out their management work. Increasingly, they also engage in managing quality, marketing, and evaluating. Individual chapters of the book are devoted to each of these activities, presenting in-depth information about each of them. A brief précis of each chapter follows.

Chapter 1, "The Work of Managers in Health Programs," contains key definitions and a background discussion of programs and program management. The work of managers is considered in terms of the core activities in which all managers engage as they do management work: developing/ strategizing, designing, and leading. Consideration of this work is extended to include managers' facilitative activities: decision making, communicating, managing quality, marketing, and evaluating. The entire set of core and facilitative activities in management work is modeled graphically in Figure 1.4. This figure is the chapter's centerpiece, depicting the core and facilitative activities of management work as an integrated and interactive set of activities. There is also a discussion of the roles played by managers and the competencies necessary to manage health programs well.

Chapter 2, "Developing/Strategizing the Future," emphasizes the initial development and strategizing that bring programs into existence. Developing a program initially simply means conceptualizing the program as a vehicle for delivering services or products that may succeed in the marketplace. In ongoing programs, development pertains to improving established services or products, or to expanding a program's portfolio of services or products. Development triggers strategizing, which is the work that managers do as they establish or revise the specific mission and objectives of a program and plan the means of achieving them.

Chapter 3, "Designing for Effectiveness," is built around discussion of the work managers do when establishing and changing the intentional patterns of relationships among human and other resources within a program, and when establishing and changing the program's relationship to its external environment, including to the larger organizational home in which it is embedded. Attention is also given to designing logic models for programs.

Chapter 4, "Leading to Accomplish Desired Results," describes leading as the work managers do when influencing other participants to contribute to the performance of a program. Emphasis is given to the fact that leading requires managers to help participants be motivated to contribute to programs in positive ways. Attention is given to specific leader behaviors that can improve management in programs.

Chapter 5, "Making Good Management Decisions," emphasizes that decision making permeates all management work. The discussion of decision making represents a turn from core management activities to facilitative activities. Decisions are divided into two subsets: problem-solving decisions and opportunistic decisions. Problem-solving decisions are made to solve existing or anticipated problems. Opportunistic decisions are typically sporadic and arise with opportunities to reshape or advance accomplishment of a program's mission and objectives. Although decision making is defined simply as making a choice from among alternatives, the decision-making process is discussed in terms of seven steps: (1) becoming aware that a decision must be made, whether it stems from a problem or an opportunity; (2) defining in as much detail as possible the problem or opportunity; (3) developing relevant alternatives; (4) assessing the alternatives; (5) choosing from among the alternatives; (6) implementing the decision; and (7) evaluating the decision, and making necessary follow-up decisions.

Chapter 6, "Communicating for Understanding," stresses that communicating activities are also ubiquitous in facilitating a manager's performance of all other management activities. Communicating is discussed as being both vital to the successful performance of management work and a challenge for managers. It is described as an activity that involves senders (individuals, groups, or organizations) conveying ideas, intentions, and information to receivers (also individuals, groups, or organizations). Communication is effective when receivers understand ideas, intentions, or information as senders intend, but several environmental and interpersonal barriers must be overcome to communicate effectively. The communicating activity is discussed as a key to managing relationships with a program's internal and external stakeholders.

Chapter 7, "Managing Quality—Totally," discusses why managers of health programs typically make effectively managing the quality of the services provided a high priority. Quality is important not only to those who use the services of a program, having an important impact on their service-seeking decisions, but also to people who work in programs. This chapter stresses that above all else, managing quality in a health program requires a systematic approach. Three components of what is called a total quality approach to managing quality in health programs are presented: patient/customer focus, continuous improvement, and teamwork.

Chapter 8, "Commercial and Social Marketing," discusses two important ways managers of health programs can use marketing to facilitate program performance. The financial or commercial success of many programs is affected by the use of commercial marketing. In addition, especially in programs focused on health promotion and education, social marketing is used in the provision of services. The classic four Ps of successful commercial marketing strategies are discussed: **p**roduct or service, **p**rice, **p**lace, and **p**romotion, with attention given to an increasingly important fifth P, **p**eople. Social marketing is discussed in terms of using some elements of commercial marketing to influence the voluntary behavior of individuals and groups for their own benefit, and in some instances for the larger society's benefit.

Chapter 9, "Evaluating," discusses health program managers' evaluating activities in terms of collecting and analyzing data and information about a program or some aspect of a program as a basis for making decisions about the program. Managers' reasons for engaging in evaluating activities are discussed, including the following: (1) improving the overall performance of programs, (2) demonstrating accountability to stakeholders and justifying the use of resources, (3) demonstrating the effectiveness of programs in terms of accomplishing missions and objectives, and (4) demonstrating the effectiveness of specific interventions undertaken by programs.

Although it is convenient for purposes of discussion and description to separate into individual chapters the core and facilitative activities that constitute management work, the danger in doing so is that it may incorrectly depict management as a series of separate activities, perhaps performed in a particular sequence. In practice, health program managers engage in these activities in a way that results in an interdependent mosaic. When managers integrate and perform this set of activities well, they are more likely to be satisfied with the performance of their programs and the results achieved. To the extent that reading this book contributes to this occurrence, I will have achieved my purpose in writing it.

An instructor's supplement is available at www.wiley.com/go/longest2e. Additional materials, such as videos, podcasts, and readings, can be found at www.josseybasspublichealth.com. Comments about this book are invited and can be sent to publichealth@wiley.com.

October 2014   Beaufort B. Longest, Jr.
                                                Pittsburgh, Pennsylvania

ACKNOWLEDGMENTS

I wish to acknowledge the contributions made by several people to this book, and to thank them for their involvement. At the University of Pittsburgh, which has been my professional home for thirty-four years, Mark Nordenberg, Arthur Levine, Don Burke, and Mark Roberts provided a supportive environment for scholarship. At Jossey-Bass, Andy Pasternack first saw the potential in this book. Following Andy's untimely death, Seth Schwartz picked up the pieces and made the book happen. I also want to thank Justin Frahm, who managed production flawlessly, and the **very thorough** Francie Jones, for contributing her professional expertise to this project. Reviewers Joseph DeRanieri and Barbara Hernandez provided insightful suggestions, which are greatly appreciated. At home, Carolyn and Butterbean continue to make joy a welcome part of life, for which I am very grateful.

THE AUTHOR

Beaufort B. Longest, Jr., is a professor of health policy and management in the Graduate School of Public Health at the University of Pittsburgh. He is the founding director of Pitt's Health Policy Institute, which he led from 1980 to 2011.

Professor Longest is a fellow of the American College of Healthcare Executives and a member of the Academy of Management, AcademyHealth, and the American Public Health Association. With a doctorate from Georgia State University, he served on the faculty of Northwestern University's Kellogg School of Management before joining the Pitt faculty in 1980. He is an elected member of Beta Gamma Sigma, the international honor society in business, and of the Delta Omega Honor Society in Public Health.

His research on modeling managerial competence, issues of governance in health services organizations, and health policymaking has appeared in numerous peer-reviewed journals, and he is author or coauthor of eleven books and thirty-two chapters in other books. His book *Health Policy-making in the United States,* soon to be published in its sixth edition, is among the most widely used textbooks in health policy and management graduate programs. His book *Managing Health Services Organizations and Systems*, coauthored with Kurt Darr, is now in its sixth edition.

He has consulted for health services organizations and systems, universities, associations, and government agencies on health policy and management issues, and he has served on several editorial and organization boards.

HEALTH PROGRAM
MANAGEMENT

CHAPTER 1

THE WORK OF MANAGERS IN HEALTH PROGRAMS

Much of the pursuit of health occurs through a variety of health programs. For example, when a young adult with type 2 diabetes leads an active and productive life, her health improvements may well be attributed to a program that helps her understand the disease and take an active role in controlling it. When the federal Center for Medicare and Medicaid Innovation established the Innovation Advisors Program, supporting individuals who test and refine new models to drive health delivery system reform, improvements in the delivery system were made more likely (Centers for Medicare and Medicaid Services 2014). When a county health department mounts a project to enroll children in an innovative insurance plan, the impact on those children may be felt throughout a lifetime of better health.

One of the distinguishing characteristics of successful programs is how well their managers perform. This book is about the work program managers do. This chapter provides an overview of management work in health programs, as well as some key definitions and concepts, all of which serve as a framework for navigating the remainder of the book. Management work is described in terms of a set of core activities managers undertake in performing their work—developing/strategizing, designing, and leading—and a set of facilitative activities that also are important to management work—communicating, decision making, managing quality, marketing, and evaluating.

As a backdrop for considering management work, it is important to know that three distinct types of work occur in health programs (Charns and Gittell 2006). Direct work entails the actual provision of services or creation of products by participants in a program. This type of work is done by counselors, nurses, therapists, physicians,

LEARNING OBJECTIVES
After reading this chapter, you should be able to:

- Define health, health programs, and management

- Understand the core and facilitative activities of managers' work

- Understand the roles managers play as they do management work

- Appreciate the underlying competencies demonstrated by managers in doing management work

- Understand the importance of applying well-developed personal ethical standards in doing management work

health educators, and others who form what Mintzberg (1992) classically termed the "operating core" of a program.

A second type of work done in health programs is support work. This work is a necessary adjuvant to the direct work. In health programs, participants performing support work are involved in such activities as fund-raising and development; recruiting patients for a clinical trial; providing legal counsel; or providing marketing, public relations accounting, or financial services for a program.

The third type of work done in health programs is management work. This work involves establishing—often with the direct involvement of others—the mission and objectives a program is intended to achieve, and creating the circumstances through which the direct work, aided by support work, can lead to the accomplishment of that mission and fulfillment of objectives.

An example will clarify the different types of work. A manager may establish one of the objectives of a program as enrolling one thousand children in an innovative insurance plan. The establishment of this objective is management work, as is the training of program participants to help parents or guardians enroll children. The act of enrolling children in the plan is some of the direct work of the program. The manager may also arrange for publicity surrounding the plan to increase awareness and encourage enrollment. The provision of publicity is support work, although arranging for the publicity is management work.

As we will see in this chapter, one useful way to assess and study management work is in terms of the activities managers engage in as they do this work. Often in the management literature the term *functions* is used instead of *activities* (Daft 2014; Marquis and Huston 2012). I will generally use the term activities, although the two words are interchangeable in this context. I will also discuss the roles that managers play in performing their work, as well as the competencies needed to do management work well.

Key Definitions

Before considering management work in more depth, it is useful to establish several key definitions to describe health and health determinants, health programs, and program management.

Health and Health Determinants

The World Health Organization (www.who.int/en/) has provided a long-standing definition of *health* as the "state of complete physical, mental, and social well-being, and not merely the absence of disease or infirmity" (World

Health Organization 1948, 100). The state of health in human beings is a function of *health determinants*, which are a "range of personal, social, economic, and environmental factors that influence health" at both the individual level and the population level (U.S. Department of Health and Human Services 2014). The wide variety of determinants means that health programs have an enormous range of possible foci.

Health determinants for individuals or populations include the physical environments in which people live and work; their behaviors; and their biology (genetic makeup, family history, and physical and mental health problems acquired during life). Health determinants also include a host of social factors, which include economic circumstances; one's socioeconomic position in society; income distribution; discrimination based on race or ethnicity, gender, sexual orientation, or some other characteristic; as well as the availability of social networks and social support. Finally, the health services to which people have access also are health determinants (U.S. Department of Health and Human Services 2014). Health programs can be focused on any of these determinants, as well as on combinations of them.

Health Programs

A *program* is generally defined as an organizational unit intended to accomplish one or more objectives through a plan of action that describes what work is to be done, by whom, when, and how, as well as what resources will be used. Programs are embedded in organizations and exist to be of benefit to the larger host organization. Figure 1.1 depicts a program embedded in a host health services organization.

Host organizations can be very large, involving thousands of participants. Expansive integrated health systems, large foundations, agencies of the federal government, or state health departments, for example, are large organizations that house numerous health programs. Interestingly, even though programs are typically much smaller than such organizations, they are in fact themselves organizations. Therefore, another way to define programs is as organizations, albeit usually small ones. They are organizations in that they meet the standard definition of an organization: groups of people and other resources formally associated with each other through intentionally designed patterns of relationships to pursue desired results. Wholey, Hatry, and Newcomer (2010, 5) defined a program as "a set of resources and activities directed toward one or more common goals, typically under the direction of a single manager or management team." Because health programs are embedded within larger organizations, it is useful to think of these programs as organizations within organizations.

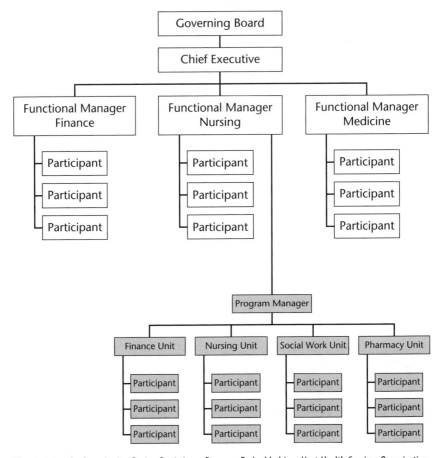

Figure 1.1   An Organization Design Depicting a Program Embedded in a Host Health Services Organization

Programs that pertain to any of the determinants of health noted earlier are by definition **health programs**. Thus health programs address some aspect of the physical environments in which people live and work, their behaviors, their biology, the social factors that affect them, or the health services they receive.

The terms *programs* and *projects* are sometimes used interchangeably, although they do not refer to the same things. The differences between programs and projects are rather subjective and pertain mostly to scope and longevity. Some people view projects as subsets of programs. For example, the Project Management Institute (2013, 165) views a program as a "group of related projects." The institute defines a project as "a temporary endeavor undertaken to create a unique product, service, or result" (168). In this view, projects are smaller and more focused than programs. In addition, projects are typically more time limited. That is, a project has a predetermined life

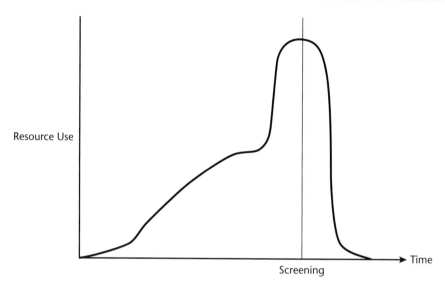

Figure 1.2   A Project's Life Cycle

cycle, and a program may have a more indeterminate life cycle. The duration of a project is scheduled at its beginning, although some run for a longer or shorter duration than originally planned because of changing circumstances.

Figure 1.2 graphically depicts a project's life cycle. Assume that the project is intended to involve conducting diabetes screenings at an annual health fair. The curve reflects the consumption of human, financial, and material resources during the life cycle of the project. A gradual buildup of activity during which arrangements are made for the conduct of the screenings precedes the peak of activity when the actual conduct of the screenings occurs, and the peak is followed immediately by the project's conclusion and termination.

Examples of Health Programs and Projects

Examples of health programs include those in cancer care, cardiac rehabilitation, data and statistics, geriatrics, health education, home care, palliative care, prevention, health promotion, research and development, substance abuse, wellness, and women's health. Less obvious examples of health programs include housing programs, job training programs, or programs to clean up the physical environment, as well as programs aimed at reducing ignorance, illiteracy, discrimination, or poverty. These less obvious examples are also health programs because they address one or another health determinant. Appendix A provides a brief description of a health program, the Global Health Program, embedded in a host organization, the Bill and Melinda Gates Foundation.

Examples of health projects include research or demonstration projects pertaining to a health determinant, as well as projects to promote seat belt use, healthier eating, or safe sex practices. Projects also may be designed to achieve some specific physical or intellectual purpose within a host program or organization, such as designing and equipping a laboratory, training a staff in a new protocol or to use some new technology, designing an information system, or developing a strategic plan or a new accounting system. Appendix B provides a brief overview of a health project, the Mass General Care Management Project, which. involves testing ways to improve coordination of care for Medicare patients.

Program Management

The definition of *program management* begins with a generic definition of *management*, and there are many. Daft (2014, 6), for example, defined management in any organizational setting as "the attainment of organizational goals in an effective and efficient manner through planning, organizing, leading, and controlling organizational resources." In another source, management is defined as "the process, composed of interrelated social and technical functions and activities, occurring within a formal organizational setting for the purpose of helping establish objectives and accomplishing the predetermined objectives through the use of human and other resources" (Longest and Darr 2014, 255).

Building on these and other similar generic definitions of management, and in light of the earlier discussion of management work in terms of the activities of managers, program management is here defined as the activities through which the mission and objectives of a program are established and pursued by means of various processes using human and other resources.

Managers, when doing management work, often with the help of other participants in a program or in the organization in which it is embedded, seek to accomplish the following tasks:

- Analyzing variables in the program's external environment, assessing their importance and relevance, and responding to them appropriately
- Determining the program's mission and objectives
- Assembling the resources necessary to achieve the desired results
- Determining the processes necessary to accomplish the mission and objectives, and ensuring that the processes are carried out effectively and efficiently
- Leading others in contributing to accomplishment of the mission and objectives

The Work of Program Managers in Terms of Core and Facilitative Activities

In performing *management work*, managers engage in an interrelated set of activities and play a variety of interconnected roles, both of which are facilitated by possession and use of certain competencies. All three perspectives on management work are considered in this chapter. Subsequently, the book itself is organized around the activities that program managers engage in as they manage. These activities are divided into a set of core activities and a set of facilitative activities that together constitute program management work.

Throughout this chapter and in the more in-depth discussions that follow in the book, the descriptions of, and prescriptions and recommendations pertaining to, the activities in which program managers engage reflect as much as possible evidence-based management, also known as EBMgt (Briner, Denyer, and Rousseau 2009; Kovner, Fine, and D'Aquila 2009; Rousseau 2014), or the more specific evidence-based health services management, also known as EBHSM (Kovner and Rundall 2006). The practice of management is not as evidence based as it should be, although it is moving in this direction. In essence, practicing evidence-based management means that managers, like clinicians practicing evidence-based medicine, ground their professional work in empirical evidence from management research (Walshe and Rundall 2001).

Core Activities in Program Management Work

All health program managers engage in three *core management activities* as they perform management work: developing/strategizing, designing, and leading. This conceptualization of management work is similar to one developed by Zuckerman and Dowling (1997), although it extends their conceptualization and applies it specifically to managing health programs. In performing these core activities, managers also engage in other activities that facilitate and support accomplishment of the core activities. These facilitative activities are briefly discussed later in this chapter, and a subsequent chapter is devoted to each of them. The core developing/strategizing, designing, and leading activities of program management work are modeled in Figure 1.3, and are discussed briefly in the following subsections as an introduction to the more detailed discussions of these activities in subsequent chapters.

All managers perform these core activities regardless of their hierarchical level in an organizational setting. There are of course differences

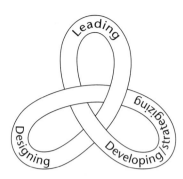

Figure 1.3   Model of the Core Activities in Program Management Work

between the work of managers at the level of programs and the work of the president or chief executive officer (CEO) of a large host organization. But the work of managers at both, and other, levels can be considered in terms of this set of core activities.

In considering management work in terms of these activities, it is convenient to separate them so that each can be discussed independently; but management work should not be viewed as a series of separate activities sequentially performed. In practice, a manager performs these activities simultaneously, not sequentially, and as part of an interdependent mosaic of activities. The separation of management activities is necessary for the purposes of our discussion, but it is an artificial treatment of the reality of managing.

Developing/Strategizing

Programs come into existence because someone develops them and strategizes their future. Developing a program initially simply means conceptualizing the program as a vehicle for delivering services or products that may succeed in the marketplace. In ongoing programs, development pertains to improving established services or products or to expanding a program's portfolio of services or products. Development triggers strategizing, which is the work that managers do as they establish or revise the specific mission and objectives of a program and plan the means of achieving them.

Although the relative degree of the work's complexity may vary, managers of all programs engage in *developing/strategizing* as part of performing their management work. This activity not only results in decisions about the existence, revision, purpose, and direction of programs but also helps managers adapt their programs to the challenges and opportunities presented by continuously and often turbulently changing external environments (Ginter, Duncan, and Swayne 2013).

The aim of developing/strategizing is to achieve an integrated set of direct, support, and management work sufficient to establish and achieve the results envisioned for a program. Effective developing/strategizing lays the foundation for designing effective relationships among people and other resources that are necessary to achieve desired results. It also provides the blueprint managers use in leading others in contributing to their achievement.

There are a number of reasons why developing/strategizing activities are so crucial to the success of health programs. Perhaps none is more important than the simple fact that developing/strategizing focuses attention on desired results. When done well, developing/strategizing activities yield statements of intended results, expressed as a mission and objectives, and help conceptualize the means through which these can be achieved. In this way, developing/strategizing contributes to the coordination and integration of the actions of all participants in a program toward shared purposes.

Another reason why developing/strategizing is important in ongoing programs is that it helps offset the pervasive uncertainty that health programs face. When managers anticipate the future and plan for contingencies that can be imagined or foreseen, they greatly reduce the possibility of being caught unprepared. Uncertainty cannot be eliminated, but it can be prepared for through developing/strategizing. Conditions of uncertainty require that programs be adaptable and flexible, which makes developing/strategizing a critical core activity in management work.

A third reason why developing/strategizing is important is that it enhances efficiency and effectiveness. By performing this activity, a manager facilitates the substitution of coordinated and integrated effort in place of random activity, controlled flow of work in place of uneven flow, and careful decisions in place of snap judgments. Growing pressure for health programs to be operated efficiently and effectively increases the importance and value of developing/strategizing as a core management activity.

Finally, developing/strategizing in health programs is important because it facilitates managers' efforts to assess and control results. Controlling relies on comparing actual results with predetermined, desired results and taking corrective action when actual results do not match desired results. Good strategizing yields statements of desired results against which actual results can be compared.

Control techniques are based on the same basic elements, regardless of whether quality, cost, participant or patient/customer satisfaction, or some other variable is being controlled. Controlling, wherever it occurs, involves four steps: (1) establishing desired results, (2) measuring performance, (3) comparing actual results with desired results, and (4) correcting deviations from desired results when they occur. As will be seen later on, the facilitative activity of evaluating is important to effective control.

Designing

Designing is the work managers do when establishing and changing the intentional patterns of relationships among human and other resources within a program and when establishing and changing the relationship of the program to its external environment, including to the larger organizational home in which it is embedded.

Designing activity permits a manager to establish an organizational structure for a program. This includes assembling the necessary inputs or resources for a program. Because human resources are key resources in all programs, the designation of individual positions and the aggregation or clustering of these positions into the work groups, teams, or other subunits of a program is a critical aspect of a manager's designing activity. The number and type of individual positions are typically determined by how a program's work is divided and specialized.

In larger programs, the designing activity may also include clustering work groups into divisions or other units, such as separate smaller projects, as well as determining how the various work groups and clusters of work groups are integrated and coordinated. A key part of designing is relating a program to its larger organizational home. For example, a program embedded in a county health department must fit within the context of that department. A program manager in such a setting reports to a superior in the larger organizational home, and in doing so makes certain that the program's mission and objectives are consistent with and supportive of those of the department in which it is embedded.

The pattern of relationships among the human and other resources that results from the designing activity forms the organization design of a program. Remember that a program is a type of organization. Further, staffing involves the specific activities of attracting and retaining people to occupy the positions in an organization design, and is thus a vital part of organizing a program.

In practice, an organization design proceeds from individual positions through a clustering of positions into work groups, which may serve as subunits of a program or may be the entire program. In the larger organizational home of a program, clustering of work groups also forms the organization design of the organization's departments and its larger subdivisions. Clustering eventually produces an entire organizational structure and perhaps even a system comprising interconnected organizations.

Successful designs in health programs, as well as in larger organizations, depend on appropriate distributions of authority and responsibility as the program or organization is built up through the successive rounds of clustering. Authority is primarily the power one derives from occupying a position in an organization design. Responsibility can be thought of as the obligation to execute work, whether it is direct, support, or management work. Every participant in a program has responsibility as a result of his or her position. The source of responsibility is one's organizational superior. By delegating responsibility to an organizational subordinate, the superior creates a relationship between superior and subordinate that is based on obligation.

Effective organization designs achieve a balance between authority and responsibility. When responsibility is given to a participant, that person must also be given the necessary authority to make commitments, use resources, and perform the actions needed to fulfill the responsibility.

Depending on the circumstances of a program, a challenge for its design can stem from the degree of coordination required among participants. There is a correlation between the degree to which a program's work is divided and the need for attention to coordination among participants. The more differentiated the work is, the more important—and often the more difficult—the coordination task is likely to be. For example, a large, comprehensive program in women's health would involve many different people—managers, physicians, nurses, and counselors, for example—each performing highly differentiated work, making coordination quite challenging.

In addition, the direct, support, and management work in most programs are highly interdependent. This condition of functional interdependence makes achieving coordination an important aspect of the organization design of a program.

Another key to successful health program organization designs is the inclusion of features that minimize and resolve conflict among participants. Individuals participating in a program may perceive the program's mission or objectives differently, or may favor various pathways to their achievement. Conflict can occur between and among any of the various participants in a program, as well as with others outside the program.

Conflict involving two or more individuals within a program, as well as conflict between a program and its organizational home or one or more other entities, may arise. In fact, both forms of conflict should be anticipated, and can be addressed at least partially through the organization design. Even such low levels of conflict as those evidenced by participants who dislike other participants or have difficulty getting along with others can reduce performance in a program. Thus, the prevention or resolution of conflict is an important aspect of successful organization designs.

Leading

The work that managers do when influencing other participants to contribute to the performance of a program is *leading*. No matter how well a manager develops/strategizes and designs, a program's success also depends on the manager's effectively leading.

In leading the other participants in a program, the manager seeks to instill in them a shared understanding of the program's mission and objectives, and to stimulate determined and sustained efforts to achieve them. As leaders, managers focus on the various decisions and actions that affect a program, including those intended to ensure its survival and overall well-being.

Leading successfully in any setting is challenging. It is especially so in settings such as health programs, where leaders must satisfy diverse constituencies. It is necessary to take into account not only the often-heterogeneous needs and preferences of a program's patients/customers but also the needs and preferences of other participants. Only rarely are the needs and preferences of all participants in a program in complete harmony.

As Figure 1.3 illustrates, the core activities of managers are interrelated. Leading is not done in isolation from designing and developing/strategizing. How well managers engage in one of the core activities affects their performance of the others. In addition to undertaking these core activities of management work, managers engage in a number of other activities that facilitate and support their performance of the core activities. These facilitative activities are examined next, when we consider a more complete model of the activities that make up management work.

Facilitative Activities in Program Management Work

Managers routinely engage in decision making and communicating as they perform the core activities of developing/strategizing, designing, and leading. Increasingly, they also engage in managing quality and marketing, and evaluating is a common activity in most programs. Thus, Figure 1.3 can be expanded into a more complete model of the activities performed in management work as a manager seeks to ensure the success of a program.

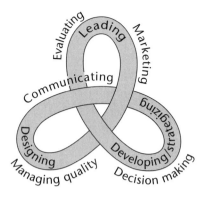

Figure 1.4   Model of the Core and Facilitative Activities in Program Management Work

Figure 1.4 shows the *facilitative management activities* of decision making, communicating, managing quality, marketing, and evaluating intertwined with the core activities involved in management work.

Decision Making

Decision making permeates all management work. Performance of the core activities of management work requires extensive *decision making*, as does performance of the other facilitative activities. Managers make decisions when they establish desired results through developing/strategizing or when they make alterations in a program's organization design. In fact, not only are designs subject to change, but all management work is performed in a dynamic context that requires continual decision making to modify such variables as missions and objectives as well as the means to accomplish them through tasks, technologies, and people.

Decision making is simply making a choice between two or more alternatives (DuBrin 2012; Dunn 2010). The myriad decisions that program managers face can be divided into two subsets: problem-solving decisions and opportunistic decisions. Problem-solving decisions are made to solve existing or anticipated problems. Opportunistic decisions are typically sporadic and arise with opportunities to reshape or advance accomplishment of a program's mission and objectives.

Communicating

Just as decision-making activities permeate all management work, *communicating* is also ubiquitous in facilitating a manager's performance of the core activities of developing/strategizing, designing, and leading (Adler and Elmhorst 2012). For example, managers who can effectively articulate and communicate their ideas and preferences have a distinct advantage in leading a program's participants. Communicating with participants is vital if they are to be involved in establishing and changing the program's organization design; and the design's details must be effectively communicated if those affected by the design are to understand it. Communicating is essential in establishing strategies for a program and in sharing the strategies with stakeholders—individuals inside as well as individuals, groups, and other organizations outside the program with significant interests in it.

Communicating involves senders (individuals, groups, or organizations) conveying ideas, intentions, and information to receivers (also individuals, groups, or organizations). Communication is effective when receivers understand ideas, intentions, or information as senders intend. Managers must be concerned with communication in two contexts: (1) communicating with a program's internal stakeholders, and (2) facilitating communication between the program and other stakeholders in its external environment.

Managing Quality

In successfully managing health programs, managers are heavily involved in *managing quality*. Not only is quality obviously important to those for whom services are provided, but also it is important to the people who work in programs. For example, it has been shown that working in an environment characterized by efforts to continuously improve quality yields higher levels of work satisfaction among participants (Berlowitz et al. 2003).

In a widely used definition, the Institute of Medicine (IOM; 1990, 128–129) defined quality as "the degree to which health services for individuals and populations increase the likelihood of desired health outcomes and are consistent with current professional knowledge." In addition to this definition of quality, the IOM (2001) also established six aims for quality improvement, saying that health care should be all of the following: safe, effective, patient centered, timely, efficient, and equitable.

The IOM's definition of quality and the six aims for quality improvement apply equally well to programs intended to serve individuals and those aimed at populations. Paying specific attention to population-based public health programs, the U.S. Department of Health and Human Services (2008) has developed the *Consensus Statement on Quality in the Public Health System,* in which quality in public health is defined as "the degree to which policies, programs, services, and research for the population increase desired health outcomes and conditions in which the population can be healthy" (1). The consensus statement also includes nine characteristics of quality in public health as follows (1):

- *Population-centered:* protecting and promoting healthy conditions and the health for the entire population

- *Equitable:* working to achieve health equity

- *Proactive:* formulating policies and sustainable practices in a timely manner, while mobilizing rapidly to address new and emerging threats and vulnerabilities

- *Health promoting:* ensuring policies and strategies that advance safe practices by providers and the population and increase the probability of positive health behaviors and outcomes

- *Risk-reducing:* diminishing adverse environmental and social events by implementing policies and strategies to reduce the probability of preventable injuries and illness or other negative outcomes

- *Vigilant:* intensifying practices and enacting policies to support enhancements to surveillance activities (e.g., technology, standardization, systems thinking/modeling)

- *Transparent:* ensuring openness in the delivery of services and practices with particular emphasis on valid, reliable, accessible, timely, and meaningful data that is readily available to stakeholders, including the public

- *Effective:* justifying investments by utilizing evidence, science, and best practices to achieve optimal results in areas of greatest need

- *Efficient:* understanding costs and benefits of public health interventions and to facilitate the optimal utilization of resources to achieve desired outcomes

In what we will call a total quality (TQ) approach in this book, managers are guided by the application of the three interrelated components as they seek to manage quality in a program: (1) focusing on the patients/customers of the program, (2) striving for continuous improvement, and (3) teamwork (Dean and Bowen 1994). Patient/customer focus means identifying what a program's patients/customers need and want, and then developing and delivering services that satisfy those needs and wants. Continuous improvement means making a commitment to ongoing efforts to examine the processes through which services are provided, in search of better ways to provide them. Teamwork is emphasized in a TQ approach because quality is a collective responsibility of all those involved in a program.

Marketing

The boundary between a program and its external environment is important territory for its manager. A manager can use *marketing* to effectively cross this boundary. Marketing is a facilitative management activity through which human and social needs can be identified and met (Kotler and Keller 2012). The purpose of marketing is to bring about voluntary exchanges with others outside a program so that the program's mission and objectives can be achieved. Others in the external environment that can be reached through marketing activities include potential patients/customers for a program's services, as well as others who can influence them. Engaging in exchanges with patients/customers is critical to the success of most programs, especially when services for sale are offered.

Successful programs also engage in voluntary exchanges with physicians and other health services providers who are positioned to refer patients/customers, and with insurers and health plans that may permit or limit use of a program's services by their subscribers or members. Similarly, voluntary exchanges are made with the organization in which a program is embedded, with potential employees, and perhaps with donors and volunteers. All of these exchanges are supported and facilitated through marketing.

Evaluating

In essence, when program managers engage in *evaluating*, they are collecting and analyzing information about a program or some aspect of a program as a basis for making decisions about the program (McNamara 2014). Program evaluation has been defined as "the application of systematic methods to address questions about program operations and results" (Wholey, Hatry, and Newcomer 2010, 5–6).

Managers engage in evaluating activities for a number of reasons, including the following: (1) to improve the overall performance of their programs, (2) to demonstrate accountability to stakeholders and justify the use of resources, (3) to demonstrate the effectiveness of their programs in terms of accomplishing missions and objectives, and (4) to demonstrate the effectiveness of specific interventions undertaken by programs.

There are many types of evaluations. Some are conducted during the development or ongoing implementation of a program, with the intent to improve the program. Other evaluations focus on the end results achieved by a program and are used to make decisions about the future of the program, including its continuation, termination, or major modification.

It is important to emphasize the interdependence among the full set of activities shown in Figure 1.4, including the core activities of management work (developing/strategizing, designing, and leading) and the facilitative activities of decision making, communicating, managing quality, marketing, and evaluating. Although it is convenient to separate these activities for purposes of discussion or description, the danger in doing so is that it may seem that managing is a series of separate activities, perhaps carried out in a particular sequence. In practice, managers do not perform the activities separately—and certainly not in a fixed sequence.

In addition to considering management work in terms of the activities described earlier, it is useful to consider this work in terms of the roles that managers play as they perform management work as well as the competencies that underpin program management work. These perspectives are described in the following sections.

Roles Played by Program Managers: The Mintzberg Model

Although it was conducted decades ago and did not focus specifically on health program managers, a historically important study of management work has direct applicability to the work of contemporary health program managers. In this seminal work, Mintzberg (1973, 1975) observed a sample of managers over a period of time, recorded and analyzed what they did, and concluded that management work can be described meaningfully in terms of three categories of interrelated *roles* that all managers play. Thus, another way to examine the work of managers is to think about the different roles they play.

Roles are the typical or customary sets of behaviors that accompany particular positions. Teachers play identifiable roles in schools, quarterbacks play defined roles on football teams, conductors play clear-cut roles in orchestras, and managers play roles as they perform management work. Mintzberg concluded that managers, simply because they are managers, must adopt certain patterns of behavior when doing management work.

He saw the work of managers in terms of three broad categories of roles—interpersonal, informational, and decisional—with each category comprising a number of separate and distinct roles as summarized in Figure 1.5.

Interpersonal Roles

In Mintzberg's (1973) view, all managers play interpersonal roles as figureheads, influencers or leaders, and liaisons. The figurehead role is played as

- **Interpersonal Roles**
  - Figurehead
  - Influencer (leader)
  - Liaison
- **Informational Roles**
  - Monitor
  - Disseminator
  - Spokesperson
- **Decisional Roles**
  - Entrepreneur
  - Disturbance handler
  - Resource allocator
  - Negotiator

Figure 1.5   The Manager's Roles

managers engage in ceremonial and symbolic activities, such as presiding over the opening of an additional site for a program or giving a speech to a graduating class of speech pathology students. Managers play the role of influencer or leader when they seek to inspire others or to help motivate them to higher levels of performance, or when they set an example through their own behavior. The liaison role involves making formal and informal contact with those inside a given program as well as with external stakeholders. Managers usually play the liaison role to establish relationships that will help them achieve a program's mission and objectives.

Informational Roles

As Figure 1.5 illustrates, Mintzberg (1973) also ascribes a category of informational roles to managers, whereby they serve as monitors, disseminators, and spokespeople. In taking on the monitor role, managers gather information from their networks of contacts (including those established in playing the liaison role), filter the information, evaluate it, and choose how to act as a result of the information. The disseminator role grows out of access to information and managers' ability to choose what to do with the information they obtain. In dissemination, managers have many choices about whom inside and outside a program they route information to. The third informational role, that of spokesperson, is related to managers' figurehead role. As spokespeople, managers communicate information about a program to internal and external stakeholders.

Decisional Roles

The third category of roles managers play in Mintzberg's (1973) model, decisional roles, includes entrepreneur, disturbance handler, resource allocator, and negotiator roles. In the entrepreneur role, managers function as initiators and designers of changes intended to improve performance in a program. When playing this role, managers are acting as change agents. In the disturbance handler role, managers decide how to handle a wide variety of disturbances that arise as they carry out their daily work routines. A program manager may face disturbances created by participants, by a regulatory agency, or by the actions of a competitor. Even a heavy snowfall that makes it impossible for key participants to come to work can be a significant disturbance. The ability to handle disturbances is an important determinant of managerial success.

In playing the resource allocator role, a manager must allocate human and other resources across alternative uses. As resources become more constrained, decisions about resource allocation become more difficult and more important. In the negotiator role, managers interact and bargain with participants, suppliers, regulators, patients/customers, and others who have some relationship to a given program. Negotiating includes deciding what objectives or outcomes to seek through negotiation, as well as deciding what techniques will be used in conducting any negotiations.

The Gestalt of Program Managers' Roles

The ten managerial roles shown in Figure 1.5 cannot really be neatly separated. In practice, they are closely intertwined into a gestalt—an integrated whole. Management work is not merely a summation of these ten roles; it is much more. When the interconnected roles are each played well, the result is synergistic. Being a good negotiator makes a manager a better disturbance handler. Playing the informational roles effectively improves performance in the decisional roles, because managers will have better information on which to base their decisions.

Most, if not all, of the activities in which managers engage as they manage their programs can be categorized into one or more of the core or facilitative activities depicted in Figure 1.4. Similarly, the roles they play are comprehensively depicted in Figure 1.5. Descriptions of these activities and roles say very little, however, about the competencies needed to perform the activities or play the roles well. Another important element in getting a sense of what management work entails is therefore to understand the competencies successful managers possess.

Competencies That Underpin Program Management Work

A *competency* is "a cluster of related skills, knowledge, and ability (sometimes referred to by the acronym SKA) that: 1) affect a major part of one's job, 2) correlate with performance on the job, 3) can be measured against well accepted standards, and 4) can be improved by training and development" (Parry 1996, 48). A similar definition of a competency is "a cluster of related abilities, commitments, knowledge, and skills that enable a person (or an organization) to act effectively in a job or situation" (BusinessDictionary 2014). The competencies required of effective managers provide another useful way to consider program management work.

The earliest studies of management competencies were conducted to investigate the skills needed by managers. For example, decades ago Katz (1974) identified three types of skills that effective managers use: technical, conceptual, and human or interpersonal skills. The technical skills of managers, like the technical skills of physical therapists or nurses, are apparent as they do their work. A manager's work in counseling a participant in a program about performance, or developing a budget, requires technical skills. Human or interpersonal skills contribute to managers' ability to get along with other people, to understand them, and to lead them in the workplace. Conceptual skills reflect managers' ability to visualize mentally all the complex interrelationships that exist in the workplace. For example, relationships exist between a program and other departments or units in its organizational home. Relationships also exist between a program and components of its larger external environment. Conceptual skills permit managers to understand how the various factors in particular situations fit together and interact with one another. Conceptual skills are clearly reflected in the appropriateness and usefulness of a program's organization design.

More recently, the Katz model of skills required of managers has been broadened into a larger set of competencies (Longest and Darr 2014). In this newer model, the competencies that are useful to program managers are (1) conceptual, (2) technical (managerial and clinical), (3) interpersonal and collaborative, (4) policy, and (5) commercial. Each is discussed in the following subsections.

Conceptual Competence

In all settings, managers must be able to envision the place and role of a given program within its larger context. This may mean envisioning its place and role in the larger society, as well as in the organizational home in which it is embedded. This competency also allows managers to visualize the complex interrelationships in the workplace—relationships among participants in a program, as well as relationships between the program and other units of its host organization or external entities with which it interacts.

In short, adequate conceptual competence allows managers to identify, understand, and interact with a program's myriad external and internal stakeholders. Conceptual competence also enhances managers' ability to comprehend the culture and historically developed values, beliefs, and norms present in a program, and to visualize its future.

Technical (Managerial and Clinical) Competence

The cluster of knowledge and associated skills that make up technical competence pertains to management work as well as to the direct work performed in a program. In health programs, direct work often involves clinical activities, such as conducting a health education session, performing a screening test, conducting a physical therapy session, or counseling a patient about nutrition. The technical aspects of management work, such as planning for a new service or facility or developing a program budget, are also crucial to a program's success. Knowledge and relevant skills in using or applying the knowledge in both clinical and management areas constitute technical competence for health program managers.

Interpersonal and Collaborative Competence

An important ingredient in managerial success is the cluster of knowledge and related skills pertaining to human interactions and relations by which managers lead others in pursuit of a program's mission and objectives. For example, a survey of managers in ambulatory health services settings intended to determine competencies most important to success in management performance found that interpersonal skills rated highest (Hudak et al. 1997). Interpersonal competence incorporates knowledge and skills useful in effectively interacting with others. It enables managers both to help participants achieve higher levels of motivation and to handle conflicts among participants.

The key elements of traditional interpersonal competence expand considerably when programs must interact with other organizational entities. This requires collaborative competence, which facilitates synergistic interaction between a program and various other organizational units. Collaborative competence is exercised, for example, when two programs are successfully merged, or when a joint venture among programs is created and operated to better serve a particular population. This competency relies on a manager's ability to build trust between a program and other organizational units, and to effectively form partnerships with other units to achieve certain purposes. It also is reflected in the manager's ability to build effective coalitions and alliances.

Policy Competence

Policy competence, defined as the dual ability to accurately assess the impact of public policies on the performance of a program and to influence public policymaking at state and federal levels (Longest 2010), is an increasingly important area of competence for program managers. Managers can influence public policy at many points in the policymaking process. For example, they can help define problems that policies might address, they can help create solutions to the problems, or they can help establish the political circumstances necessary to advance solutions through the policymaking process (Kingdon 2010).

Program managers are often in an excellent position to have firsthand knowledge about particular health problems because they deal with them daily. And by permitting a program to serve as a demonstration site for assessing possible solutions, they can play an important role in identifying feasible solutions to problems.

Based on their knowledge and expertise in addressing particular health issues, managers can participate in drafting legislative proposals and testify at legislative hearings. They can also influence the rule-making process. Procedurally, rules are made to guide the implementation of public policies. The process of rule making is designed to include input in the form of formal comments on proposed rules from those who will be affected by them.

Commercial Competence

In any setting, commercial competence refers to managers' ability to establish and operate value-creating situations in which economic exchanges between buyers and sellers occur. Value in services produced by health programs has a specific meaning, and it requires that buyers and sellers think about both quality and price. Value is quality divided by price. Today, managers of health programs are being challenged at unprecedented levels to deliver value, which is created when services have more quality attributes desired by buyers than do the services of competitors, or when services can be provided with a comparable set of quality attributes at a lower price compared to the services of competitors (Burns, Bradley, and

Weiner 2012). The commercial success of health programs may be essential for their survival, requiring managers to possess commercial competence.

Managers' Use of Different Mixes of Competencies

All managers need the full set of competencies—conceptual, technical (managerial and clinical), interpersonal and collaborative, policy, and commercial—to perform management work effectively. Not all managers use the various competencies to the same degree, however, or in the same mix. For example, the management work that takes place in a very large program providing health education services could require three different levels of management and three different mixes of competencies. The program manager would be vitally concerned about the overall performance of the program and how it fit within its larger environment. If this program were housed in a hospital, for example, the manager would be concerned about how the program fit into the total picture of the hospital and its plans, including how the program might grow in the future. Such concerns would require a heavy dependence on conceptual, policy, and commercial competencies.

The large health education program might have major subdivisions—such as one focusing on services offered to individual clients and another focusing on offering services to employers for their employees—each with its own division director. These middle-level managers would rely more on their technical (managerial and clinical) competence and their interpersonal and collaborative competencies than on conceptual, policy, or commercial competencies, although like all managers they would use all the competencies to a degree. In this program the division managers would spend much of their time troubleshooting the health education services provided by their respective divisions of the program and might be constantly required to make decisions based on technical knowledge.

In contrast to the program manager and the two division directors, a health educator who is the account manager in charge of a team of educators providing a single employer with services might use a considerable amount of technical (managerial and clinical) competence, because in addition to being a first-level manager, or supervisor of direct work, this individual would have to provide health education services. This manager, more than either the program manager or the division directors, would also be required to use interpersonal and collaborative competence on the job, because almost all of this person's work would involve direct contact with the other educators on the team. The variation in the mixes of these five types of competencies used in management work can be seen in Figure 1.6.

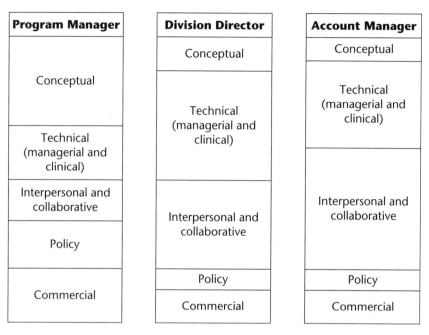

Program Manager	Division Director	Account Manager
Conceptual	Conceptual	Conceptual
	Technical (managerial and clinical)	Technical (managerial and clinical)
Technical (managerial and clinical)		
Interpersonal and collaborative	Interpersonal and collaborative	Interpersonal and collaborative
Policy		
Commercial	Policy	Policy
	Commercial	Commercial

Figure 1.6   Relative Mixes of Competencies Needed for Effective Management Work in a Large Program

The work of program managers has been viewed from the perspective of the activities managers engage in as they do their work (see Figure 1.4), from the perspective of the managerial roles they play in doing management work (see Figure 1.5), and from the perspective of the competencies needed to perform this work well (see Figure 1.6). Each perspective contributes to an understanding of program management work. In addition, it is important to consider the ethical aspects of management work.

Managing Health Programs Ethically

The beginning of an appreciation for the extent to which ethics affects management work rests in the recognition that all decisions and actions in health programs include ethical dimensions, whether they are clinical or management decisions, or some combination of these. Managers, if they are to behave ethically, must first recognize ethical issues, and then act on them.

Managers routinely make decisions and perform actions that have consequences for their programs, as well as for these programs' internal and external stakeholders. As a foundation for their decisions and actions, managers need well-developed personal *ethical standards*. These standards must be applied in the context of the philosophy and culture of a given program, as well as in the context of the philosophy and culture of the organization in which the program is embedded. Compatibility between the personal ethical standards of managers and those of the programs and organizations within which they work is important, and both sets of standards should be built on four key ethics principles: respect for persons, justice, beneficence, and nonmaleficence.

Respect for Persons

The principle of respect for persons has four elements: autonomy of persons, truth telling, confidentiality, and fidelity. The concept of autonomy recognizes that individuals have the right to their own beliefs and values, and that they have the right to make the decisions and choices that further those beliefs and values. Specifically, autonomy pertains to individuals' right to independent self-determination in regard to how they live their lives; it also pertains to the rights of individuals concerning what happens to them in health care situations.

In health programs, honoring the autonomy of patients/customers means not only following their wishes about their care but also letting them be involved in their care to the extent that they choose to be. It also means that when its patients/customers either are children or are adults with diminished competence due to a physical or mental condition, a program has special procedures to allow for surrogate decision making or substituted judgments.

The principle of respect for persons is especially important in regard to its effect on consent and the use of confidential patient information in health programs. Respect for persons as autonomous beings implies honesty in relationships with them. Closely related to honesty in such relationships is the element of confidentiality. Confidences broken will impair the performance of management work.

A third element of respect for persons is fidelity. This means doing one's duty and keeping one's word. Fidelity is often equated with promise keeping. When managers tell the truth, honor confidences, and keep promises, they are behaving in an ethically sound manner.

Decisions and actions that reflect the principle of respect for persons can sometimes be better understood in contrast to those reflecting its opposite—paternalism. Paternalism means that one thinks one knows what is best for someone else. Decisions and actions guided by a preference for autonomy limit paternalism. One of the most vivid examples of the application of this principle in health care is the 1990 Patient Self-Determination Act (PL 101-508). This public policy is designed to uphold individuals' right to make decisions concerning their health care, including the right to accept or refuse treatment and the right to formulate advance directives concerning their care. These directives are a means by which competent individuals give instructions about their health care that are to be implemented at some later date, should they lack the capacity to make these decisions. In concept, this policy allows people to exercise their right to autonomy in advance of a time when they might no longer be able to actively exercise that right.

Justice

A second principle of significant ethical importance to managers and their work in programs is justice. The concept of justice has a direct impact on management work because justice, in the context of ethics, is defined as fairness (Rawls and Kelly 2001). The principle of justice also includes the concept of desert: justice is done when a person receives that which he or she deserves (Beauchamp and Childress 2012). The key ethical question in many of the decisions and actions of managers, deriving from attention to the principle of justice, is, of course, what is fair in this situation?

The principle of justice provides the underpinnings for many ethically sound decisions and actions concerning the allocation of resources. Decisions about resource allocation that adhere closely to the principle of justice are made under the provisions of a morally defensible system rather than being arbitrary or capricious. The application of justice in making decisions in health programs, as well as in other settings, is in part ensured by the existence of the legal system, which serves as an appeals mechanism for those who believe they have been done an injustice.

Beneficence and Nonmaleficence

Two other ethics principles that are of direct relevance to managers in health programs are beneficence and nonmaleficence. Beneficence means acting with charity and kindness. This principle is incorporated into acts through which services or products are provided that are beneficial to people, including the services of health programs. The principle of beneficence also includes, however, the more complex concept of balancing benefits and harms, which may require using the relative costs and benefits of alternative decisions and actions as one basis on which to choose from among alternatives.

The growing emphasis on cost-effectiveness in health care will increasingly bring into play the principle of beneficence in the conduct of management work in health programs. Managers who are guided by the principle of beneficence feel a positive duty to contribute to the welfare of patients/customers. This inclination is rooted in the Hippocratic tradition and has a long and noble history in the health professions and in health services settings, including health programs.

Nonmaleficence, a principle with deep roots in medical ethics, is exemplified in the dictum "Primum non nocere," or "First, do no harm." Managers who are guided by the principle of nonmaleficence try to make decisions that minimize harm. Harm can be mental as well as physical, and it can be caused through such acts as violating the privacy of patients/ customers. Whereas beneficence is a positive duty involving taking action to do good, nonmaleficence involves refraining from doing something that harms. The principles of beneficence and nonmaleficence are reflected in actions and decisions involving the assurance of the quality of the services of a program, and in managers' exercise of their fiduciary duties, their use of confidential information, and their resolution of conflicts of interest.

Supporting Ethical Behavior in Health Programs

Health programs by nature routinely involve people providing health services. In these situations, the service providers face a set of ethical obligations that stem from their roles as health professionals. These obligations may be summarized as follows:

- *Obligations between professionals and patients/customers.* As fiduciaries for their patients/customers, professionals must be honest, candid, competent, loyal, fair, and discreet in these relationships.

- *Obligations to third parties.* In many health programs, other people or organizations (for example, parents or other family members, employers, teachers, or insurance plans) have interests in the professional-patient/customer relationship. The ethical issues that arise from these obligations usually have to do with confidentiality and the protection of privacy. These issues also often involve compliance with laws, such as the Health Insurance Portability and Accountability Act (HIPAA). They may also involve responding to court orders. HIPAA includes privacy provisions that generally limit the use or disclosure of protected health information to a minimum necessary standard. It also gives patients the right to see and receive copies of their records, request amendments to their records, and learn details about disclosures of their records.

- *Obligations between professionals and their employers.* Obligations exist between professionals and the health programs that employ them. Ethical issues that arise from these obligations involve due process, confidentiality, and professional support. Professionals, as participants in programs, have obligations to their employers that include being honest, candid, competent, loyal, fair, and discreet.

* *Obligations to the profession.* The professionals that work in health programs have obligations to their profession that include advancing knowledge, reforming the profession, and respecting the profession.

A number of codes of ethics have been developed for individual professions, as well as for various health services organizations. For example, the American Hospital Association has produced a prototype code of ethics for hospitals. It includes sections on the community roles and responsibilities of these institutions, on patient care therein, and on organizational conduct. The American Public Health Association has produced a code of ethics to guide the practice of public health. The American Association for Health Education offers a code of ethics for health educators. The American Medical Association adopted the first version of its *Principles of Medical Ethics* at its founding in 1847. The American Nurses Association has developed a code for nurses. The American College of Healthcare Executives provides a code of ethics to guide its members. Similarly, other health professions have developed codes. In fact, a code of ethics is a hallmark of any profession. Beyond these codes, many individual health services organizations develop their own. Such codes often provide very visible evidence of the commitment of organizations to ethical behavior; programs embedded in such organizations are also expected to follow these codes of ethics.

In addition to relying on codes of ethics developed by others, participants can follow the guidelines of a program-specific code of ethics. Program managers can support ethical behavior in other ways as well, such as by developing a culture or climate that minimizes ethical ambiguity and continuously reminds participants to make ethical decisions and take ethical actions (Martin and Cullen 2006). Ethical climates "influence both decision making and behavioral responses to ethical dilemmas, which then go on to be reflected in various work outcomes" (Simha and Cullen 2012, 20–21).

Managers can also reward ethical behavior and create a climate in which people are free to challenge standards or practices they consider unethical. Finally, managers can encourage ethical behavior by providing training in applied ethics to increase awareness of the ethical dimensions of decisions and actions, encourage critical evaluations of values and priorities, and help program participants integrate ethics considerations into their decisions and actions.

Managers and the Success of Programs

In concluding this introductory chapter, it is important to emphasize the significant impact that managers can have on their programs. The manager, more than anyone or anything else, establishes a program's work climate. A work climate is defined as comprising "the shared perceptions of procedures, policies, and practices [of a program], both formal and informal" (Simha and Cullen 2012, 20). Work climates are known to influence the behaviors of program participants to a great degree (Tsai and Huang 2008).

Health programs are not random groups of people assembled by chance interactions. Instead, they are consciously formed for the purpose of achieving a mission and specific objectives. From this fact stems the overarching purpose of all program management work, which is to facilitate the achievement of a program's intended results—that is, to accomplish its mission and fulfill its objectives.

The contributions managers make to the degree to which desired results are successfully achieved can be measured along many dimensions. Measuring managers' contributions to success may involve measuring a program's results in terms of counts of services and productivity levels, the quality of services, and patient/customer satisfaction. For example, the number of services rendered can be counted and compared to established targets. Productivity can be measured in terms of resources used per unit of service. The quality of the services provided by a program can be measured in terms of clinical outcomes achieved, as well as in terms of process measures (such as adherence to protocols) and input measures (such as the credentials of staff). Patient/customer satisfaction levels can be measured by surveys, and by loyalty demonstrated by continued use of services. Success can also be measured through such outcomes as changes in the attitudes, behaviors, health status, or level of functioning of patients/customers. Finally, managers' contributions can be measured in terms of the impact of a program on the overall health status of a community.

There is no universally accepted formula by which managers maximize their contributions to program effectiveness. There is, however, a correlation between a program's success and how well its manager performs the core activities of developing/strategizing, designing, and leading. Similarly, the manner in which a manager makes decisions, communicates, manages quality, markets the program, and evaluates the program has a direct bearing on success.

There is also a correlation between how well managers play their interpersonal, informational, and decisional roles and the level of performance a program attains. Similarly, it matters to performance whether or not a program's manager possesses and uses appropriate conceptual, technical (managerial and clinical), interpersonal and collaborative, policy, and commercial competencies. Effective managers, by creating conditions that are conducive to superior performance, make vital and unique contributions to the programs they manage. The remaining chapters in this book are intended to help program managers maximize their contributions to successful programs.

Summary

Definitions of health, health programs, and program management are provided in this chapter. Following the World Health Organization's (1948) view, health is defined as the "state of complete physical, mental, and social well-being, and not merely the absence of disease or infirmity." Health is discussed as a function of a number of health determinants, which for individuals or for populations include the physical environments in which people live and work; their behaviors; and their biology (genetic makeup, family history, and physical and mental health problems acquired during life). Health determinants also include a host of social factors, such as economic circumstances; one's socioeconomic position in society; income distribution; discrimination based on race or ethnicity, gender, sexual orientation, or some other characteristic; and the availability of social networks and social support. Further, the health services to which people have access also are health determinants. The variety of health determinants means that health programs can have a wide array of foci.

The work of health program managers is considered in terms of the core activities in which all managers engage as they do management work: developing/strategizing, designing, and leading. Consideration of this work is extended also to include the facilitative activities of management work: decision making, communicating, managing quality, marketing, and evaluating. The entire set of core and facilitative activities in management work is modeled graphically in Figure 1.4.

As an adjunct to the discussion of the activities in management work, Mintzberg's model of the roles that managers play in doing management work is also presented. Figure 1.5 summarizes these roles in interpersonal, informational, and decisional categories. There is also a discussion of the conceptual, technical (managerial and clinical), interpersonal and collaborative, policy, and commercial competencies necessary to manage health programs well.

The chapter acknowledges the growing impact that ethics considerations have on all actions and decisions in health programs in both the clinical and managerial spheres of activity. The ethics principles of respect for persons, justice, beneficence, and nonmaleficence are discussed as the basis for the construction of personal ethical standards for managers.

REVIEW QUESTIONS

1. Define health, health programs, and program management.
2. Discuss how the determinants of health shape the focus of health programs.
3. Briefly describe the core activities of management work.
4. Briefly describe the facilitative activities of management work.
5. Discuss the Mintzberg model of the roles managers play in doing their work.
6. Discuss the competencies that are useful to managers in performing their work, including the different mixes of competencies that would be appropriate in different circumstances.
7. Why is it important for managers to develop personal ethical standards? Discuss the principles on which such standards should be based.
8. Discuss the overall contributions managers make to the success of the health programs they manage.

KEY TERMS AND CONCEPTS

communicating	health programs
competency	leading
core management activities	management
decision making	management work
designing	managing quality
developing/strategizing	marketing
ethical standards	program
evaluating	program management
facilitative management activities	roles
health	
health determinants	

References

Adler, Ronald B., and Jeanne Marquardt Elmhorst. *Communicating at Work: Principles and Practices for Business and the Professions*, 11th ed. New York: McGraw-Hill Higher Education, 2012.

Beauchamp, Thomas L., and James F. Childress. *Principles of Biomedical Ethics*, 7th ed. New York: Oxford University Press, 2012.

Berlowitz, Dan R., Gary J. Young, Elaine C. Hickey, Debra Saliba, Brian S. Mittman, Elaine Czarnowski, Barbara Simon, et al. "Quality Improvement Implementation in the Nursing Home." *Health Services Research* 38, no. 1 (February 2003): 65–83.

Bill and Melinda Gates Foundation. "What We Do." Accessed May 9, 2014. http://www.gatesfoundation.org/What-We-Do.

Briner, Rob B., David Denyer, and Denise M. Rousseau. "Evidence-Based Management: Concept Cleanup Time?" *Academy of Management Perspectives* 23, no. 4 (November 2009): 19–32.

Burns, Lawton Robert, Elizabeth H. Bradley, and Byran J. Weiner. *Shortell and Kaluzny's Health Care Management: Organization Design and Behavior*, 6th ed. Clifton Park, NY: Delmar, Cengage Learning, 2012.

BusinessDictionary. "Competence." Accessed May 8, 2014. http://www.businessdictionary.com/definition/competence.html.

Centers for Medicare and Medicaid Services. "Innovation Advisors Program." Accessed May 7, 2014. http://innovation.cms.gov/initiatives/Innovation-Advisors-Program/index.html.

Charns, Martin P., and Jody Hoffer Gittell. "Work Design." In *Healthcare Management: Organization Design and Behavior*, edited by Stephen M. Shortell and Arnold D. Kaluzny, 5th ed., 212–236. Clifton Park, NY: Thomson Delmar Leaning, 2006.

Daft, Richard L. *Management*, 11th ed. Mason, OH: South-Western, Cengage Learning, 2014.

Dean, James W., Jr., and David E. Bowen. "Management Theory and Total Quality: Improving Research and Practice through Theory Development." *Academy of Management Review* 19, no. 3 (July 1994): 392–418.

DuBrin, Andrew J. *Essentials of Management*, 9th ed. Mason, OH: South-Western, Cengage Learning, 2012.

Dunn, Rose T. *Dunn and Haimann's Healthcare Management*, 9th ed. Chicago: Health Administration Press, 2010.

Ginter, Peter M., W. Jack Duncan, and Linda E. Swayne. *Strategic Management of Health Care Organizations*, 7th ed. San Francisco: Jossey-Bass, 2013.

Hudak, Ronald P., Paul P. Brooke, Jr., Kenn Finstuen, and James Trounson. "Management Competencies for Medical Practice Executives: Skills, Knowledge, and Abilities Required for the Future." *Journal of Health Administration Education* 15 (Fall 1997): 219–239.

Institute of Medicine. *Medicare: A Strategy for Quality Assurance*. Washington, DC: National Academies Press, 1990.

Institute of Medicine. *Crossing the Quality Chasm: A New Health System for the 21st Century*. Washington, DC: National Academies Press, 2001.

Katz, Robert L. "Skills of an Effective Administrator." *Harvard Business Review* 52 (September-October 1974): 90–102.

Kingdon, John W. *Agendas, Alternatives, and Public Policies*, 2nd ed. Upper Saddle River, NJ: Pearson, 2010.

Kotler, Philip, and Kevin Keller. *Marketing Management*, 14th ed. Upper Saddle River, NJ: Prentice Hall, 2012.

Kovner, Anthony R., David J. Fine, and Richard D'Aquila. *Evidence-Based Management in Healthcare*. Chicago: Health Administration Press, 2009.

Kovner, Anthony R., and Thomas G. Rundall. "Evidence-Based Management Reconsidered." *Frontiers of Health Services Management* 22, no. 3 (Spring 2006): 3–22.

Longest, Beaufort B., Jr. *Health Policymaking in the Untied States*, 5th ed. Chicago: Health Administration Press, 2010.

Longest, Beaufort B., Jr., and Kurt Darr. *Managing Health Services Organizations and Systems*, 6th ed. Baltimore: Health Professions Press, 2014.

Marquis, Bessie L., and Carol J. Huston. *Leadership Roles and Management Functions in Nursing: Theory and Application*, 7th ed. Philadelphia: Lippincott Williams & Wilkins, 2012.

Martin, Kelly D., and John B. Cullen. "Continuities and Extensions of Ethical Climate Theory: A Meta-Analytic Review." *Journal of Business Ethics* 69 (2006), 175–194.

Massachusetts General Hospital. *Fact Sheet–Phase One MGH Medicare Demonstration Project for High-Cost Beneficiaries*. Accessed May 9, 2014. http://www.massgeneral.org/News/assets/pdf/CMS_project_phase1FactSheet.pdf.

McCall, Nancy, Jerry Cromwell, and Carol Urato. *Evaluation of Medicare Care Management for High Cost Beneficiaries (CMHCB) Demonstration: Massachusetts General Hospital and Massachusetts General Physicians Organization (MGH)*. Final Report, RTI Project Number 0207964.025.000.001. Research Triangle Park, NC: RTI International, September 10, 2010.

McNamara, Carter."Basic Guide to Program Evaluation." Accessed May 26, 2014. http://managementhelp.org/evaluation/program-evaluation-guide.htm.

Mintzberg, Henry. *The Nature of Managerial Work*. New York: Harper and Row, 1973.

Mintzberg, Henry. "The Manager's Job: Folklore and Fact." HBR Classic. *Harvard Business Review* 68 (March-April 1990): 163–176. First published 1975.

Mintzberg, Henry. *Structure in Fives: Designing Effective Organizations*. Upper Saddle River, NJ: Prentice Hall, 1992.

Parry, Scott B. "The Quest for Competencies." *Training* 33 (July 1996): 48.

Project Management Institute. *The Standard for Program Management*, 3rd ed. Newton Square, PA: Project Management Institute, 2013.

Rawls, John, and Erin Kelly. *Justice as Fairness: A Restatement.* Cambridge, MA: Harvard University Press, 2001.

Rousseau, Denise M., ed. *The Oxford Handbook of Evidence-Based Management.* New York: Oxford University Press, 2014.

Simha, Aditya, and John B. Cullen. "Ethical Climates and Their Effects on Organizational Outcomes: Implications from the Past and Prophecies for the Future." *Academy of Management Perspectives* 26, no. 4 (November 2012): 20–34.

Tsai, Ming-Tien, and Chun-Chen Huang. "The Relationship among Ethical Climate Types, Facets of Job Satisfaction, and the Three Components of Organizational Commitment: A Study of Nurses in Taiwan." *Journal of Business Ethics* 80 (2008): 565–581.

U.S. Department of Health and Human Services. *Consensus Statement on Quality in the Public Health System.* Washington, DC: U.S. Department of Health and Human Services, Office of Public Health and Science, 2008. http://www.hhs.gov/ash/initiatives/quality/quality/phqf-consensus-statement.html.

U.S. Department of Health and Human Services. "Determinants of Health." Accessed May 7, 2014. http://healthypeople.gov/2020/about/DOHAbout.aspx.

Walshe, Kieran, and Thomas G. Rundall. "Evidence-Based Management: From Theory to Practice in Health Care." *Milbank Quarterly* 79, no. 3 (September 2001): 429–457.

Wholey, Joseph S., Harry P. Hatry, and Kathryn E. Newcomer. *Handbook of Practical Program Evaluation*, 3rd ed. San Francisco: Jossey-Bass, 2010.

World Health Organization. Preamble to the Constitution of the World Health Organization as adopted by the International Health Conference, New York, June 19–22, 1946; signed on July 22, 1946, by the representatives of sixty-one states (Official Records of the World Health Organization, no. 2, 100) and entered into force on April 7, 1948.

Zuckerman, Howard S., and William L. Dowling. "The Managerial Role." In *Essentials of Health Care Management*, edited by Stephen M. Shortell and Arnold D. Kaluzny, 34–62. Clifton Park, NY: Delmar, 1997.

EXAMPLE OF A HEALTH PROGRAM: THE GLOBAL HEALTH PROGRAM OF THE BILL AND MELINDA GATES FOUNDATION

This example is described in terms of the host organization (the Bill and Melinda Gates Foundation) and one of that organization's programs (the Global Health Program).

The Host Organization

The Bill and Melinda Gates Foundation is a private organization with 501(c)(3) charitable exemption status granted by the Internal Revenue Service. With an endowment of more than $40 billion, it is the largest private foundation in the world. Founded in 1994, the organization works to help all people lead healthy, productive lives. It is led by a CEO under the direction of its three trustees: Bill Gates, Melinda Gates, and Warren Buffett. With a staff of about 1,200 people, the foundation is headquartered in Seattle, Washington, and maintains offices in Washington, DC; Delhi, India; Beijing, China; and London, United Kingdom.

In 2012 the foundation awarded grant payments of about $3.4 billion. It operates four programs, each with its own team and budget (Bill and Melinda Gates Foundation 2014):

- The Global Development Program seeks "to help the world's poorest people lift themselves out of hunger and poverty."

Much of the information presented in this appendix was obtained from the following source: Bill and Melinda Gates Foundation. "Foundation Fact Sheet." Accessed May 9, 2014. http://www.gatesfoundation.org/Who-We-Are/General-Information/Foundation-Factsheet.

- The Global Health Program seeks "to harness advances in science and technology to save lives in developing countries."

- The United States Program seeks "to improve U.S. high school and postsecondary education and support vulnerable children and families in Washington State."

- The Global Policy & Advocacy Program seeks "to build strategic relationships and promote policies that will help advance [its] work."

The Global Health Program

The Global Health Program is organized as a division of the foundation and focuses on saving lives in developing countries by harnessing advances in science and technology. The program invests heavily in vaccine research to prevent infectious diseases, including HIV, polio, and malaria. It also supports development of health improvements through family planning, nutrition, maternal and child health, and mosquito control. Global Health structures its activities around a number of more focused program areas, including the following (Bill and Melinda Gates Foundation 2014):

- Discovery & Translational Sciences, which seeks "to direct scientific research toward areas where it can have the most impact and to accelerate the translation of discoveries into solutions that improve people's health and save lives."

- Enteric and Diarrheal Diseases, which seeks "to eliminate the gap in mortality from enteric and diarrheal diseases between developed and developing countries and to significantly reduce impaired development associated with these diseases in children under age 5."

- HIV, which seeks "to significantly reduce the incidence of HIV infection and extend the lives of people living with HIV."

- Malaria, which seeks "a world free of malaria."

- Neglected Infectious Diseases, which seeks "to reduce the burden of neglected infectious diseases on the world's poorest people through targeted and effective control, elimination, and eradication efforts."

- Pneumonia, which seeks "to significantly reduce childhood deaths from pneumonia."

- Tuberculosis, which seeks "to accelerate the decline in tuberculosis incidence worldwide."

EXAMPLE OF A HEALTH PROJECT: THE MASS GENERAL CARE MANAGEMENT PROJECT

The Centers for Medicare and Medicaid Services (CMS), the federal agency responsible for Medicare, supports numerous demonstration projects intended to improve Medicare. One of these projects—the Mass General Care Management Project—is at Massachusetts General Hospital (MGH) in Boston. The project was originally approved for three years in 2006, and was renewed for another three years in 2009. At renewal, the project was expanded beyond MGH to include Brigham and Women's Hospital and North Shore Medical Center. The project is testing strategies to improve the coordination of Medicare services for high-cost, fee-for-service beneficiaries.

Operationally, the Mass General Care Management Project provides highly integrated care management services through the use of practice-based case managers, individualized plans of care, twenty-four-hour access to care managers, and electronic medical records. Under the terms of this demonstration project, CMS pays MGH a monthly fee per Medicare patient to coordinate that person's care. If there are savings from the project, MGH and CMS share them.

The project is described as a provider-based care management project "intended to provide an enhanced level of care to a high risk patient population through comprehensive outpatient practice based case management" (McCall, Cromwell, and Urato 2010, 4). The project was structured to facilitate communication "(a) between patients and case managers, (b) between patients and physicians, (c) between case managers and physicians, and (d) among case managers" (5).

As is typical with demonstration projects funded by outside agencies or foundations, CMS commissioned an independent evaluator, Research Triangle Institute (RTI), to assess the performance of the Mass General Care Management Project. Comparing the results achieved for the patients enrolled in the project to those of a comparison group, RTI found MGH's project to be successful along several dimensions (McCall, Cromwell, and Urato 2010). The hospital summarized the achievements of the project as follows (Massachusetts General Hospital, 2014 1):

Successful Enrollment and High Satisfaction

- 87 percent of eligible beneficiaries enrolled

- Improved communication between patients and health care team

- High patient and physician satisfaction

Improved Patient Outcomes

- Hospitalization rate among enrolled patients was 20 percent lower than comparison

- Emergency department visit rates were 13 percent lower for enrolled patients

- Annual mortality 16 percent among enrolled versus 20 percent among comparison group

Achieved Savings Target

- 12.1 percent in gross savings among enrolled patients

- 7 percent in annual net savings among enrolled patients after accounting for the management fee paid by CMS to MGH

- Return on investment—for every $1 spent, the project saved at least $2.65

CHAPTER 2

DEVELOPING/STRATEGIZING THE FUTURE

All programs have a beginning, and this is an appropriate place to begin thinking about the activities that constitute management work in programs. The initial development of a program involves someone envisioning the program as a vehicle for delivering services or products that may succeed in the marketplace or meet some unmet need, even if it is not a commercial success. In effect, someone theorizes about a program in the beginning.

As noted in Chapter 1, once the initial development of a program occurs, further developing activities pertain to improving established services or product, or to expanding a program's portfolio of services or products. Development triggers strategizing, which is the work that managers do as they establish or revise the specific mission and objectives of a program and make plans to achieve them.

All program managers engage in ***developing/strategizing*** as part of performing their management work, along with the other two core activities of designing and leading (see Figure 1.3). Developing/strategizing results in critical decisions about a program's existence, revision, purpose, and direction. Through developing/strategizing activities, managers lay a foundation for designing the intentional patterns of relationships among the human and other resources within the program. The mission and objectives established through developing/strategizing, along with the operational plans as to how to accomplish them, also inform managers about where they should be leading other participants.

Developing/strategizing for a nascent program requires managers to engage in activities different from those needed when developing/strategizing for an ongoing program. Both situations are covered in this chapter, although the more common situation of developing/strategizing in an ongoing program receives more attention. The special circumstance

LEARNING OBJECTIVES
After reading this chapter, you should be able to:

- Understand the developing/ strategizing activities of program managers

- Understand the underlying theory and logic model of a program

- Understand how to conduct internal and external situational analyses

- Formulate and reformulate statements of the mission and objectives for a program

- Model the operational planning process and understand the steps in the process

- Understand how to assess and control performance and evaluate results to achieve the desired results established for a program

of the initial round of developing/strategizing for a new program being developed is discussed in terms of preparing a business plan for the program. Developing/strategizing for any program, however, whether it is new or ongoing, should be based on an underlying theory of how the program should operate.

Developing the Underlying Theory of a Program

Any program can be conceptualized as a ***program theory***, which is simply a model of how it is intended to work (Funnell and Rogers 2011). A good program theory is one that is plausible and sensible. The theory underlying a particular program can be expressed as follows: if inputs or resources a, b, and c are assembled; and processed by doing m, n, and o with the resources; then the results will be x, y, and z.

Using as a guideline a program's underlying theory (or its hypothesis, as the theory is sometimes called), any program can be described in terms of the relationships among the resources available for it to use, the work processes it undertakes with the resources, and the results it achieves by processing the resources. As will be seen in this discussion, this way of conceptualizing or thinking about a program can be very useful to its manager and to its other internal and external stakeholders.

The term ***logic model*** derives from the fact that implicit in the theory on which a program is based is an underlying logic or rationale (Knowlton and Phillips 2013). This logic is expressed in terms of how resources are processed to achieve desired results in the form of fulfilling the program's mission and the more specific objectives established for it.

Adapting the most widely used definition of a logic model, one developed by the W. K. Kellogg Foundation (2004), the logic model of a program is simply a schematic, visual way to present the relationships among the resources available to the program, the work processes planned and undertaken with the resources, and the results intended to be achieved through operating the program. These relationships can be drawn for any program. Figure 2.1 depicts a basic logic model for a program. More will be said about designing logic models for programs in Chapter 3, and their role in managers' evaluating activities is discussed in depth in Chapter 9. For now, however, a few critical aspects of logic models as a basis for developing/strategizing are discussed.

The feedback loops from desired results to resources and work processes indicate that adjustments are likely to be needed in an ongoing

External environment of the program (with cultural and social, competitive, demographic, economic and financial, ethical and legal, policy, and scientific and technological dimensions)

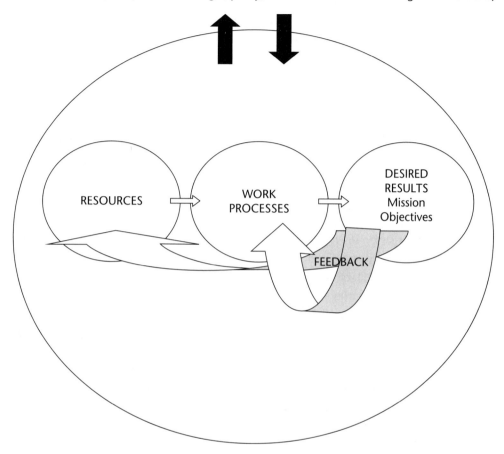

Figure 2.1   Logic Model of a Program

program's resources and work processes. It is important to note that Figure 2.1 shows a program existing within its external environment.

As discussed later in this chapter, the external environment of a program includes many variables that can influence its performance. These are illustrated in Figure 2.1 by the arrow that flows from the environment into the program's logic model. Important aspects of the external environment include cultural and social, competitive, demographic, economic and financial, ethical and legal, policy, and scientific and technological dimensions, as well as the priorities and resources of the host organization in which the program is embedded.

External variables can influence almost everything about a program, including whom it seeks to serve, the extent of patients/customers' need for its services, and the resources available to it. A program cannot be isolated from its external environment. All programs are affected by and affect their respective external environments. The results accomplished by a program flow out into its external environment, as shown by the arrow flowing out of the logic model and into the external environment in Figure 2.1. This arrow means that the results achieved by a program affect the individuals and populations that it serves, as well as other program stakeholders.

Using Program Theory and Logic Models in Establishing and Maintaining Effective Stakeholder Relationships

Health programs typically have a variety of **stakeholders**, the individuals, organizations, or groups with a stake or significant interest in the program. Internal stakeholders are the participants in a program, whereas external stakeholders include existing and potential patients/customers; public and private funders; as well as accrediting agencies, competitors, government bodies (as both payers and regulators), insurance plans, the media, and suppliers, among many others. Stakeholders are critical to a program's success, sometimes even to its existence, and a program's underlying theory and logic model provide a useful way of explaining the program to its stakeholders. When stakeholders understand a program, it is more likely that effective **stakeholder relationships** can be established and maintained.

Relationships between a program and its stakeholders can be along a continuum of positive to neutral to negative, with positive and negative relationships varying in intensity. The patterns of relationships with stakeholders are unique for each program, depending on its situation. It is important to note that managers can alter these relationships (for example, from negative to neutral or positive). Further, the intensity of positive and negative relationships varies, and managers seek to cultivate strongly positive relationships with stakeholders. Because neutral relationships are better than negative relationships, but not as good as positive relationships, it is desirable to convert neutral stakeholders to positive ones. A comprehensive logic model can aid in these efforts.

As program managers seek to establish and maintain highly positive relationships with stakeholders, they must accomplish two things: (1) achieve widespread understanding and acceptance of the desired results established for the program in the form of its mission and objectives among internal and external stakeholders, and (2) garner support for and resource contributions toward achievement of these desired results from external stakeholders, and secure internal stakeholders' effective direct involvement in the operation of the program's work processes.

The clearer and more comprehensive a program's underlying theory and logic model are, the more useful they can be in helping stakeholders understand the program—and understanding can increase support. A good program theory and logic model can also assist managers in their efforts to shift stakeholder relationships from negative to neutral or positive. At a minimum, a program's theory and logic model can help its manager explain the results the program seeks to achieve and the resources and work processes necessary to achieve the desired results.

For example, internally, a theory and logic model can help a manager explain the roles that individual participants play in a program's overall operation. Work processes used within the program are less likely to be viewed as mysterious or trivial by participants when their roles can be linked to specific desired results. It is easier to motivate participant behaviors that contribute positively to desired results—behaviors such as cooperating, supporting fellow participants, protecting property, avoiding waste, and generally going beyond the call of duty—when participants understand a program's organization and operation thoroughly, including their roles in the work processes that lead to results.

When participants can connect their performance and contributions to accomplishment of a program's desired results, and if they are properly rewarded for good performance as discussed in Chapter 4, they are more likely to be motivated to make positive contributions. This is especially true when participants have been involved in determining and specifying the desired results. Such involvement encourages participants to identify more closely with the program and to more enthusiastically perform their work to accomplish its mission and objectives. In addition, when managers encourage and facilitate program participants' involvement in designing work processes, they enable a wider range of ideas, experiences, and expertise to be brought to bear on developing effective processes. Participants involved in conceptualizing and developing work processes are also more committed to performing well within the constructs of those processes.

A good program theory and comprehensive logic model can also be very useful in managing relationships with a program's external stakeholders, such as foundations, accrediting and regulatory agencies, and the general public. Adjustments in a program's logic model can serve as a basis for seeking and defending new proposals and requests for support. Similarly, a logic model can be useful when a program's manager is explaining details to superiors in the host organization or comprehensively reporting perform-ance results to various stakeholders. Further, a priori statements of desired results become benchmarks against which actual performance can be measured and reported. Finally, when desired results are not fully realized, a logic model can help explain causes and offer ideas for corrective actions.

Developing/Strategizing Activity

Assuming an underlying theory and logic model are in place for an ongoing program, managers continue their developing/strategizing work by determining the current situation of the program. A program's current situation is the basis for all other aspects of developing/strategizing and must be determined carefully. Developing/strategizing also involves managers' consideration of how they want the program to change in the future, usually in the coming year or perhaps during a five-year period.

Programs do not exist in a static world, and change is inevitable. When changes in a program's mission and objectives occur, managers must then consider how the revised desired results will be accomplished. This involves them in operational planning. To bring the developing/strategizing activities full circle, managers must also monitor progress toward achieving the new or modified desired results. This involves them in evaluating aspects of their programs and assessing and controlling performance.

This chapter provides information about how managers can systematically determine the current situation of a program. This will be discussed in terms of the conduct of internal and external situational analyses for a program, as well as the development of an inventory of the desired results established for it. The chapter also addresses how managers reconsider and revise the desired results established for a program, and how they successfully pursue accomplishment of revised desired results—a discussion that includes a description of managers' operational planning activities. Finally, this chapter addresses how managers use techniques of assessing and controlling performance and evaluating results to assure themselves that the desired results—both continuing and revised—are being accomplished.

Health programs typically exist within the context of an extremely turbulent external environment, and managers must be prepared to accept uncertainty as the inevitable consequence of operating in such a dynamic world. Managers have a responsibility, however, to try to reduce the uncertainty and prepare their programs to cope with it. As managers seek to reduce and otherwise contend with uncertainty, effective developing/strategizing is often their most useful and powerful tool. As noted earlier, assuming that a program theory and a logic model are in place, developing/strategizing activity in an ongoing program begins with determining the program's current situation.

Situational Analysis: Determining a Program's Current Situation

Effective developing/strategizing in an ongoing program should be based on the periodic conduct of a thorough *situational analysis*, in which available information about the program's current situation is collected and analyzed. The eventual effectiveness of developing/strategizing activity is dependent on the quality and quantity of the information generated through situational analysis. In practice, situational analysis is ongoing, although it is useful to complete an entire analysis at least once during each year of operation. A thorough situational analysis for a program includes three components: (1) an external situational analysis, (2) an internal situational analysis, and (3) an inventory of the desired results established for the program.

A manager's complete situational analysis considers the desired results intended for a program in relation to the opportunities and threats it faces from the external environment, and also in relation to the internal strengths and weaknesses of the program. Sometimes the internal and external situational analyses are said to constitute a SWOT analysis, which is conducted to determine a program's **s**trengths, **w**eaknesses, **o**pportunities, and **t**hreats. A SWOT analysis is among the most widely used analytical tools in developing/strategizing because it is intuitive and relatively simple to use (Heuer and Pherson 2011).

The order in which the external and internal analyses are conducted in the situational analysis is important, because many internal strengths and weaknesses can be identified only in relation to the external environment. For example, a health program's physical location can be considered one of its strengths if there is ample demand for its services in the area, and if it enjoys a strong market share compared to its competitors. In other instances, physical location may be a weakness for a program, such as when the program is located in an area experiencing severe population loss. Answering the question, what is the current situation of our program? should begin with the external situational analysis.

External Situational Analysis

A program's external environment produces combinations of cultural and social, competitive, demographic, economic and financial, ethical and legal, policy, and scientific and technological information that, depending on circumstances, may be relevant to the program's future. All health programs can be influenced, sometimes dramatically, by what goes on in their respective external environments. External environments can provide health programs with both opportunities and threats, which must be recognized and responded to for effective developing/strategizing to take place.

The relevant external environment includes all the factors outside a program's boundaries that can influence its manager's decisions and actions. In addition to the general environmental factors listed earlier, important aspects of the external environment may include complementary or competitive programs; the organizational home in which the program is embedded; as well as patients/customers, suppliers, regulators, insurers, accrediting agencies, and so on with which the program has direct interactions.

The conduct of an *external situational analysis* includes five interrelated steps: (1) scanning to identify relevant information (trends, developments, or possible events that represent either opportunities or threats for the program); (2) monitoring or tracking the relevant information identified through scanning; (3) forecasting or projecting how relevant information might change in the future; (4) assessing the implications of the information for the program; and (5) using and disseminating the information to those who can use it to guide decisions and actions (Ginter, Duncan, and Swayne 2013). Each of these steps is discussed next.

Scanning

Scanning the external environment of a program involves acquiring and organizing information that can affect its future. The information might be relevant to the resources needed by the program, for example. Information can even change the desired results established for a program. An objective of reducing teenage pregnancy rates, for example, could be affected when demographic shifts in a program's community result in fewer teenagers.

Determination of what is important to scan is often a matter of judgment. For this reason, it is useful to have more than one person making these judgments. For example, a manager might rely on a group of participants in a program to decide what to scan. The group would probably include some members from the program's organizational home. Another useful approach is to use outside consultants to provide expert opinions and judgments.

Although the determination of what is important to scan is specific to a particular program, there are models that can help guide the conduct of situational analyses. For example, one that is especially useful in conducting a situational analysis or assessment at the level of an entire community is the

Mobilizing for Action through Planning and Partnerships (MAPP) model. This model, which has been developed by the National Association of County & City Health Officials (NACCHO) in cooperation with the Public Health Practice Program Office of the Centers for Disease Control and Prevention, can be reviewed at www.naccho.org/topics/infrastructure/ mapp/framework/mappbasics.cfm. As noted on this Web site, the MAPP model relies on four different assessments to gather situational information at the level of a community (NACCHO 2014, 1):

- *The Community Themes and Strengths Assessment* identifies themes that interest and engage the community, perceptions about quality of life, and community assets.

- *The Local Public Health System Assessment* measures the capacity of the local public health system to conduct essential public health services.

- *The Community Health Status Assessment* analyzes data about health status, quality of life, and risk factors in the community.

- *The Forces of Change Assessment* identifies forces that are occurring or will occur that will affect the community or the local public health system.

After it has been decided what to scan, the process moves to the next step: monitoring.

Monitoring

Effectively scanning the external environment of a program helps a manager identify and organize specific information about trends, developments, and events that represent either opportunities or threats. Information about these opportunities and threats requires continued attention through monitoring. Monitoring is more than scanning. It involves tracking or following important information over time.

Aspects of the external environment are monitored or tracked because they are thought to be relevant to the program's future. Monitoring these aspects of the environment, especially when there is ambiguity as to their importance to the program's future, permits more information to be assembled about trends, developments, and events, which helps clarify their importance or determine the rate at which they may be becoming important.

Monitoring has a much narrower focus than scanning because the purpose of monitoring is to build a base of data and information around the set of important or potentially important aspects of the external environ- ment that were identified through scanning or verified through earlier monitoring. Usually far fewer aspects of a program's external environment are monitored than are scanned.

Monitoring is vital because it is so often difficult to determine whether information concerning trends, developments, or events actually represents either real opportunities or threats for a program. Under conditions of certainty, managers would fully understand the information and all its consequences for their decisions and actions. But uncertainty characterizes much about the external environments of programs, and uncertainty cannot be removed completely. Uncertainty can, however, be significantly reduced by the acquisition of more detailed and sustained information through effective monitoring. As with scanning, techniques that feature the acquisition of multiple perspectives and expert opinions can be helpful. Careful monitoring and tracking provide the background for the next step in analyzing a program's external environment: forecasting changes in that environment.

Forecasting

Scanning and monitoring cannot, in and of themselves, provide managers with all the information they need about a program's external environment. Often, if they are to use this information effectively in developing/strategizing, they need forecasts of future conditions or states, which may give them time to adjust statements of the program's mission or objectives or to formulate and implement successful operational plans in response to the forecasted conditions.

Scanning and monitoring external environments involves searching for early signals that portend strategically important trends, developments, and events. Forecasting involves extending information beyond its current state.

Forecasts of some types of information can be made by extending past trends or by applying a formula of some kind. In other situations, forecasting must rely on conjecture, speculation, and judgment. Sometimes even sophisticated simulations can help in forecasting the future. However, none of these methods can eliminate uncertainty. It is especially difficult to reconcile any of these approaches with the fact that few strategically important pieces of information exist in a vacuum. There are almost always multiple variables at work simultaneously, and no forecasting techniques or models have been developed to fully account for this reality.

Two widely used forecasting techniques are described in the following subsections. Each can be useful in a program manager's efforts to forecast relevant external environmental changes.

Trend Extrapolation   A widely used forecasting technique is *trend extrapolation* (Morlidge and Player 2010). When properly used, this technique can be remarkably effective, and it is relatively simple to apply. Trend extrapolation is nothing more than tracking information and then using the tracking results to predict future states. It works best to predict general trends, such as the number of patients/customers who will be served by a program or the program's reimbursement rate for certain services from Medicare or Medicaid. For example, if the number of patients/customers has increased by 5 percent for each of the past five years, it may be reasonable to assume a 5 percent increase in the next year. Similarly, if reimbursement rates have increased by 2 or 3 percent for several years, this information suggests a continued rate of increase of 2 or 3 percent.

Scenario Development   Another useful forecasting technique is *scenario development* (Wade 2012). A scenario is a plausible prediction about the future. This technique is especially appropriate for analyzing environments that include many uncertainties and imponderables, as is the case with the external environments many health programs face.

The essence of scenario development is to define several alternative future states. These predictions can be used as the basis for making contingency plans; alternatively, a manager can use the set of scenarios to select what he or she considers to be the most likely future, the one on which developing/strategizing the future will be based. A common mistake in using scenario development, however, is to envision too early in the process one particular scenario as the correct picture of the future.

Assessing

Scanning and monitoring information that is relevant to developing/strategizing the future, and making accurate forecasts of the information, are each important steps in conducting an external situational analysis. But managers must also concern themselves with the specific and relative strategic importance—and the implications—of the information they are analyzing.

Making these assessments is not an exact science. More than anything else, it relies on the judgment of the people making them. Even so, there are several bases on which the strategic importance of information in an external environment can be considered. Prior experience with similar information is frequently a useful basis for assessing the importance of information. Other bases include intuition or best guesses about what particular information might mean to a program, as well as advice and insight from others who are well informed and experienced. When possible, quantification, modeling, and simulation of the potential impacts of information can be useful, but these techniques are often beyond the resources of a program.

It is rarely a simple task to accurately determine acquired information's relevance and importance to the future of a program. Aside from the difficulties encountered in collecting and properly analyzing enough information to fully inform the assessment, sometimes there are problems that derive from the influence of the personal preferences and biases of those conducting the external situational analysis. Such problems can result in assessments that fit preconceived notions about what is strategically important rather than reflecting the realities of the impact of particular information. As with other steps in an external situational analysis, obtaining multiple judgments about the strategic importance of information can help avoid the problem of bias.

Using and Disseminating

The final step in analyzing a program's external situation involves using the acquired information and forecasts in developing/strategizing activities, which may include disseminating or spreading the information to all those whose decisions and actions might be affected by it. This step is frequently undervalued as part of the conduct of an external situational analysis; it may even be overlooked. But unless information is disseminated to and used by all who need it, it does not matter how well the other steps in the analysis have been performed.

Managers must base their developing/strategizing on valid information about a program's external environment if this core management activity is to be properly performed. In many cases, managers need to share the information with others as well. For example, in a large program, there may be subdivisions with managers of their own who must engage in developing/strategizing. Managers can disseminate the strategically important information obtained through the conduct of an external situational analysis in the following three ways:

- Dictating or requiring use of the information, perhaps resorting to coercion or sanctions to see that the information is used in all the appropriate places in the program

- Persuading others to use the information by reasoning with them

- Educating others as to the importance and usefulness of the information in their own developing/strategizing activities

In dictating use, managers simply rely on the power associated with their position to require that the information be used. Other participants in the program are expected to carry out the dictates by using the information in their own developing/strategizing. There are times when such dictates are appropriate. For example, an abrupt and surprising change in a state's reimbursement policy for Medicaid services might require an immediate shift in how a program operates, leaving little time for anything but an edict to ensure the use of this information in revising operational plans. Dictates have the advantage of being fast and easy for managers to issue, although major drawbacks are their disruptiveness and recipients' feelings of nonparticipation in important decision making in which they were not involved.

The more participative persuasion and education approaches work better when time permits their use. These approaches are greatly facilitated when those who will end up using the information from an external situational analysis participate in its production. Participation can be achieved through such devices as membership on committees or teams charged to conduct the scanning, monitoring, forecasting, and assessing aspects of the assessment.

Using and disseminating the strategically important information about a program's external environment brings the process of conducting an external situational analysis to completion. Overall, the extent to which any program's manager and other participants are appropriately knowledgeable about and comfortable with the external environment depends very heavily on the quality of the external situational analysis.

The external situational analysis, no matter how well it is conducted, is only part of a complete situational analysis of a program. A complete analysis also requires information about the internal situation of the program, as well as an inventory of the desired results established for it.

Internal Situational Analysis

The second component of conducting a complete situational analysis is an *internal situational analysis*, involving cataloguing both strengths and weaknesses inherent in a program. This analysis provides managers with an inventory of the program's resource base for use in developing/strategizing the future. To ensure the development of a systematic inventory, a framework should guide the internal situational analysis, including at least the following components:

- A *financial analysis* covering the program's financial condition, trends in its financial performance, revenue streams, and funding sources. This information may include how a program compares to industry norms or to similar programs.

- A *human resource analysis* covering the program's capabilities in regard to performing its direct, support, and management work. This analysis should provide information on the adequacy of participants, in terms of numbers and credentials, both for present activities and for possible future development. This analysis sometimes covers cultural aspects of a program. Cultural aspects include participants' shared beliefs (such as in the centrality of patient care, the importance of medical research, and the primacy of quality in health services delivery) and shared values (such as duty, integrity, trust, and fairness). Shared beliefs and values help guide the behavior of participants. Although this part of a human resource analysis may involve a degree of subjectivity, it can be an important component of a complete internal situational analysis.

- A *marketing analysis* covering all aspects of the program's ability to distribute its services. This analysis should identify the program's target markets and its competitive position (market share) within these markets.

- An *operations analysis* covering the program's various production or service delivery activities. This analysis should cover activities in the direct work of the program, but it should also cover support and management operations.

Inventory of Desired Results

The third component of a complete situational analysis is an ***inventory of desired results*** established for a program. These should exist as written statements of the program's ***mission*** and ***objectives***.

A mission statement typically is a broad, general expression of a program's overall purpose or purposes. For example, the expressed mission of the California Breast Cancer Research Program (2014), the largest state-funded breast cancer research effort in the nation, is "to prevent and eliminate breast cancer by leading innovation in research, communication, and collaboration in the California scientific and lay communities." Similarly broad and qualitative, the mission of the Central Florida Immunization Coalition (2014) is to "improve the health of Central Floridians from birth through adulthood by promoting immunizations that prevent diseases." These statements each contain the key element of a useful mission statement: what the program intends to do.

Most mission statements are inherently qualitative, although some do incorporate more quantitative terms. Even when a mission statement does include quantification, the mission may not be expressed with a high degree of precision. Mission statements are important expressions of what programs intend to accomplish. They are usually too general, however, to fully guide the work done in programs. Thus, the more concrete, quantified statements of objectives are very important.

Objectives express the specific, quantified desired results established for a program. For example, objectives might be to increase service sessions by 10 percent in the coming year and to enroll five hundred patients/customers in the next three months. Objectives can also be expressed in terms of desired changes in the patients/customers served by a program. Examples are changes in behavior, knowledge, health status, or level of functioning brought about in patients/customers through the services of the program. Objectives can also be expressed in terms of desired changes in the operation of the program. Examples are objectives expressing a desire to attain a quality level consistent with best practice guidelines, to have all patients/customers treated in a culturally sensitive manner, or to produce a new educational brochure.

Statements of objectives for a program should, to the extent possible, be concrete and specific. This means the objectives should be quantified and related to a time frame. For example, an objective to achieve one hundred units of a service provided in a six-month period is more useful as a guide to action than an objective to achieve one hundred units of a service, but with no time frame specified. Stated objectives should be realistic, achievable, and understandable to the participants responsible for their accomplishment.

Quantifying objectives facilitates pinpointing accountability for their accomplishment. Every participant in a program who has responsibility for accomplishing specific objectives, and who is given the resources to do so, can and should be held accountable for the results. Accountability for results is clearer if the results are measurable.

Objectives are not chiseled in stone. They should be flexible, because circumstances change, which may necessitate changing stated objectives. For example, a program's manager may have established an objective to hold payroll expenditures for the year below a certain level. But if the number of patients/customers increases above that which was projected when the objective was developed, then the objective may have to be altered to remain appropriate in the new circumstances.

When missions and objectives for programs do not exist in writing, preparing written statements becomes a critical task in effective developing/

strategizing. These statements of desired results are necessary in determining the current situation of a program.

The information collected through conducting external and internal situational analyses, along with the inventory of desired results established for a program, provides a solid foundation for the other aspects of developing/strategizing, which are (1) reconsidering and revising the program's current state and developing operational plans to achieve the revisions, and (2) evaluating performance, which involves both assessing progress toward and controlling performance related to accomplishing the revised desired results. We will consider first the manager's tasks of determining how the program should be changed and developing operational plans to accomplish the changes.

Reconsidering and Revising a Program's Current Situation

Using the information obtained in conducting the situational analysis just discussed, a program's manager has a starting point for developing/strategizing the program's future. This begins with considering whether or not something about the program should be changed. The manager must establish a blueprint for the program's future state. This blueprint reflects how the manager wants the program to be situated in the future (usually in the next year, although developing/strategizing can also be done in multiyear increments). It is not unusual, for example, for a program to have a five-year plan or strategy. The blueprint can contain changes in the desired results established for the program, as well as changes in how the desired results can be accomplished.

Reconsidering and Revising Statements of Missions and Objectives

In determining how a program should be situated in the future (assume the next year), those who are involved in developing/strategizing its future must reconsider and revise statements of desired results, whether the mission, the objectives, or both. They can add new statements as well as delete or modify existing statements as they choose. By reconsidering and revising the statements of desired results, they restate what they intend for the program to accomplish in the future.

The reconsideration and revision necessary in determining a preferred future state for a program do not end merely with changes in statements of desired results. Managers must determine whether new resources, such as additional funding or people with different educational backgrounds and credentials, are needed to accomplish new desired results. They might consider possible changes in existing resources, such as redirecting existing funding or retraining existing staff. They must also consider changing existing processes used in conducting the program's direct work, either by addition, deletion, or modification. These changes can be made to accomplish new desired results, but they can also be made to improve the efficiency or quality of work processes intended to attain the existing mission and objectives.

Although changes in resources and processes typically are necessary if new desired results are to be attained, it is well documented in health services settings that changes in work processes are difficult to establish and maintain. The inertia built into established patterns of work and the effort necessary to implement new work processes make changing them very challenging (Daft 2014; Ham, Kipping, and McLeod 2003).

Changing the desired results for a program can also be difficult. Managers sometimes find it challenging to establish a new objective, for example, when its selection means giving up a previously established objective. When a decision is made to pursue a new objective and commit resources to achieving it, this may mean other alternatives must then be foregone. Some managers may find it difficult to accept the fact that their program cannot achieve all the results that are important to them, and may therefore be reluctant to make firm commitments to specific statements of desired results to avoid the painful consequence of giving up pursuit of other desirable results.

Another problem that affects some managers at the point of establishing or revising a program's desired results is their concern that they might fail to accomplish the intended results. Whenever a manager sets a clear-cut desired result—whether in the form of a mission or objectives—there is an accompanying risk that the result will not or cannot be achieved. Concerns about such failure prevent some managers from establishing definitive statements of desired results against which their performance can eventually be judged. Those who lack confidence in their ability to attain results or who are highly risk averse may be reluctant to establish statements of desired results that may be difficult to accomplish.

In spite of such difficulties, however, managers must be explicit in stating desired results for a program if these decisions are to serve as a guide in moving to a desired future state. Similarly, managers must consider the resource and work process implications of revising the desired results. They must develop operational plans for accomplishing these changes.

Developing Operational Plans to Accomplish Missions and Objectives and Changes in Them

The accomplishment of desired results in a program, including moving to a new or revised preferred future state, depends on developing and implementing a good *operational plan*. A program's mission and objectives can be thought of as the ends toward which those involved in a program work; operational plans represent the detailed means of accomplishing those ends.

Once decisions about ends have been made, decisions about means can be addressed. In operational planning, managers develop and assess alternative means of achieving established ends, selecting the specific manner in which the ends will be pursued. Much of the day-to-day management work in programs consists of finding effective ways to accomplish the established ends reflected in missions and objectives.

Although there is no formula by which the most appropriate means to accomplish ends are selected, once alternative ideas about the means to accomplish ends have been placed on a menu for consideration, their relative advantages, disadvantages, and potential effects and implications can be assessed. The manager's task is to assess the available alternatives relative to each other and select those thought to give the best chance of accomplishing the desired results.

In some situations, operational planning can influence decisions about ends. An objective established for a program that cannot be achieved should be reconsidered. Therefore, although we are discussing ends and means in this order, in reality decisions about each influence the other.

If a manager concludes that a particular objective cannot be achieved with available or obtainable resources and work processes, then the objective must be modified or abandoned. Similarly, a manager choosing between two equally attractive ends for a program—when both cannot be achieved simultaneously—can readily make the choice if operational planning determines that one attractive end will cost significantly more or less than another equally attractive end. Great care must be exercised, however, in permitting assessments of means to influence decisions about ends. In general, means are not as important as ends. Means are but ways to achieve the ends of a program. A program's ends in the form of its mission and objectives are the reason it exists.

Choosing from among the Alternatives in Developing an Operational Plan

Armed with comparative information based on assessments of alternatives, managers can choose from among their alternatives in an informed way as they develop operational plans. As with other types of management decisions, selection of the means to accomplish a program's ends can be based on experience, on intuition, on advice from consultants or colleagues, on systematic analyses to identify the alternative that most closely fits a set of criteria, or on some combination of these bases. In making these decisions, managers can also be guided by the information provided in Chapter 5, "Making Good Management Decisions," including that pertaining to decision grids, payoff tables, decision trees, and cost-benefit analysis. The program evaluation and review technique, or PERT as it is often called, can be especially useful in assessments of the timing of elements in operational plans.

Managers, as they actually choose from among alternatives in developing an operational plan, face some of the same difficulties that all decision makers face at the point of decision. For example, they may hesitate because they are not certain they have assembled all the relevant information. The process of collecting and analyzing information in the situational analysis is often difficult, and there is the persistent problem of knowing when enough information has been considered to ensure a well-informed planning process. This problem exists in most decision-making circumstances. In addition, managers can be indecisive or impulsive, just as decision makers in other situations can be.

The difficulties inherent in making the choices necessary in formulating operational plans are not insurmountable, and in general they are reduced as managers gain experience with operational planning. In addition, managers who have the opportunity to receive coaching and counseling from more experienced managers are better able to develop their operational planning capabilities and to enhance other aspects of their developing/strategizing activities.

Coaching and counseling can occur quite naturally in most programs, because programs are embedded in larger organizations. A manager's immediate superior in an organization can provide training and guidance in establishing statements of desired results and in developing suitable operational plans to achieve results. In addition, recognition and rewards for success that the superior provides can reinforce learning, and constructive and supportive critiques of mistakes can provide less-experienced managers with valuable learning opportunities.

Managers who lack confidence in their ability to develop good operational plans can benefit from participating in management development programs. One of the important purposes of such programs is to enhance the capabilities of managers in regard to making better decisions, including those made within the context of developing/strategizing. When programs are embedded in an organization that offers management development opportunities, that has a well-understood approach to developing/strategizing, and that devotes sufficient resources to the activity, it is easier for all managers to effectively develop/strategize. In the absence of such organizational support, managers must seek to develop and enhance their capabilities by drawing on the resources of a program, or through participation in outside management development opportunities provided through professional associations and universities, including online opportunities.

Implementation Considerations in Operational Planning

The development of good operational plans includes paying careful attention to factors that will affect their implementation, including available resources, attitudes about the plans, and other operational plans being implemented simultaneously. Operational plans, no matter how carefully crafted, do not implement themselves. Attention must be given during their formulation to the challenges likely to arise in implementing them.

A good operational plan is formulated with attention to a program's capabilities for implementing the plan. Ideally, managers recognize the connection between plans and implementation capabilities and factor this into operational planning decisions. When mismatches occur between operational plans and implementation capabilities, problems invariably arise. Such mismatches can be overcome in two ways: (1) a particular operational plan can be changed, and (2) a program's capabilities in regard to implementing a particular operational plan can be changed. In the latter case, resources can be redirected; participants can be provided with additional training and education; and new participants can be brought into the situation to support implementation.

Even when there is a close match between operational plans and implementation capabilities, implementation requires that managers also be effective at designing and leading. For example, in the staffing aspect of organization design, attracting and retaining participants with the skills and abilities needed to implement operational plans are crucial to the successful implementation of plans. Similarly, leading other participants in doing their part in implementation is also vital to success.

When a manager knows the current situation of a program, has a clear vision of how the program should change in the future, and has developed appropriate operational plans for moving to the new state, the developing/strategizing challenge moves to one of assessing or evaluating performance and controlling performance related to moving to the new desired state.

Assessing and Controlling Performance to Achieve Desired Results

The developing/strategizing activity in management work is brought full circle through (1) determining whether or not acceptable progress is being made toward achieving a program's mission and objectives, and (2) taking corrective steps if needed. In undertaking both of these tasks, managers increase the likelihood that desired results will eventually be achieved.

Controlling Defined and Modeled

Technically, *controlling* in work situations is regulating actions and decisions in accordance with the stated desired results—whether in the form of missions or objectives—and the standards of performance established in operational plans. The word *control* often carries a negative connotation. People tend to think of it as referring to a sinister activity involving surveillance, correction, or even reproach. But control is a normal part of most human endeavors.

Monitoring the results accomplished and feeding this information back to those who can influence future results constitute a normal, pervasive, and natural phenomenon in work settings, including health programs. Chefs watch their hollandaise sauces carefully, nurses monitor the condition of patients in their care, manufacturers check the quality of products coming off their assembly lines, and soccer coaches watch the scoreboard and clock. All this monitoring is done so that deviations can be detected and corrected in time to favorably affect results.

Controlling expenditures, quality of services, participants' morale, or anything else involves monitoring performance, comparing actual results with previously established desired results and standards, and correcting deviations that are found. Figure 2.2 illustrates these interrelated parts of controlling applied to assessing and controlling performance in the laboratory of a program designed to screen for HIV infection. Note that the work of this laboratory is modeled in terms of the resources required, work processes used, and objectives achieved (see the shaded portion of the figure). The elements necessary for assessing progress and controlling performance are also shown (see the box labeled "Monitoring Results and Comparing Them to Objectives and Standards" and the box labeled "Adjusting and Correcting Performance").

In this model, it is assumed that objectives have been established earlier in developing/strategizing for this program's laboratory. Objectives are, in effect, the targets or ends desired for a program, or in this case a unit of a

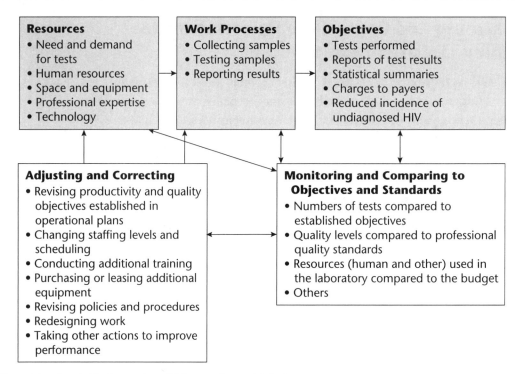

Figure 2.2   Control of Performance in an HIV Screening Program's Laboratory

program. Standards are typically established by professions, regulators, and accrediting agencies. Together, the objectives and standards become the criteria against which performance can be compared and judged.

To be most useful in controlling, both objectives and standards should be expressed in terms against which actual performance can be measured. Examples include quantity, cost, time, attitude, or quality measures. Controlling is facilitated when the criteria against which performance will be assessed are expressed in concrete terms, although this works better in some situations than in others. For example, an objective of high morale among participants may be more difficult to specify in concrete terms than an objective of not exceeding an established operating budget in a given year. However, ways of subjectively determining whether movement is toward or away from achievement of an objective of improved morale can be devised and used.

Monitoring and Comparing

In monitoring and comparing, actual performance is measured. There is no substitute for direct observation and personal contact by managers as they monitor performance, although such techniques are inefficient. Thus, some monitoring is typically done through other means. Written reports on performance can be especially useful for managers with a large or diverse domain of responsibility. To monitor performance in a large program, managers may have to rely almost exclusively on written or verbal reports provided by others. In some instances, managers prefer to receive performance reports only when established desired results or standards are not being met, relying on what is called the exception approach to monitoring.

Program managers also may find an *information system (IS)* useful in their controlling efforts (Smaltz, Glandon, and Slovensky 2013). Such a system can be designed so that information relevant to controlling can be collected, formatted, stored, and retrieved in a timely way to support the monitoring and comparing aspects of controlling. It is important to make a distinction between data and information because, although different, both are important in monitoring and comparing. *Data*, on the one hand, is "information in raw or unorganized form (such as alphabets, numbers, or symbols) that refer[s] to, or represent[s], conditions, ideas, or objects" (BusinessDictionary 2014a). *Information*, on the other hand, is "data that is (1) accurate and timely, (2) specific and organized for a purpose, (3) presented within a context that gives it meaning and relevance, and (4) [possibly leading] to an increase in understanding and decrease in uncertainty" (BusinessDictionary 2014b). For managing purposes, including use in monitoring and controlling, information is far better than raw data. This means that attention must be given to converting data into information, and an IS can do this.

An IS can be relatively simple or very elaborate. If it is to be useful, however, an IS should show deviations at critical points. Effective control requires attention to those factors that actually affect a program's performance. A good IS will show deviations promptly and contain information that is understandable to those who use the system. Finally, a good IS will contain information that permits a manager to see where possible corrective action is needed. An IS that detects deviations from the accomplishment of objectives or from adherence to relevant standards will be little more than an interesting exercise if it does not show the way to corrective action. A good IS will disclose where failures are occurring and who is responsible for them, so that corrective action can be taken.

Adjusting and Correcting

When the process of monitoring and comparing reveals deviations from the accomplishment of objectives or from adherence to chosen standards, adjustments should be made, or corrective actions should be taken. These adjustments and corrective actions are intended to curb undesirable results and bring performance back in line. Knowing what actions to take, however, can be a challenge for managers.

Because so many underlying factors can be involved, it is often difficult to determine the flaws in operational plans or to ascertain why implementation falters. Are the established objectives reasonable? Are the operational plans developed to accomplish them adequate? Is the implementation of operational plans going smoothly? Are there adequate resources, and are participants properly trained to implement the operational plans?

Managers should base their decisions about adjustments and corrective actions on a careful analysis of the situation, starting with consideration of the objectives and standards against which they are monitoring performance. After all, the objectives or even a program's mission may have been poorly conceived; or conditions may have changed, rendering them inappropriate. Too, standards undergo revisions from time to time. When desired results or standards are changed, adjustments may be necessary in resources or work processes used.

Only after a thorough analysis of the reasons for a deviation will a manager be in a position to take effective corrective action that will secure improved results in the future. Such corrective action may consist of revising the mission or objectives, changing a work process, redeploying resources, having a simple discussion with participants about their work, employing a change in technology, increasing training, upgrading equipment, budgeting more time, creating a new schedule, or doing anything else to rectify the situation.

Budgets and Effective Control

Managers need effective control systems or techniques to support their efforts to assess and control performance in a program. These techniques should assist managers in detecting discrepancies between objectives and actual performance, and in taking corrective action. Managers of health programs routinely employ *budgets*, the most widely used control systems, in their efforts to control performance.

Budgets reflect projected activities of programs, or subunits within them, in numerical terms covering a specified period of time. Their use as control systems derives from the fact that budgets reflect preestablished objectives or standards against which actual operating results can be compared and adjusted through the exercise of control.

Budgets provide information that enables managers to take corrective action when necessary to bring results into conformity with targets. Although budgets often are expressed in monetary terms, they can be expressed in other terms as well. Personnel budgets, for example, indicate the number of people needed at various skill levels and the number of person-hours allocated for certain activities.

For most programs, an operating budget, which is a combination of a revenue budget and an expense budget, may be the only budget required for controlling purposes. Exhibit 2.1 contains the annual operating budget for a large program designed to provide a range of health services on a fee-for-service basis for patients/customers who use the program, and to also provide services for an enrolled population that includes twelve thousand members. These services are provided under contract on a capitated, or per person, basis.

EXHIBIT 2.1 A Program's Operating Budget for Year X

Part I Volume Assumptions

A.	Fee-for-service (FFS)	20,000	visits
B.	Capitated lives (plan members)	12,000	members
	Number of member-months	144,000	
	Expected use per member-month	0.20	visits
	Number of visits	28,800	visits
C.	Total expected visits	48,800	visits

Part II Revenue Assumptions

A.	FFS	$ 110	per visit
		× 20,000	visits
		$2,200,000	
B.	Capitated lives	$ 11	per member per month
		× 144,000	member-months
		$1,584,000	
C.	Total expected revenues	$3,784,000	

(continued)

EXHIBIT 2.1 (Continued)

Part III   Cost Assumptions

    A.   Variable costs

Staffing (26,000 hours at $77 per hour)	$2,002,000	
Supplies	247,500	
Total variable costs	$2,249,500	
Variable cost per visit	$ 46.09	($2,249,500 ÷ 48,800 visits)

    B.   Fixed costs

Overhead, depreciation, and leasing	$1,100,000	
C. Total expected costs	$3,349,500	

Part IV   Pro Forma Profit and Loss (P&L) Statement

Revenues		
FFS	$2,200,000	
Capitated	1,584,000	
Total	$3,784,000	
Variable costs	$2,249,500	
Contribution margin	$1,534,500	($3,784,000 − $2,249,500)
Fixed costs	1,100,000	
Projected profit	$ 434,500	

The construction of an operating budget for this program requires volume projections or estimates as a starting point. Based on past experience, the manager estimates that 20,000 visits to the program will be made by FFS patients/customers in Year X. In addition, the capitated population has averaged 0.20 visits per member-month. Therefore, the manager calculates that in Year X the capitated population will produce 12,000 × 12 = 144,000 member-months. The manager uses the historical average of 0.20 visits per member-month to calculate an estimated number of visits by the capitated population as follows: 144,000 × 0.20 = 28,800 visits. Estimated total volume expressed as the number of visits to the program for services for Year X is 20,000 + 28,800 = 48,800 visits. (These volume assumptions are shown as Part I in Exhibit 2.1.)

To calculate the revenue budget, the manager assumes that the program's net collection for the FFS visits will average $110 per visit. Some visits will produce more revenue, some less. On average, however, past experience yields an estimate of $110 per visit from the FFS patients/customers. Thus, the manager estimates FFS revenues as 20,000 visits × $110 = $2,200,000 for Year X. Using the contract premium established for the capitated population of $11 per member per month, the manager can calculate revenue from this source as $11 × 144,000 member-months = $1,584,000 for Year X. Combining FFS and capitated patients/customers, the manager can estimate total revenue for the program in Year X as $2,200,000 + $1,584,000 = $3,784,000. These revenue assumptions are shown as Part II in Exhibit 2.1. It should be emphasized that this is an estimate of the program's revenues; conditions could change, making the estimate inaccurate.

Part III of the operating budget shown in Exhibit 2.1 contains information on the program's estimated expenses for Year X. The manager, again relying on past experience with the program's operations, estimates that the anticipated 48,800 visits will require a combined staffing cost of $41.02 per visit. This amount accounts for staff involved in direct, support, and management work in the program, and is calculated as follows: 26,000 hours of estimated staff time × $77 per hour on average = $2,002,000. Thus, staff costs per visit are expected to average $2,002,000 ÷ 48,800 visits = $41.02. Although not all costs are variable for staff shown in Exhibit 2.1 doing direct and support work, the use of part-time staff and the payment of some staff on the basis of productivity permit the manager to closely tie the number of hours of estimated staff time to the number of estimated visits.

The other portion of estimated expenses is for supplies. The manager estimates that medical and administrative supplies will cost $247,500 in Year X, based on past patterns of these expenses and the estimated volume of activity. This means that supply costs will average $5.07 per visit ($247,500 ÷ 48,800 visits). Thus, the program's combined cost for staffing and supplies per visit in Year X is estimated to be $41.02 + $5.07 = $46.09.

Finally, as can be seen in Part III, the program is expected to incur $1,100,000 of fixed costs in Year X. These expenses include overhead costs, as well as depreciation of equipment and the cost of leasing the program's space to serve the program's anticipated 48,800 visits by its patients/customers in Year X. Variable costs are expected to total $2,249,500 ($2,002,000 in staffing and $247,500 in supplies), plus $1,100,000 in fixed costs, for a total of $3,349,500.

Part IV of Exhibit 2.1 shows the determination of the program's pro forma (projected) profit and loss statement. The P&L statement is the heart of an operating budget. The difference between projected revenues of $3,784,000 and projected variable costs of $2,249,500 produces a total contribution margin of $1,534,500. Deducting the forecasted fixed costs of $1,100,000 yields a budgeted profit for the program of $434,500.

Budgets are merely guides for managers, not substitutes for good judgment. Effective budgets afford managers the necessary latitude and flexibility to accomplish the objectives established for their programs when conditions change within the periods the budgets cover. To keep budgets from becoming too restrictive, enlightened managers ensure flexibility in the use of budgets by monitoring operating conditions and revising budgets when conditions appreciably change. Additional information on budgeting can be found in the work of Gapenski (2011) and Nowicki (2011).

The Link between Developing/Strategizing and the Performance of Programs

Effective developing/strategizing is crucial to the overall performance of programs, beginning with the focus on desired results that good developing/ strategizing requires. Developing/strategizing yields appropriate statements of mission and objectives, and it supports managers in developing operational plans for accomplishing the desired ends. In this way, developing/ strategizing contributes to focusing on desired ends and coordinating the use of a program's resources and work processes toward achieving them.

Developing/strategizing also contributes to performance by helping managers at least partially offset the effects of pervasive uncertainty. When managers think about the future in systematic ways and plan for contingencies, they greatly reduce the likelihood of being caught unprepared.

Through developing operational plans and assessing and controlling performance, managers also enhance operational efficiency and effectiveness. As noted in Chapter 1, developing/strategizing affords managers opportunities to substitute integrated effort for random activity, controlled flow of work for uneven flow, and careful decisions for snap judgments. These and other results of effective developing/strategizing contribute directly to operational efficiency in programs and to the effectiveness of direct, support, and management work.

Finally, effective developing/strategizing facilitates not only the continual assessment of progress toward accomplishment of the desired results established for a program but also the exercise of control over the performance of direct, support, and management work in pursuit of these ends. This is increasingly important as those who pay for health services, whether payment is provided through public programs, such as Medicare and Medicaid, or by private employers through their insurance mechanisms, require greater accountability from those who provide these services.

The required accountability goes beyond cost to include both the quality of services and the manner in which they are delivered (Smith et al. 2012, 5–7). The trend toward more accountability and the concurrent necessity of control that it implies will become increasingly important in all health services settings. The relationship between increased pressure for accountability and managers' efforts to control performance for which they are responsible is a primary argument for effective developing/strategizing in health programs.

Before concluding this chapter, two additional topics related to developing/ strategizing are covered in the following sections: business plans and interventional planning. The unique circumstances associated with the initial development of a new program are discussed in terms of writing a business plan for the program. A business plan is also useful as a precursor to a major change in an existing program, such as the addition of a new service line.

Also discussed is interventional planning, which is the application of planning techniques to the development, implementation, and evaluation of the interventions that many health programs undertake to address one or more health determinants that affect the patients/customers they serve. Interventional planning differs from the core developing/strategizing activity as well as from operational planning. The success of most interventions or initiatives that a program undertakes depends heavily on effective use of this type of planning.

Writing a Business Plan

One of the most important stages in the life of any program is its original conceptualization and then development into a concrete, well-formed idea. At this beginning point, a program may be nothing more than an idea or a concept in the imagination of someone who thinks it can meet a real need. An early task in the life of any program is for those who support it to demonstrate that the idea is viable. Thus, an initial round of developing/strategizing for a program is required. This is termed business planning, and results in a document called a **business plan** (Abrams and Doerr 2010).

The concept of business plans emerged in the entrepreneurial world, where anyone with an idea for a new business has to make a convincing case to banks, venture capitalists, and other potential investors to attract the necessary capital to get the business to an operational stage. The business plan in this context is a written document describing the nature of the business and how the entrepreneur intends to start and operate it.

The Small Business Administration (2014), a federal agency that supports the establishment and operation of small businesses in the United States, has noted that a business plan "is an essential roadmap for business success. This living document generally projects 3–5 years ahead and outlines the route a company intends to take to grow revenues."

Writing a business plan helps managers step back and think objectively about the key elements of a planned business venture and informs their decision making. Because business planning is so ubiquitous, there are many consulting firms—such as Palo Alto Software (www.paloalto.com/business_plan_software/)—available to assist in the process.

A business plan for a nascent health program is developed as a means of making a convincing case to all those who must approve its initiation. This is especially important for the organizational superiors who must approve the program's initiation.

Although business plans vary in content, it is useful to include the following components:

- A summary description of the program, including resources needed, work processes, and desired results stated as a mission and objectives

- An explanation of why the program is needed and why it will succeed in its target market(s)

- A description of the target market(s) for the program, with projections of the need and demand for its services and, as appropriate, projections of sales and market share for the first five years of operation

- A description of how the program will be managed, including information on the qualifications of key participants

- A description of how the clinical services (if applicable) of the program will be provided, including information on the qualifications of key participants

- A detailed operating budget, usually projected for the first year of the new program and also projected through the first five years of operation

- A detailed description of space and equipment needed for the first five years of operation

- A description of funding sources for the program, including revenues expected from operations, grants, contracts, and other sources of funding

- An analysis of the major risks or challenges the program is likely to face in its first five years, and a description of how these will be addressed

- A timetable of key events and accomplishments expected for the program in its first five years

Comprehensive business plans for new programs cannot guarantee their success. They can, however, ensure that careful thought is given to the development and early operational phase of a program, and to preparing to meet the challenges that can be foreseen in this special form of developing/strategizing the new program's future.

Planning for Interventions Undertaken by Programs

Another form of planning that falls under the overall heading of developing/strategizing is *interventional planning*, which involves the application of planning techniques to the development, implementation, and evaluation of interventions undertaken by programs as part of their direct work.

In small, highly focused programs—those intended to engage in one specific intervention, such as a program in which participants conduct a single highly focused health education intervention or activity—making a distinction between overall developing/strategizing and interventional planning, especially distinguishing between operational planning and interventional planning, may not be possible or relevant. That said, in larger programs there are important distinctions between the overall developing/strategizing done for an entire program, operational planning in the interest of accomplishing the program's mission and objectives, and the interventional planning that is done for specific interventions developed and provided within the program. An example will help distinguish between interventional planning, operational planning, and the more general developing/strategizing activities in which program managers engage.

The example is of a successful health education program established by and embedded in a county health department that has served a number of clients for several years. Among the clients are groups of citizens of the county with various demographic characteristics (the elderly, minorities, female teenagers); clinical conditions (diabetes, obesity, drug abuse); and affiliations (elementary school students, eldercare program participants). All of the health education interventions for these clients are paid for through public funds made available to the health department or through grants from foundations.

In *developing/strategizing* this program's future, its manager determined that it was important to enhance the resources available to the program by adding private, paying clients. The manager envisioned many benefits available to the program from broadening the base of financial support through the addition of corporate clients that would pay for services.

The *operational planning* as to how to accomplish the desired enhancement of the program's resources led some of the program's health educators to visit the benefits managers at local companies and other businesses to explain the advantages of sponsoring various health education interventions for their employees. This resulted in two new clients—a large financial services company and the local plant of an international manufacturing firm.

Good developing/strategizing, including effective operational planning, paid off for this health education program, but the success achieved by adding the new clients triggered the need for *interventional planning*. The program manager assigned a health educator to each of the new corporate clients to do the interventional planning necessary to guide the provision of health education services. Interventional planning is typically undertaken in a series of six steps, as shown in Figure 2.3. Described next is the health educators' respective roles in each step in the interventional planning for each client.

Step 1: Building Knowledge of the Client

The health educators each met separately with a key representative of the new client to which they had been assigned. One met with the benefits manager at the plant, and the other met with the vice president of human resources at the financial services company. These meetings were held to obtain the views of these representatives as to what an intervention might accomplish. In each case, information about the organization, including information about how employees and their family members used health benefits, was reviewed. Later, in building knowledge of each client, the corresponding health educator interviewed groups of employees and family members. For each client, a health education committee was formed whose members included managers and other employees representing the client.

Step 2: Assessing the Client's Needs

In each situation, with the help of the health education committee, the health educator conducted a needs assessment (Gilmore 2011; McKenzie,

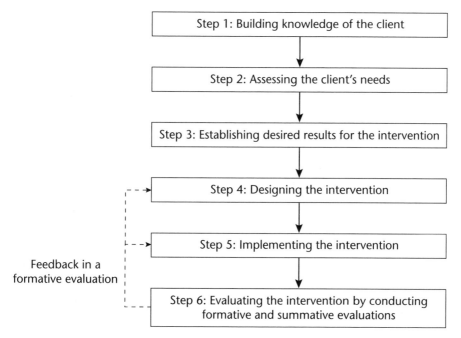

Figure 2.3 Model of Interventional Planning

Neiger, and Thackeray 2013; Petersen and Alexander 2001), including a survey of behavioral risk factors completed by samples of employees and their family members. In addition, there were several focus group meetings to explore possible needs on which to focus the intervention. Each committee also reviewed insurance claims data, without identifiers, for its firm's employees and their dependents over several years, as well as the Healthcare Effectiveness Data and Information Set (HEDIS) made available by the National Committee on Quality Assurance (NCQA) for the health plans in which employees and their families were enrolled. (Information is available on NCQA and HEDIS at www.ncqa.org.)

The assessment in both situations identified several areas of need for a health education intervention. At the financial services company, the most compelling problem in need of intervention was that employees and their spouses were experiencing a significantly higher rate of type 2 diabetes than would be expected in a population of this age and gender makeup. At the plant, the most compelling problem had to do with the prevention of injuries among employees—especially back injuries caused by lifting.

Step 3: Establishing Desired Results for the Intervention

With the involvement of the health education committees, the health educators developed statements of the desired results of the interventions.

An objective for the financial services company was to eventually reduce the incidence of type 2 diabetes among employees and their spouses to a level consistent with that expected in a group with this age and gender makeup. An objective for the plant was to reduce the incidence of injuries to a rate no greater than the industry average. In both cases, it was anticipated that the objective would take many years to achieve, and would not occur until well after the intervention had been completed.

Other objectives for the intervention at the financial services company included a specific number of face-to-face health education sessions to expose employees and spouses to information about diabetes, and the production and distribution of printed information about the disease, including its prevention, diagnosis, and appropriate treatment. Another objective for the financial services company intervention was to include information about diabetes on the company's Web site. The health education committee also established an objective that following the intervention, all employees with type 2 diabetes would have appropriate hemoglobin A1c (HbA1c), lipids (LDL-C), and kidney disease monitoring (microalbuminuria testing), as well as annual eye examinations. Appropriate objectives also were established for the health education intervention at the plant, although the financial services company will be used as the example for the remainder of this discussion.

Step 4: Designing the Intervention

The health educator assigned to the financial services company designed the intervention to include a number of specific educational activities. The design was influenced heavily by the authoritative recommendations of the National Diabetes Education Program (www.ndep.nih.gov), which is a partnership of the National Institutes of Health, the Centers for Disease Control and Prevention, and more than two hundred public and private organizations.

The design of the intervention also was guided by the health educator's use of the design features of a number of well-established health education planning models, including the following:

- The Assessment Protocol for Excellence in Public Health Model (Sharma and Romas 2012)
- The PRECEDE-PROCEED Model for Health Promotion Planning and Evaluation (Green and Kreuter 2004)
- The Model for Health Education Planning (MHEP; Sharma and Romas 2012)

- The Model for Health Education Planning and Resource Development (MHEPRD; Sharma and Romas 2012)

- The Multilevel Approach to Community Health (MATCH; Simons-Morton, McLeroy, and Wendel 2012)

- CDCynergy, a tool for planning, managing, and evaluating public health communication programs (www.cdc.gov/healthcommunication/CDCynergy)

- The Social Marketing Assessment and Response Tool (SMART; Thackeray and Neiger 2003)

- The Planning, Program Development, and Evaluation Model (PPDEM; Timmreck 2002)

- The Generalized Model for Program Planning (GMPP; McKenzie, Neiger, and Thackeray 2013)

Step 5: Implementing the Intervention

The health educator implemented the intervention by carrying out the activities called for in its design, including distributing a diabetes information sheet along with each employee's paycheck. Over the course of the implementation, this was followed up with additional information sheets in employee pay envelopes about aspects of diabetes. Two articles about diabetes were written for and included in the company newsletter, and information about the disease was featured on the company's Web site. Posters about the disease were used throughout the company to enhance awareness.

Employees and their family members with diabetes received special mailings with information about how to interact effectively with their physicians. They were provided with information produced by the National Diabetes Education Program about specific questions to ask their physicians, including (1) "What are my blood sugar, blood pressure, and cholesterol numbers?" (2) "What should they be?" (3) "What actions should I take to reach these goals?"

The employees and their family members were also given wallet cards on which to record and track these numbers.

Step 6: Evaluating the Intervention by Conducting Formative and Summative Evaluations

All interventions should be evaluated, although the extent of the evaluation can vary depending on the importance of its results and the available resources. Remember from the discussion in Chapter 1 that when program managers engage in evaluating activities they are "collecting information about a program or some aspect of a program in order to make necessary decisions about the program" (McNamara 2014). Evaluating, which is shown as one of the facilitative activities of management work in Figure 1.4, is an integral part of management work and serves a number of purposes. The discussion here is limited to the specific purpose of evaluating interventions undertaken by programs. The broader subject of program evaluation is discussed in Chapter 9. Additional useful information for conducting evaluations can be found in a comprehensive approach developed by the Centers for Disease Control and Prevention at www.cdc.gov/eval/index.htm.

In this context of evaluating interventions undertaken by programs, an evaluation is an analytical process involving the collection and analysis of information that allows managers to improve an intervention while it is in progress and to measure the degree to which the desired results have been achieved after its conclusion (Rossi, Lipsey, and Freeman 2004; Wholey, Hatry, and Newcomer 2010). There are therefore two purposes for evaluating interventions, with the fulfillment of each driving the use of somewhat different methodologies. A *formative evaluation* is intended to help improve an intervention as it takes place. A *summative evaluation* is intended to prove whether an intervention accomplished the objectives established for it. The health educator assigned to the financial services company determined that both purposes were relevant to evaluating the health education intervention, and undertook both formative and summative evaluations of the intervention.

Formative Evaluation   A formative evaluation is much like the determination of whether or not acceptable progress is being made toward achieving a program's desired results as part of the more general developing/strategizing activity. In fact, application of the control model shown in Figure 2.2 can help guide the formative evaluation of an intervention. During a formative evaluation, questions are asked about results as they are occurring. This type of evaluation entails monitoring the progress being made in an intervention and making midcourse corrections as needed to keep the intervention on track.

The health educator, in conducting the formative evaluation of the intervention at the financial services company, gathered information to determine progress toward the desired results established for the intervention in Step 3. As is typical of formative evaluation, the focus was on the specific objectives established for the intervention. The educator periodically assessed progress toward achieving the objectives by determining the number of face-to-face education sessions that had been conducted and by monitoring the production and distribution of printed information about the prevention, diagnosis, and appropriate treatment of type 2 diabetes. The educator also tracked progress toward the desired outcome of having all of the employees and spouses with the disease receiving appropriate HbA1c, LDL-C, and microalbuminuria testing, as well annual eye examinations, by the conclusion of the intervention.

When there was inadequate progress toward accomplishment of any of the objectives established for this intervention, the health educator made the necessary adjustments. This is shown conceptually in Figure 2.3 as the feedback loop between the evaluating and the designing and implementing steps of the model.

Summative Evaluation   Summative evaluations tend to be "before and after" snapshots, reported after the conclusion of an intervention. Their purpose is to prove or document whether or not an intervention worked as intended, and perhaps to summarize the lessons learned from making the intervention. Although in many cases ultimate results or impact will not be felt until well past the conclusion of the intervention, the health educator conducting the summative evaluation for the intervention at the financial services company was able to evaluate key results of the intervention. The educator had, among these results, specific information about the number and proportion of the company's employees and their spouses who had type 2 diabetes who were receiving appropriate HbA1c, LDL-C, and microalbuminuria testing, as well the number and proportion having an eye examination during the period of the intervention. It would, however, be some years before anyone could determine if the intervention had achieved its objective of reducing the incidence of type 2 diabetes among the employees and spouses to a level consistent with what would be expected in a group of this age and gender structure.

Both formative and summative evaluations were performed because each served a different purpose. The formative evaluation of the implementation of the intervention involved collection and analysis of information that permitted the health educator to assess ongoing progress in the conduct of the intervention and to make improvements in its implementation. The results of ongoing formative evaluation, as well as the actions taken in response to them by the health educator, were reported to the program manager.

The conduct of the summative evaluation of the intervention required the health educator to collect and analyze information to determine how well the intervention worked in terms of achieving its desired results—at least to the extent that the information was available at the time of the summative evaluation. The results of the summative evaluation were reported to the program manager, who also shared the results with the client company. By providing the results of the intervention, a good case was made for the conduct of further health education interventions for the financial services company.

The conduct of formative and summative evaluations can be quite complicated, in which case it can be very helpful to use consultants. Generally, however, managers and other participants can conduct useful evaluations by focusing on progress toward accomplishing the objectives of an intervention. Whether evaluations are simple or complex, however, good interventional planning comes full circle with the completion of the evaluating step shown in Figure 2.3.

Summary

This chapter describes developing/strategizing as one of the core activities of management work, along with designing and leading. Developing activities refer to the initial development of a program, which involves someone envisioning the program as a vehicle for delivering services or products that may succeed in the marketplace. Developing activities, after the initial development of a program occurs, pertain to improving established services or products or expanding a program's portfolio of services or products.

Developing triggers strategizing, which is the work that managers do as they establish or revise the specific mission and objectives of a program and make plans to achieve them.

The discussion of strategizing activities is structured around how managers do three things:

1. Determine the current situation of a program through the conduct of a thorough situational analysis, including inventorying desired results

2. Reconsider the desired results established for the program, and determine how they might successfully accomplish continuing and revised desired results

3. Use techniques of assessing and controlling performance and evaluating results to assure themselves that desired results—both the original and the new or revised—are being accomplished

The chapter discusses the three components of a situational analysis: an inventory of the desired results established for a program, as well as internal and external situational analyses of the program. The inventory of desired results is discussed as comprising a mission and objectives.

The conduct of an external situational analysis is discussed in terms of its five interrelated steps: (1) scanning, (2) monitoring or tracking, (3) forecasting or projecting, (4) assessing, and (5) using and disseminating.

The conduct of an internal situational analysis is discussed in terms of a financial analysis, a human resource analysis, a marketing analysis, and an operations analysis. Properly conducted, these analyses provide a catalogue of both the strengths and weaknesses inherent in a program.

The discussion of developing/strategizing is brought full circle by considering how to determine whether or not acceptable progress is being made toward achieving a program's desired results. Controlling is described as the regulation of actions and decisions in accord with the stated objectives and the standards of performance established in operational plans. The roles of information systems and budgets in control are discussed.

The writing of a business plan for a program at the point of its original development into a concrete, well-formed idea, or perhaps at the introduction of a major service addition in an ongoing program, is discussed, as are the contents of a good business plan.

Interventional planning is described as a form of planning that takes place within the overall developing/strategizing activities of managers. This form of planning involves the application of planning techniques to the development, implementation, and evaluation of interventions undertaken by programs. A six-step model of interventional planning (see Figure 2.3) is presented.

REVIEW QUESTIONS

1. Define developing/strategizing and interventional planning. Distinguish between the two.

2. What three things must a manager do to successfully strategize the future of a program?

3. What are the components of a complete situational analysis for a program?

4. What are the steps in conducting an external situational analysis?

5. What should be included in an internal situational analysis?

6. What should be included in an inventory of a program's desired results?

7. Discuss the role of controlling in developing/strategizing.

8. Discuss the role of budgets in controlling.

9. What should be included in a business plan?

10. Discuss the steps in interventional planning.

KEY TERMS AND CONCEPTS

budgets

business plan

controlling

data

developing/strategizing

external situational analysis

formative evaluation

information

information system (IS)

internal situational analysis

interventional planning

inventory of desired results

logic model

mission

objectives

operational plan

program theory

scenario development

situational analysis

stakeholders

stakeholder relationships

summative evaluation

trend extrapolation

References

Abrams, Rhonda, and John Doerr. *The Successful Business Plan: Secrets and Strategies*, 5th ed. Palo Alto, CA: Running 'R' Media, 2010.

BusinessDictionary. "Data." Accessed May 30, 2014a. http://www.businessdictionary.com/definition/data.html.

BusinessDictionary. "Information." Accessed May 30, 2014b. http://www.businessdictionary.com/definition/information.html.

California Breast Cancer Research Program. "About Us." Accessed May 12, 2014. http://cbcrp.org/about/.

Central Florida Immunization Coalition. "Mission Statement." Accessed May 12, 2014. http://www.cficoalition.org/.

Daft, Richard L. *Management*, 11th ed. Mason, OH: South-Western, Cengage Learning, 2014.

Funnell, Sue C., and Patricia J. Rogers. *Purposeful Program Theory: Effective Use of Theories of Change and Logic Models*. San Francisco: Jossey-Bass, 2011.

Gapenski, Louis C. *Healthcare Finance: An Introduction to Accounting and Financial Management*, 5th ed. Chicago: Health Administration Press, 2011.

Gilmore, Gary D. *Needs and Capacity Assessment Strategies for Health Education and Health Promotion*, 4th ed. Burlington, MA: Jones & Bartlett Learning, 2011.

Ginter, Peter M., W. Jack Duncan, and Linda E. Swayne, *Strategic Management of Health Care Organizations*, 7th ed. San Francisco: Jossey-Bass, 2013.

Green, Lawrence W., and Marshall W. Kreuter. *Health Promotion Planning: An Educational and Ecological Approach*, 4th ed. New York: McGraw-Hill, 2004.

Ham, Chris, Ruth Kipping, and Hugh McLeod. "Redesigning Work Processes in Health Care: Lessons from the National Health Service." *Milbank Quarterly* 81, no. 3 (September 2003): 415–439.

Heuer, Richards J., Jr., and Randolph H. Pherson. *Structured Analytic Techniques for Intelligence Analysis.* Washington, DC: CQ Press, 2011.

Knowlton, Lisa W., and Cynthia C. Phillips. *The Logic Model Guidebook*, 2nd ed. Thousand Oaks, CA: Sage, 2013.

McKenzie, James F., Brad L. Neiger, and Rosemary Thackeray. *Planning, Implementing, and Evaluating Health Promotion Programs: A Primer*, 6th ed. San Francisco: Benjamin Cummings, 2013.

McNamara, Carter. "Basic Guide to Program Evaluation." Accessed May 26, 2014. http://managementhelp.org/evaluation/program-evaluation-guide.htm.

Morlidge, Steve, and Steve Player. *Future Ready: How to Master Business Forecasting.* West Sussex, UK: Wiley, 2010.

National Association of County & City Health Officials. "MAPP Basics—Introduction to the MAPP Process." Accessed May 12, 2014. http://www.naccho.org/topics/infrastructure/mapp/framework/mappbasics.cfm.

Nowicki, Michael. *Introduction to the Financial Management of Healthcare Organizations*, 5th ed. Chicago: Health Administration Press, 2011.

Petersen, Donna J., and Greg R. Alexander. *Needs Assessment in Public Health: A Practical Guide for Students and Professionals.* New York: Kluwer Academic/Plenum, 2001.

Rossi, Peter H., Mark W. Lipsey, and Howard E. Freeman. *Evaluation: A Systematic Approach*, 7th ed. Thousand Oaks, CA: Sage, 2004.

Sharma, Manoj, and John A. Romas. *Theoretical Foundations of Health Education and Health Promotion*, 2nd ed. Burlington, MA: Jones & Bartlett Learning, 2012.

Simons-Morton, Bruce G., Kenneth R. McLeroy, and Monica L. Wendel. *Behavior Theory in Health Promotion Practice and Research.* Burlington, MA: Jones & Bartlett Learning, 2012.

Small Business Administration. "Create Your Business Plan." Accessed May 13, 2014. http://www.sba.gov/category/navigation-structure/starting-managing-business/starting-business/how-write-business-plan.

Smaltz, Detlev H., Gerald L. Glandon, and Donna J. Slovensky. *Information Systems for Healthcare Management*, 8th ed. Chicago: Health Administration Press, 2013.

Smith, Mark, Robert Sanders, Leigh Stuckhardt, and J. Michael McGinnis, eds. *Best Care at Lower Cost: The Path to Continuously Learning Health Care in America.* Washington, DC: National Academies Press, 2012.

Thackeray, Rosemary, and Brad L. Neiger. "Use of Social Marketing to Develop Culturally Innovative Diabetes Interventions." *Diabetes Spectrum* 16, no. 1 (January 2003): 15–20.

Timmreck, Thomas C. *Planning, Program Development, and Evaluation: A Handbook for Health Promotion, Aging, and Health Services*, 2nd ed. Burlington, MA: Jones & Bartlett Learning, 2002.

Wade, Woody. *Scenario Planning: A Field Guide to the Future*. Hoboken, NJ: Wiley, 2012.

Wholey, Joseph S., Harry P. Hatry, and Kathryn E. Newcomer. *Handbook of Practical Program Evaluation*, 3rd ed. San Francisco: Jossey-Bass, 2010.

W. K. Kellogg Foundation. *Logic Model Development Guide*. Battle Creek, MI: W. K. Kellogg Foundation, 2004.

CHAPTER 3

DESIGNING FOR EFFECTIVENESS

As discussed in Chapter 1, managers engage in three highly interrelated core activities in doing management work: developing/strategizing, designing, and leading (see Figure 1.3). Through *designing*, the topic of this chapter, managers establish and revise the intentional patterns of relationships among human and other resources within their programs. These patterns of relationships are called *organization designs*.

Specifically, the patterns of relationships among human and other resources established by managers are *formal* organization designs. This distinction is important because coexisting with formal organization designs are *informal* designs that exist because people working together in organizations, with their formal designs, also invariably establish relationships and interactions that are not included in the formal structure. All organization designs have both formal aspects, which are developed by managers, and informal aspects, which reflect the wishes and preferences of other participants (Schermerhorn 2013). This chapter considers both *formal and informal organization designs*.

Designing activities are an ongoing part of management work because the organization designs of programs undergo continual revision. Designing for effectiveness means structuring the relationships among human and other resources within a program in ways that facilitate the accomplishment of the mission and objectives established through developing/strategizing activities. Increasingly, it also means designing a program to be a *learning organization* (Smith et al. 2012). This means that the program's manager and other staff "systematically collect data, learn what works and does not work in [the program], and use

LEARNING OBJECTIVES

After reading this chapter, you should be able to:

- Understand the origination and revision of organization designs
- Appreciate the historical roots of key organization design concepts
- Understand the key organization design concepts, including the following:
  - Division of work and specialization of workers
  - Authority and responsibility relationships
  - Clustering or departmentalization
  - Span of control
  - Coordination
- Distinguish between formal and informal aspects of organization designs
- Understand the development and revision of logic models as part of designing
- Understand the concept of learning organizations
- Understand the staffing process as part of designing

this information to improve their organizational capacity and services provided" (Wholey, Hatry, and Newcomer 2010, 5).

Creating Organization Designs

Formal organization designs begin with the designation of individual positions. Positions are subsequently staffed as individuals are attracted to occupy them. Individual positions are the basic building blocks of organization designs, although they are typically clustered into teams or work groups. In larger programs with multiple work groups, issues of how the various work groups and clusters of work groups are integrated and coordinated become important design concerns. Designing activities also involve relating a program to the larger organizational home in which it is embedded. For example, a screening program embedded in a county health department must fit within its larger organizational home. A program manager in such a setting will report to a superior in the larger organizational home.

Within the larger organizational home of a program, organization design continues with clustering work groups into departments and other subdivisions of the organization, and then grouping and arranging the work groups and clusters of work groups to form the entire organization. At the highest level of organization design, individual organizations can be further clustered into systems or alliances of organizations (see Figure 3.1).

Managers at the various levels depicted in Figure 3.1 are concerned with different design issues. For example, top-level managers in the organizational home of a program are concerned with such design issues as establishing appropriate relationships between and among work groups

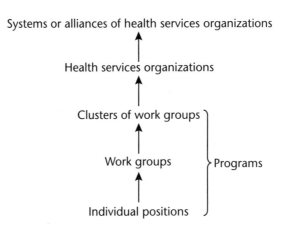

Figure 3.1   Hierarchy of Organization Design

and clusters of work groups in the organization and searching for the synergies that might exist within the organization when all of its parts work together well. They might also be involved in forming a system of organizations or in building alliances with other organizations of which their organization is a participating member. In essence, top-level managers are concerned with how effectively the entire organization is designed to achieve its mission and objectives.

Middle-level managers in large organizations are concerned with organizing work groups and clusters of work groups into effective units and divisions. First-level managers in such organizations, including those who manage a program within them, are directly concerned with establishing and staffing individual positions, and with clustering these participants and other resources into the organization design of the program. In all organization designs, the fundamental building block is the individual position and the participant who fills the position. Individuals are the starting point from which, through clustering, entire designs are elaborated. Thus, staffing the individual positions in a design is an important part of the program manager's designing activity. We will discuss the staffing process more thoroughly later in this chapter.

Key Concepts in Formal Organization Design

Before discussing the specific nature of creating formal organization designs, it will be useful to provide a brief history of the contemporary concepts that guide designs for programs, and for many other types of organizations. For those who prefer contemporary things and ideas, it is sometimes difficult to appreciate old ideas and concepts. It would be a mistake, however, to overlook the historical roots of what is known about formal organization design. Because concerns about the designing activity in management work have been relevant for a long time, some of the historical work on this topic may seem outdated to you. But rest assured, the concepts selected for inclusion and described here are as relevant as they were when first considered decades ago.

Although they have been modified over the years, many of the fundamental organization design concepts that guide how most health programs are structured can be traced back to the early twentieth century. The concepts are based on the work of such people as French industrialist Henri Fayol (1949) and German sociologist Max Weber (1947). The work of these and other organization and management theorists of the period, such as Luther Gulick and Lyndall Urwick (1937) and James Mooney and Alan Reiley (1931), resulted in what are now considered the classical concepts of formal organization design. These people are considered classical theorists. Perhaps the fact that so many basic design characteristics of contemporary health programs—indeed, of all types of organizations—are rooted in conceptualizations that are nearly a century old reflects the wisdom that went into the development of the classical concepts.

Every organized human activity, whether a Little League baseball team or Google, has two fundamental and opposing requirements: division of the work to be performed on the one hand, and coordination or integration of the divided work on the other. The classical theorists recognized the relationship between dividing work and the concomitant need to coordinate the divided work if satisfactory results are to be achieved. They developed views on both division and coordination of work, as well as other design concepts. In the following subsections, attention is given to the division of work and the closely associated specialization of workers. Other sections cover authority and responsibility relationships, clustering or departmentalization, span of control, and the coordination or integration of the work that has been consciously divided and performed by specialized workers.

Because the classical concepts strongly influence the design of almost all contemporary organizations, including health programs, their role in creating effective contemporary designs must be understood. That being said, the applications of these ideas and concepts have evolved over time. The following subsections therefore present the classical concepts of formal organization design that are most relevant to health programs, along with a contemporary perspective on each of the classical concepts.

Division of Work and Specialization of Workers

Mintzberg (1992) pointed out that the individual positions in organization designs form the foundation on which all designs—including those of entire organizations and systems of organizations—are ultimately constructed. Before Mintzberg and other contemporary thinkers, however, the classical theorists (and even before them the economist Adam Smith ([1776] 2009), who wrote *The Wealth of Nations*) saw the potential inherent in paying attention to individual positions in organization designs. These theorists recognized the benefits to be gained from dividing work in ways that maximize the ability of workers occupying individual positions to gain proficiency through specialization.

Technically, ***division of work*** means dividing the work to be performed in a program (or in any organization) into specific positions, each consisting of specified activities. The work content of a position is determined by the activities a person occupying the position is to accomplish. For example, the position of pharmacist in a drug counseling program can be described in terms of the activities a person in this position is expected to accomplish, which are different from those expected of someone occupying the position of nurse, program manager, or social worker.

Much of the work done in health programs is performed by people who are trained through education and experience to do particular work. Their specialized capabilities are often reflected in professional licensure and in accreditation rules and policies that require the programs that hire them to employ people who are properly credentialed for the work they are to do. *Specialization*, including but not limited to that which is documented by licensure or certification, implies expertise based on education, experience, or both in the activities of a position or particular job. Health programs are often structured to accommodate the specialties of the participants who work in them through clustering groups of participants according to specialty.

Division of work and specialization of workers enhance managers' ability to select, train, and equip people to do the work of programs. Division of work also affords managers a greater degree of control over work because they can more easily standardize and monitor specialized work and workers. Increased division of work has a negative side, however. People who perform highly specialized work may at times find it repetitive, monotonous, and unfulfilling.

In response, such contemporary developments as cross-training (equipping people with skills that permit them to perform more than one job); job enlargement (combining tasks to create a new job involving a broader set of activities); and job enrichment (expanding responsibilities so work becomes more challenging and satisfying) permit managers to minimize the negative effects of division and specialization. For example, some health services organizations have adopted the use of integrated patient care teams. Such teams reflect job enrichment efforts that involve each member in making team decisions and in the total care of patients. Cardiac rehabilitation teams, for example, work together to diagnose, treat, rehabilitate, and provide extended care, from the point of a patient's initial incident through recovery.

Authority and Responsibility Relationships

Growing directly out of the division of work in creating organization designs is the need to assign *responsibility* for and *authority* over the performance of the work. Authority is the power derived from a person's structural position in an organization design. Organizational authority permits managers to give orders and to expect that orders will be carried out.

Responsibility is the obligation to perform certain activities or to achieve certain results and, like authority, is derived from one's position in the organization design.

Authority and responsibility are delegated downward, resulting in a scaling or grading of levels of authority and responsibility. The authority and responsibility of a program's manager are different from those of managers of its subdivisions, as well as those of individual participants.

Vertical layers in an organization design are the clearest evidence of the delegation of authority and responsibility. The process of delegation results in what is called a scalar chain of command within the organization design. Individuals higher up in the chain have more authority than those lower in the chain. This scalar chain helps define authority and responsibility relationships from the manager down to the level of individual participants.

Classical theorists were obsessed with the roles of authority and responsibility in organization designs. In their view, the assignment of authority and responsibility held organizations together. Furthermore, they believed that the rights attached to one's organizational position were the only important sources of power or influence in organizations. The effect of these beliefs was that managers were viewed as all-powerful in their organizations. This might have been true one hundred years ago, but no longer. Now, authority, especially positional authority, is seen as just one element in the larger concept of power in contemporary organization designs.

There are numerous sources of **interpersonal power**, which has been defined as the ability to influence others in all types of organizational settings, including health programs. The authority that derives from one's formal position is only one source of power. French and Raven (1959) conceptualized interpersonal power as having five distinct bases in organization designs: legitimate, reward, coercive, expert, and referent. Only the first three bases derive from a manager's formal position in a design.

Legitimate power, or positional power, is clearly derived from one's position in an organization design. This formal authority resides in managers and exists because organizations find it advantageous to assign power to individuals so they can perform their work effectively. All managers have some legitimate power or authority based on position.

Managers also have reward power, which is based on their ability to reward desirable behaviors and stems from the legitimate power granted to them. Because of their position, managers control such rewards as pay increases, promotions, and flexible work schedules, and this reward power buttresses their legitimate power. Also based on their position, managers have coercive power, the opposite of reward power. Coercive power is based on the ability to punish someone or prevent him or her from obtaining desired rewards.

By definition, the legitimate, reward, and coercive sources of power in organization designs are restricted to managers, but other sources of power not restricted to managers are quite important in health programs and have the effect of spreading power and influence beyond the managers.

One of the most important forms of power in many programs is expert power, which is derived from having knowledge that is valued within a program, or by the organization in which the program is embedded. Expert power is specific to the person who has the expertise. It is therefore different from legitimate, reward, and coercive power, which are prescribed by the organization design, even though persons may be granted these types of power because they possess expert power. For example, health professionals with expert power often rise to a management position in their area of expertise. In addition, in programs where work is highly technical or professional, expert power alone can make certain people powerful. In any program, participants with expertise that is scarce in the program will typically have more expert power than people whose expertise is more readily replicable.

Referent power results when someone engenders admiration, loyalty, and emulation to the extent that he or she gains the power to influence other people. Sometimes called charismatic power, this form of power is certainly not limited to managers. In some health programs, charismatic individuals wield considerable influence. As with expert power, referent power cannot be given by the organization in the way that legitimate, reward, and coercive power can.

Authority and responsibility considerations heavily influence the design of contemporary organizations, including health programs. The contemporary view continues the classical conceptualization that power or authority derives primarily from managerial position, but emphasizes that positional authority is only one of several sources of power. In this perspective, with expertise and charisma being more important, interpersonal power is definitely not limited to managers. A broader discussion of power and influence can be found in Chapter 4.

Clustering or Departmentalization

The process of clustering or grouping work and workers into manageable units (again, see Figure 3.1) heavily influences organization designs. The classical theorists saw *clustering*—or, as they preferred to call it, *departmentalization*—as a natural consequence of division and special-ization of work. In their view, because it is rational to specialize work, it is also rational to place similar workers together in work groups. In turn, these groups are grouped into clusters of related work groups until the organiza-tion design has a superstructure.

Gulick and Urwick (1937), among other classical theorists, noted four bases for clustering work and workers: purpose, process, persons and things, and place. Other factors on which clustering can be based have emerged. Mintzberg (1979), for example, suggested the following six bases for group-ing workers into units and units into larger units:

- *Specialized knowledge and skills.* A health program might group nurses in one unit and social workers in another.

- *Functions or processes performed.* A large program might have market-ing, finance, and clinical services units.

- *Timing of their work.* A program that operates twenty-four hours per day might group workers according to day, evening, and night shifts.

- *Outputs of their work, whether services or products.* A program might group workers by whether they provide inpatient or outpatient services.

- *Clients or patients they serve.* Programs, such as geriatric or women's health programs, might be established based on the age or gender of patients.

- *Place or physical location of their work.* A program might operate ambulatory clinics in a downtown location as well as in the city's suburbs.

A single large health program might use several of these bases for grouping workers to create an effective organization design. Larger organi-zational homes of programs use many if not all of these bases for clustering to create their designs.

No matter which basis is used, the clustering of work and workers into manageable units helps establish the means by which workers' work can be integrated and coordinated, both within and across work groups. Mintzberg (1979) suggested that clustering has at least four important implications for participants and the organization designs within which they work:

- *Clustering sets up a system of common supervision.* Once participants are clustered into a group, a manager can be appointed to integrate and control the work of that group.

- *Clustering facilitates sharing resources.* People in a work group share a common budget, facilities, and equipment.

• *Clustering typically leads to common measures of performance.* Shared resources on the input side and group-level outputs allow group members to be evaluated based on common performance criteria. Common performance measures encourage group members to integrate their work.

• *Clustering encourages communication.* Shared resources and shared desired results, along with close physical proximity, promote communication. They also facilitate integrating the work of group members.

Health programs and the larger organizations in which they are embedded use all six of the previously discussed bases for clustering work and participants, including doing so by function, the basis most favored by the classical theorists. This functional basis, reinforced by the specialized knowledge and skills of many participants in health programs, is clearly visible in large health programs where nurses are in one cluster, pharmacists are in another, and social workers are in yet another. In smaller programs, this basis is less frequently used, and clustering is more likely to be based on patients/customers served, or on physical location.

One important contemporary development in the organization designs of many health programs—as well as of the organizations in which they are embedded—is the increased focus on patients/customers as the basis for clustering participants. This is one result of the increased competition for patients/customers. For example, as the leaders of health services organizations seek to devise business strategies to increase their organization's market share, many have initiated geriatric and women's health programs and comprehensive cardiac care programs.

As Figure 3.1 indicates, the first level of clustering in an organization design occurs when individual participants are grouped into work groups, or teams as they are often called. In almost all projects and in smaller programs, this first level of clustering is vitally important because the projects or small programs are typically organized as teams. The participants often form a single team, which may even be called the project team. Larger programs may contain a number of teams.

Groups and teams are established within organization designs for many purposes. For example, large organizations establish management teams, governing boards, and standing committees. Some groups, ubiquitous in health services settings, are assembled for specific problem-solving purposes or to pursue improvements in quality or productivity. More is said about teams and teamwork in Chapter 7, where the role of teamwork in managing quality is discussed. The focus here, however, is on the formal work teams made up of the participants in programs.

Because work teams are vital to the success of a program, a manager should view team building or team development as an important responsibility (Dyer, Dyer, and Dyer 2013; *Harvard Business Review* 2011). Team building or team development includes enhancing the ability of individual participants to contribute to team performance through education and training, through increasing their motivation to perform as individuals and as team members, and through enhancing their ability to perform as a team.

An important aspect of building and developing work teams is the reality that all teams form in a series of evolving stages (Fallon, Begun, and Riley 2013; Fried, Topping, and Edmondson 2012). Although not all teams evolve in precisely the same manner, typically the evolution of a work team involves several discernible stages, beginning with a formation stage that occurs when a team is first established. Team participants in this stage sort out their own roles and those of the other participants as they begin to identify themselves as part of a team and try to determine what is acceptable within the group.

The formation stage is followed by a stage variously characterized as the storming, disequilibrium, or differentiation stage. In this stage there are real and potential conflicts among team participants. A manager can play an important role in moving a team beyond this stage by building trust and respect among participants and by clarifying the roles of individuals and of the entire team. Some teams never emerge from this stage, and this stage, as its name suggests, is always "stormy."

For teams that do progress, the next stage is characterized as the norming, integrating, or achieving role clarity stage. Agreement is reached in regard to roles, and cohesion among team participants increases significantly. Team members begin to identify with the desired results established for the team and the program within which the team works, and they start to develop or reaffirm shared values. Communication flows relatively easily within the team as participants gain trust in and familiarity with each other.

Successful teams evolve further and enter the maturity stage, or what is sometimes called the performing stage. In this stage, the organization design as it pertains to team participants is well established, and participants are concerned about the team and its effectiveness. Team members at this stage are able to effectively accomplish the team's work and to deal with conflicts within the team. Participants are aware of one another's strengths and weaknesses and accept each other's differences. They typically experience satisfaction with their work; enjoy high levels of cooperation, mutual trust,

and support among team members; and experience pride in the accomplishments of the team.

It is important to note that a team's maturity is not an end point. A team's effectiveness—in terms of both work accomplishment and participant satisfaction—must be maintained, which can be thought of as a new stage. Or perhaps it is more accurate to say that this is not so much a new stage as a continuation of the maturity or performing stage, accomplished through significant and ongoing efforts to maintain the team's effectiveness.

A work team's final evolutionary stage is reached when the team dissolves or adjourns. The adjournment or dissolution stage for a team may result from changes in the strategies of a program or the organization in which it is embedded, perhaps driven by changes in the target markets for services, or from changes in reimbursement policies. Dissolution may also result from a program's failure to achieve its mission or objectives. Some programs simply fail and are terminated. Teams within such programs would also dissolve.

Span of Control

An organization design question of concern to the classical theorists was how large a cluster of workers a single manager could effectively manage. A related question had to do with the bases on which to make decisions about the size of a cluster. In considering these questions, classical theorists developed the organization design concept of *span of control*, which refers to the number of organizational subordinates reporting directly to an organizational superior, typically a single manager. Classical theorists generally agreed that managers should have a limited number of people reporting directly to them, a conclusion that was based on their view of managers' ability to exercise the necessary degree of control over those whom they managed.

Spans of control significantly affect organization designs. As seen in Figure 3.2, narrow spans of control produce tall organization designs, and wider spans produce flat organization designs. The tall and flat structures in Figure 3.2 have equal numbers of positions; but the tall structure has four levels, whereas the flat structure has two. Complex health organizations, such as hospitals or large health departments, typically have a tall structure, resulting from extensive division of work and concurrent specialization of workers into numerous and varied departments and units. This structure results from the need for managers to have limited spans of control when

A Tall, Complex Organization

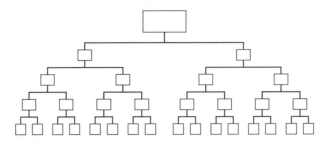

A Flat Health Program

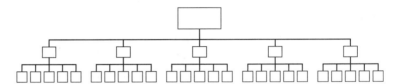

Figure 3.2   Contrasting Spans of Control

work is highly divided and performed by specialized workers. In contrast, health programs typically have a flat design.

The factors contemporary managers use to determine an appropriate span of control include the following:

• *The level of professionalism and training of participants.* Participants who are professional and highly trained (characteristics often prevalent among participants in health programs) require less supervision, which permits a wider span of control.

• *The level of uncertainty in the work being done.* Complex and varied work requires close supervision when compared to simple and repetitive work. Close supervision requires a narrow span of control.

• *The degree of standardization of work.* Standardized and routinized work requires less direct supervision. The span of control for standardized work can be wider than that for less standardized work.

• *The degree of interaction required between managers and other participants.* Work situations in which more interaction is needed between managers and other participants necessitate a narrower span of control, because effective interactions take time.

• *The degree of task integration required.* If the work being done by participants must be carefully coordinated or integrated, or if the various aspects of work are interdependent, a narrower span of control may be needed.

The classical concept of span of control remains highly relevant to the design of health programs, although several contingencies must be considered when applying it in the contemporary work situation. For example, the managers in a large program with four or five separate units must apply this concept flexibly. For the program manager, the heads of the four or five units, with each unit performing different work, might constitute an appropriate span of control. But at levels of the program where work is more standardized and routine, a manager of one of the units could appropriately handle a much wider span of perhaps ten or twelve participants.

Another determining factor in span of control decisions is the nature of the work. It is usually easier to supervise ten coders than five drug counselors. Also, the abilities and availability of managers must be taken into account. The training and personal qualities of some managers enable them to manage a broader span of control than others can. Similarly, better training and higher potential for self-direction among those being managed help reduce the need for them to have a relationship with their manager and widens the span of control the manager can handle.

Coordination or Integration

The terms *coordination* and *integration* are used interchangeably in the organization design literature. Whichever term is used, the concept pertains to processes intended to achieve unity of effort among the various component parts in an organization design in the accomplishment of the organization's desired results. Although the focus here is on integration within programs, the concept applies to the entire hierarchy of organization designs shown in Figure 3.1.

As was noted previously, health programs often exhibit high degrees of division of work and specialization of workers. When they do, there is a greater need for effective coordination. Although in some situations it is possible to separate work so as to minimize the degree of coordination needed, health programs typically require much coordination if their mission and objectives are to be achieved. It is important to recognize the interaction between (1) the need to divide, specialize, and cluster work and participants, and (2) subsequent requirements for coordination. More differentiation of work and greater specialization of participants increases the need for coordination.

The necessity of effective coordination is also influenced by the type of *interdependence* existing among participants in a program. Thompson

(1967) identified three forms of interdependence, all of which are found in health programs: pooled, sequential, and reciprocal. Pooled interdependence occurs when individual participants or work groups are related, but not very interactively. They simply contribute separately in some way to the larger whole. For example, several geographically dispersed units of a health education program housed in a single health department can be viewed as linked largely in the sense that each contributes to the overall success of the program; however, they have very little direct interdependence. They operate as separate entities for all practical purposes.

Sequential interdependence occurs when individual participants or work groups bear a close and sequential connection. For example, patients/customers enrolled in a large multiservice program become the focal point for extended chains of sequentially interdependent activities. The program's intake office enrolls them and schedules an initial evaluation of their status and needs. This may trigger separate appointments with a nurse, social worker, and physical therapist, all occurring in a sequentially interdependent manner.

The third type of interdependence, reciprocal interdependence, occurs when individual participants or work groups bear a close relationship and the interdependence moves in both directions. For example, a hospice program exists to serve patients of a particular health services organization or system. The hospice relies on the organization as its source of patients, and the organization relies on the hospice as a place to refer appropriate patients. The interdependence is reciprocal because it moves in both directions.

As interdependence moves from pooled, to sequential, to reciprocal, managers typically must pay greater attention to issues of coordination. Health programs often exhibit very high levels of internal interdependence among their component parts, usually of a sequential or reciprocal nature. Some also have a high level of interdependence with the organization in which they are embedded. Thus, the need for effective coordination is usually significant in health programs.

Mechanisms for Achieving Coordination

The *coordinating mechanisms*—the techniques and processes that managers use to achieve coordination—are diverse and result in different levels of success, depending on characteristics of specific situations. No single coordinating mechanism is best for all situations. Managers need to match the most appropriate coordinating mechanism to a given situation, recognizing that often a combination of mechanisms is required.

Managers can select from a large menu of coordinating mechanisms, typically choosing and applying several of them simultaneously. A number of categorizations of these mechanisms have been developed, one of which (Litterer 1965) outlines three ways for managers to achieve coordination:

• Using an organization design's hierarchical structure

• Relying on administrative systems and procedures, such as reporting arrangements

• Relying on participants to voluntarily coordinate their work as needed

Hierarchical coordination relies on having the various participants in a program placed under a single line of managerial authority. In small and relatively simple organization designs, typical of many programs, this form of coordination is very effective. In large, complex programs, however, and in other larger organization designs with multiple organizational levels and many subdivisions, it becomes more difficult to rely on hierarchical coordination.

Although a program's manager is a focal point of authority, it may be impossible for one person to cope with all the coordination problems that might arise in the hierarchy. Therefore, coordination through the hierarchical structure is almost always supplemented by other mechanisms.

A second coordinating mechanism suggested by Litterer (1965) is the incorporation of formal procedures and administrative systems into a program's organization design. Such procedures and systems can be as simple as routing certain information to the set of participants whose work is to be coordinated. To the extent that administrative procedures can be programmed or made routine, they are easy to use. For nonroutine and nonprogrammable events, other administrative procedures, such as establishing committees, may also facilitate coordination within a program.

A third type of coordinating mechanism in Litterer's (1965) view is participants' voluntary actions undertaken to ensure coordination in a program. In many health programs, much of the coordination does in fact depend on the willingness and ability of participants to voluntarily find ways to integrate or coordinate their activities with those of other participants.

Managers can facilitate voluntary coordination by providing participants with information concerning specific problems of coordination. If this information can be coupled with the motivation to do something about coordination problems, voluntary coordination will routinely occur. In part, such motivation stems from the professionalism of so many of the participants in health programs. Their value systems, which are supportive of patients/customers' welfare, facilitate voluntary coordination.

In a second important categorization of coordinating mechanisms available to managers, Mintzberg (1992, 5) identified the following five mechanisms:

- Mutual adjustment

- Direct supervision

- Standardization of work processes

- Standardization of work outputs

- Standardization of worker skills

In mutual adjustment, which is quite similar to the voluntary actions identified by Litterer (1965), coordination is achieved through the willingness of participants to coordinate work by mutually adjusting to each other's needs. Managers facilitate this mechanism by encouraging communication among those whose work must be coordinated. This mechanism to achieve coordination is especially useful in self-directed work teams.

In direct supervision, which is similar to the hierarchical coordination identified by Litterer (1965), coordination is achieved by having certain participants take responsibility for the work of others, including issuing instructions to them and monitoring their actions. This occurs as a matter of course in the relationships between managers and those they manage.

In standardization of work processes, the content of work is programmed or specified in advance. Health programs routinely standardize many of their work processes, such as intake procedures for patients/customers. They also standardize work processes through the establishment of patient care protocols or clinical pathways for guiding the provision of services.

The standardization of work outputs as a coordinating mechanism involves the specification of the products or outputs of work, with determination of how to perform the work left to the worker. Professional work is often more readily coordinated through mechanisms that standardize outputs than through attempts to standardize the work processes.

Finally, when neither work processes nor outputs can be standardized, coordination can, according to Mintzberg (1992), be achieved through standardization of worker skills, which is accomplished through training, education, and experience. This coordinating mechanism is frequently used in health programs in which the complexity of much of the work does not allow standardization of work processes or outputs. In such situations, standardization of participant skills and knowledge can be an excellent coordinating mechanism. It is routine for teams of physicians, nurses, and other clinicians to coordinate their care of patients largely through this mechanism. It also helps explain why membership on such teams is highly interchangeable.

Hage (1980) offered a third useful categorization of coordinating mechanisms, which includes these four:

- Programming (developing rules and prescriptions for how to do things)
- Planning
- Customs
- Feedback

In Hage's (1980) view, managers use programming to accomplish coordination by specifying what work is to be done in each individual position in a program, as well as how it is to be done. They can also specify the relationships among clusters of individual positions, up to the level of an entire organization or system. With such guidance, participants can conduct their work in a coordinated manner. The programming in an organization design is accomplished through rules, manuals, job descriptions, personnel procedures, promotion policies, and so on. This type of coordinating mechanism is quite similar to Litterer's (1965) use of administrative systems and procedures and to Mintzberg's (1992) standardization of work processes and worker skills. These coordinating mechanisms are pervasive in many health programs.

The usefulness of planning as a coordinating mechanism is obvious when viewing plans for one part of a program in relation to plans for its other parts, or when viewing plans for an entire program in relation to those for its organizational home. For example, the plans of a program must take into account the expansion plans of its organizational home. Similarly, subunit plans within a large program must take into account the plans of the entire program. Coordination is facilitated when managers make sure their plans are compatible with all other relevant plans.

Customs are a frequently overlooked coordinating mechanism. Yet many managers rely heavily on the history and customs of a program, or of the organization in which it is embedded, as a coordinating mechanism. For example, it may be customary in a particular long-term care organization to use the holiday season as an occasion to invite the families of residents into the facility for a meal and social interaction. Advanced knowledge of this custom permits the various departments and programs to begin to prepare for this event well in advance and facilitates the coordination of their various contributions to its success. Customs alone, however, are rarely sufficient to fully meet the coordination challenge.

The final mechanism in Hage's (1980) categorization, feedback, may indicate when a program, or some component of it, is not functioning well; feedback can trigger renewed efforts to coordinate work. Feedback often takes the form of written reports on operations and activities in health programs, but it also includes verbal exchanges that occur among participants. All forms of effective communication include feedback, as discussed in Chapter 6.

Feedback often occurs in the context of committees or teams, which actually form another coordinating mechanism. Some of these groups are made up of participants from subunits of a large program, established for the specific purpose of achieving coordination among the subunits through better communication among them. Using committees or teams for purposes of coordination is a well-established approach. Of course, committees and teams serve other purposes besides coordination, including performing services and filling advisory or decision-making roles.

Selecting from the Menu of Coordinating Mechanisms

As can be seen from the preceding discussion, managers have available a rich menu of mechanisms to achieve coordination within a program. Managers can select from the following:

- Administrative systems and procedures
- Committees and teams
- Customs
- Direct supervision
- Feedback
- Hierarchy
- Mutual adjustment
- Planning
- Programming
- Standardization of work processes, work outputs, or worker skills
- Voluntary action

As noted earlier, managers almost always use various combinations of these mechanisms to achieve coordination, often using several of them concurrently. Depending on the circumstances inherent in different situations, various packages of these mechanisms can be tailored appropriately. A manager concerned about how a program is coordinated with other parts of the organization in which it is embedded might select a particular package of coordinating mechanisms. For example, the manager of the program depicted in Figure 1.1 might rely heavily on administrative systems and procedures and planning to coordinate with the larger host organization in which the program is embedded. The program manager would rely on direct supervision, the hierarchy, and feedback to coordinate across the program's units. The managers of the units of this program, concerned about coordination among the units, would choose a different package of mechanisms, perhaps relying on planning, committee, and mutual adjustment mechanisms. The manager of one of the units, say the pharmacy unit in Figure 1.1, concerned about coordination issues involved in properly dispensing pharmaceuticals, might select yet another set of mechanisms, emphasizing direct supervision, standardization, and reliance on the voluntary actions of professional pharmacists.

Application of the Key Organization Design Concepts

The influence of the design concepts examined previously—division of work and specialization of participants, authority and responsibility relationships, clustering or departmentalization, span of control, and coordination or integration—on the actual organization designs of contemporary health programs is readily seen in the schematic representation of an organization design known as an organization chart. For example, the simplified organization chart in Figure 3.3 reflects the consequences of applying the

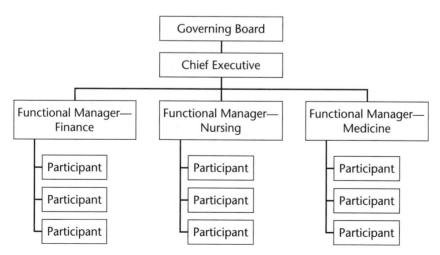

Figure 3.3   Simplified Organization Design of a Functionally Organized Health Services Organization

organization design concepts to a health services organization. The result is the classic functional organization chart so ubiquitous in business, government, academia, and health services.

Each unit in the chart represents a division of work and suggests that participants in each unit do work for which they are specialized. The chart also reflects authority and responsibility relationships, with lines showing these relationships between organizational superiors and subordinates. The vertical dimension of the organization chart shows who has authority over and responsibility for whom and what. Participants who are higher in the chart generally have authority over those in lower positions. Participants on the same level generally have equal amounts of authority and responsibility.

The chart also depicts clustering of individual participants into units, with the clustering being based primarily on functions of finance, nursing, and medicine. The chart permits an assessment of the span of control at various points simply by counting the participants reporting to any manager. Finally, because there are multiple interdependent or interrelated units depicted, this organization chart points to the importance of coordinating among the units. The chart does not, however, suggest what coordinating mechanisms might be used.

Figure 3.4 illustrates that the organization design of a program can also be a functionally designed structure. Finally, to complete the picture of this organization chart, the program can be shown as embedded in its organizational home, as was done previously in Figure 1.1.

There are organization designs in which almost all work is done through programs or projects. Many architectural, engineering, and consulting firms are organized into projects and derive their revenues from carrying out these projects for clients. Other organizations, including certain construction firms, defense contractors, and other government contractors, are organized

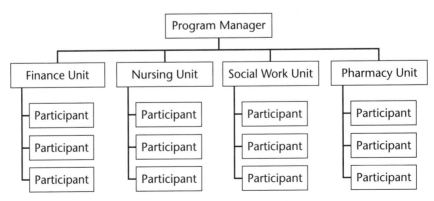

Figure 3.4   Simplified Organization Design of a Functionally Organized Program

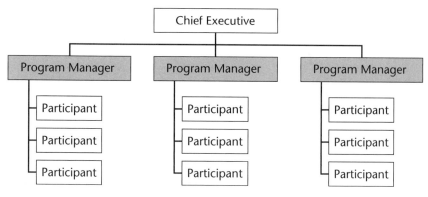

Figure 3.5   Programmized Organization Design

into programs. Figure 3.5 illustrates the extreme form of what might be called a "programmized" organization design.

The ***matrix organization design*** shown in Figure 3.6 blends elements of the functional designs depicted in Figure 3.3 and Figure 3.4 and the programmized design shown in Figure 3.5. This organization design is used for some health programs.

To illustrate an example of a matrix organization design, consider how a health services organization might design a comprehensive home

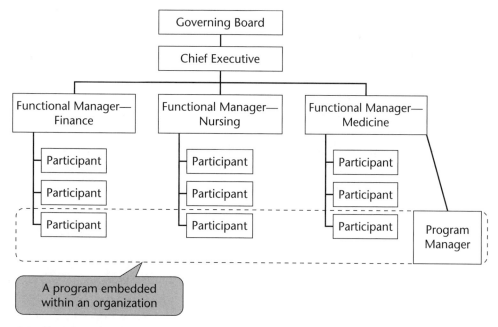

Figure 3.6   Matrix Organization Design

health program for the chronically ill. This would require a work group organized around the focus of the program. Participants in the group could be drawn from a variety of functional units of the host organization, including nursing, social services, respiratory therapy, occupational therapy, pharmacy, and physicians specializing in chronic disease. To market the program and to handle finance and reimbursement issues, participants with such expertise could be drawn from the marketing and finance areas of the host organization, respectively. A program manager would be named and given authority over and overall responsibility for the program. The manager would report to a superior in the larger organization.

Health services organizations create matrix organization designs when they superimpose programs on their existing functionally clustered designs. The programs do not replace the components of a functionally organized design; they organically complement the more mechanistic functional structure and help eliminate some of its rigidity in certain circumstances. Matrix organization designs are particularly useful for projects, which tend to have a limited scope and finite life (for example, projects to design and implement a system of electronic medical records or to design an off-site clinic).

Contemporary health services organizations contain a variety of organization designs, most of which are functionally organized designs. Some of the programs embedded within them may also have a functional design. Others may use a matrix organization design. As was noted earlier in this chapter, however, no matter how a manager builds the formal organization design of a program, coexisting within the formal organization design will be an informal structure.

Managers neither establish nor fully control the informal aspects of organization designs. Instead, the other participants, according to their preferences and wishes, inevitably establish informal relationships and activities that are not prescribed by the formal structure. Thus, it is important for program managers to understand both the formal and the informal aspects of organization designs.

Informal Aspects of Organization Designs

The informal relationships that occur within formal organization designs are characterized by dynamic behavior and interactions resulting from people working with other people across formal design parameters. Informal relationships are established as people in organizational settings

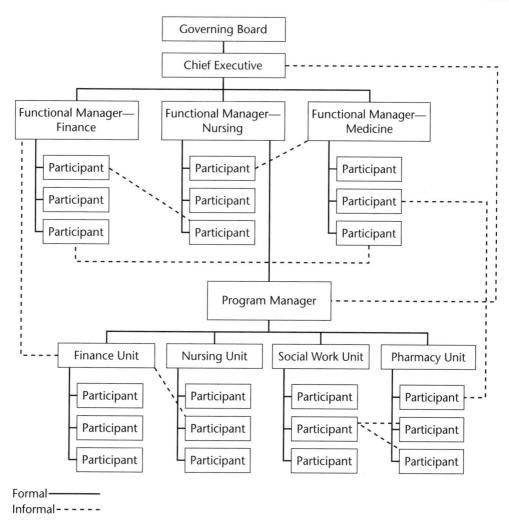

Figure 3.7 A Contact Chart

interact to accomplish work within the context of the formal organization design, as well as for other more personal reasons, such as a desire for friendships and social interaction.

Figure 3.7 illustrates some of the actual contacts that might occur between participants in an organization design. As can be seen, not all contacts follow the formal paths. In some of the contacts levels of the organization are bypassed; in others there is cross contact from one chain of command in the organization to another. Although contact charts do not show the reasons for informal relationships, they do reflect the nature of the informal relationships that can arise within organization designs.

Informal Groups within Organization Designs

Fully drawn contact charts often show, in addition to the one-to-one, informal relationships depicted in Figure 3.7, a type of clustering that occurs within a formal organization design. *Groups* within organization designs can be either formally or informally established. As was discussed previously in the subsection on clustering, managers intentionally cluster participants into formal groups, such as teams, departments, or committees, as a means of achieving certain purposes. In contrast, informal groups arise from the propensity of people to form social groups on their own (Fried, Topping, and Edmondson 2012).

People seek to fulfill a variety of their needs through work and in the context in which the work is performed. If formal organization designs satisfied all the needs of participants, there would be no reason for them to establish or engage in informal relationships. Basically, informal interactions occur because participants' needs are not fully met by the formal organization design. In fact, many needs can best be met in the context of informal relationships and groups.

Interpersonal contacts within small, informal groups provide relief from the boredom, monotony, and pressures of the workplace. In groups, people can be with others with similar values and interests. Groups may accord their members status, which may be little more than a sense of belonging to a group that is more or less exclusive. Informal group membership also provides a degree of personal security; the group member feels acceptance by peers as an equal and feels secure in their company. Group membership permits the individual to express views to sympathetic listeners. He or she may even find an outlet for a leadership drive. Finally, group membership assists people in securing information, at least information of a certain type. The grapevine—the flow of communication through informal channels as described in Chapter 6—is a phenomenon known to all participants in organizations. The common denominator in all these reasons for group membership is the satisfaction of specific needs of members that are not fully met by the formal organization design. It is very important for managers to understand that informal groups arise and persist within organization designs because these groups perform desired functions for their members.

An informal group that forms within a formal organization design tends to develop a complex structure of relationships of its own. This structure is determined by different possible status positions of a group's members: group leader, primary group member, fringe group member, and member in out status. For example, Figure 3.8 shows the informal structure of a group of nine

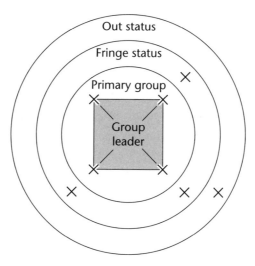

Figure 3.8 Informal Group Structure

people working in one section of a large health program. The shaded square in the center represents the group leader. Clustered around the leader are the other four members of the primary group. This close association is characterized by extensive interaction and communication. The three people in fringe status are likely to be newcomers who are, in effect, being evaluated by the primary group and who may become full members. If not accepted, they move to out status. One person is already in out status. This has significant implications if the person in out status wants to belong to the primary group. Being a participant in the formal organization design of this program is no substitute for full membership in the informal group.

An important parameter of how informal groups function is their leadership, even if it is unofficial or unsanctioned within the formal organization design. Informal group leaders emerge from within groups because they serve several functions. The leader not only initiates action and provides direction but also resolves differences of opinion on group-related matters and conflicts between the group's members. Furthermore, the leader can communicate group values and feelings to representatives of the formal organization design. The informal group leader role is retained only as long as the role is performed well: a group's members grant the leader role, and they can take it away.

Balancing the Informal and Formal Aspects of Organization Designs

Because the informal relationships within organization designs are not established by managers, and because managers cannot control these informal relationships to the extent that they can control the various formal aspects of a design, managers sometimes view informal aspects of designs as a problem. Informal aspects can indeed be problematic, but they can also serve useful purposes for managers. They can be blended with the formal organization design of a program to help facilitate the accomplishment of the program's mission and objectives with quality and efficiency.

Formal organization designs sometimes are too inflexible to meet the needs of a dynamic situation. Thus, the more flexible and spontaneous characteristics of informal relationships—such as the speed of communication through the grapevine—can have advantages. In emergencies, for example, the informal relationships and arrangements existing within a formal organization design may protect the organization from the harm that could result from strict adherence to formal channels of communication or literal obedience to the rules and regulations governing who does what.

Another potential advantage of informal relationships is that when informal group support is available to the manager, management work is easier. Managers can delegate and decentralize authority and responsibility more easily when informal groups are cooperative. The converse of this is also true; in the absence of informal group support, management work is more difficult. To protect themselves and to make their work situation acceptable, people typically resist what they perceive as autocratic management. The resistance often takes place in the context of informal relationships and arrangements, and may take the form of such undesirable behaviors as reducing effort or slowing the pace of work, insubordination, or disloyalty.

The level of performance achieved by any program is affected by its participants' willingness to grant cooperation and enthusiasm. Managers who understand this, and who understand that the coexistence of the formal and informal aspects of organization design is a fact of life, will take steps to balance those aspects. A suitable balance may be difficult to achieve, but managers can do two things to move toward this balance.

First, they can seek to understand the informal relationships and arrangements that exist among the participants in a program, and they can demonstrate their understanding and acceptance of them. Particularly important for managers in conveying acceptance is minimizing the negative effects of their decisions and actions on the often-fragile informal relationships and arrangements. Above all, managers should realize that attempting to suppress informal relationships and arrangements creates destructive and dysfunctional situations.

Second, managers can integrate the formal and informal aspects of an organization design. In so doing they should avoid formal organization design features that unnecessarily threaten or diminish the quality of informal relationships and arrangements. In effect, blending the informal relationships and arrangements that exist within an organization design with formal elements helps establish the program's culture.

Overall, the informal relationships among participants in programs are important to the participants and to the programs as well. Such informal aspects deserve the attention of managers because they can contribute to the effectiveness of formal organization designs.

Designing Program Logic Models

When managers establish the desired results for a program, expressed as its mission and objectives, as discussed in Chapter 2, the designing of its *logic model* is under way. Desired results are an integral component of the logic model for any program (see Figure 2.1), dictating to a large extent how the other components of the logic model are designed. These other components are expected to help accomplish the desired results. In designing logic models, managers must carefully consider the work processes through which resources are used to produce the desired results.

In designing the resources component of a logic model, attention is given to the human, financial, technological, and organizational inputs necessary for a program to achieve its desired results. Depending on the situation of a particular program, it is likely to require a unique package of resources, typically including some mix of human resources in the form of paid staff and perhaps volunteers, funding, potential collaborators, technology, organizational or interpersonal networks, physical facilities, equipment, and supplies.

In designing the work processes component of a logic model, attention is given to the activities, events, procedures, and techniques used to perform the direct, support, and management work necessary for a program to achieve its mission and objectives. Every program, depending on its specific circumstances, requires a unique mix of various work processes to achieve its desired results. For example, service provision processes differ in many ways across programs focused on cancer care, cardiac rehabilitation, geriatrics, health education, home care, palliative care, prevention of some disease or disorder, promotion of some aspect of health, research and development, substance abuse, wellness, and women's health. The differences in service provision processes may be even greater across housing programs, job training programs, and programs intended to clean up the physical environment.

Although work processes often differ depending on the nature of a program, there are commonalities. For example, many programs share such processes as intake and initial screening of new patients/customers, budget preparation, and interventional planning, and carry them out in essentially the same way. An increasingly important and widespread aspect of designing work processes in health programs is ensuring the cultural and linguistic appropriateness of services. The U.S. Department of Health and Human Services, Office of Minority Health (2014, 1), has recommended as a national standard that all programs providing health services ensure that all patients/customers receive from all participants "effective, equitable, understandable, and respectful quality care and services that are responsive to diverse cultural health beliefs and practices, preferred languages, health literacy, and communication needs." Commonalities aside, each program requires a unique mix of work processes if its desired results are to be achieved. Different work processes require different activities, events, procedures, and techniques. Depending on their processes, programs will engage in different mixes of such activities as diagnosis and treatment of illness, counseling, provision of day care, and provision of information and other educational modalities, among many others.

One challenge in designing work processes that form part of a program's logic model is choosing the basic methods through which services will be provided. Will services be offered to individual patients/customers, for example? Will services be provided in a group setting or even in the homes of patients/customers? For each service a program offers, there is a specific set of tasks that determines how the service is provided. For example, provision of counseling services in a drug treatment program could involve the following tasks for a given patient/customer:

- Intake and screening of the patient/customer
- Case planning by a counselor
- Implementation of the case plan
- Monitoring of service provision processes by the manager
- Evaluation of the effects of services for the patient/customer
- Termination of the patient/customer from services at completion
- Follow-up concerning the patient/customer's status and progress

Designing the work processes component of a program's logic model is a complicated undertaking. Adding to this task the design of resources and the determination of desired results in the form of a mission and more specific objectives suggests the extent of the challenge in designing a complete logic model as depicted in Figure 2.1. This challenge is further extended by the fact that logic models are not static; they undergo continual revision throughout the life of a program. Complexity aside, however, thinking of a program in terms of a logic model can be a very important adjuvant to the more traditional perspective on organization design presented earlier in this chapter.

The Staffing Process in Health Programs

As was noted earlier in this chapter, *staffing*, which is the process of filling the individual positions established in an organization design with participants, is an important part of the designing activity of a program manager. Fortunately, because programs are embedded in larger organizational homes, they can often take advantage of the specially trained human resource professionals who typically orchestrate this highly specialized organizational process. Because all managers have staffing responsibilities, however, the process cannot be left entirely to others.

The staffing process consists of a set of interrelated steps through which vacant or newly created positions in an organization design are filled (see Figure 3.9). Although a full discussion of this process is beyond the scope of this book, you will find excellent, in-depth discussions of general human resource management in such textbooks as those by Mondy (2013), Pynes (2013), and Fried and Fottler (2011). An overview of the steps in the staffing process is provided in the subsections that follow.

Human Resource Planning

The first step in the staffing process, *human resource planning*, involves gathering and analyzing information to identify human resource needs as well as planning to meet those needs. This planning is influenced by environmental conditions affecting a program. It begins with profiling human resource needs at some future date. Short-term (one-year) and long-term (five-year) profiles can be useful, allowing the manager to anticipate the program's ability to meet the demands of these profiles and to make concrete plans for overcoming any shortfalls.

The way a program's future has been developed/strategized (see Chapter 2) is very important to its human resource plans. For example, plans to diversify into new activities (such as providing a wellness program) or to significantly increase the provision of current services will directly affect the human resource profile. Does the expertise necessary to operate a wellness program exist within the program, or will new participants need to

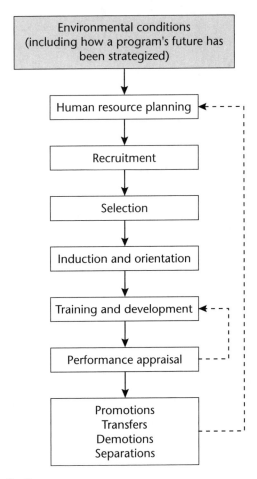

Figure 3.9   The Staffing Process

be recruited? Can current participants be retrained for the new work? And so on. An important part of this planning is maintaining up-to-date job descriptions, based on careful job analysis, for all current and anticipated positions in the program.

Recruitment

Guided by the provisions of a human resource plan, recruitment of prospective participants is undertaken by human resource professionals to develop a pool of job candidates. Candidates are usually attracted through advertisements placed in newspapers, in professional journals, via social media; through the efforts of employment agencies; and through recruiting visits to education programs that prepare health professionals.

Selection

Selection involves evaluating and choosing from among job candidates. Application forms, résumés, interviews, and reference checks are standard selection tools or techniques. A program functions through its participants, and new participants are selected in the belief that they will benefit the program. Wise selections can result in a range of outcomes, spanning from simply an absence of problems with new participants to genuinely excellent results in the form of their contributions to fulfilling the program's mission and objectives (Schmitt 2014).

Induction and Orientation

Induction and orientation are activities in the staffing process through which a new worker is introduced to his or her colleagues and to a program's history, culture, and organization design. An important part of this introduction is a thorough discussion of the mission and objectives established for the program, and of the new participant's expected part in achieving these desired results. The participant should become acquainted with his or her responsibilities and be made to feel welcome in the new workplace.

Training and Development

These activities in the staffing process are intended to increase the ability of a program's participants to contribute to achieving its desired results. Training usually is specific to job skills currently needed by participants, whereas development activities are designed to prepare participants beyond the requirements of their present position so that they can advance, or to prepare them for new work. Training and development, as illustrated by the feedback loop in Figure 3.9, are partially guided by the results of performance appraisals.

Performance Appraisal

The performance appraisal step involves periodic review and evaluation of the performance of individual participants, and in some cases the performance of teams. Appraisals serve two purposes, both of which are very important to managing effectively. Appraisals serve an administrative purpose in that the information from performance appraisals is taken into account in decisions about compensation, promotion, and termination. Appraisals also serve a developmental purpose by helping identify strengths and weaknesses among participants, which can be used to guide training and development activities (again, see the feedback loop in Figure 3.9).

Effective performance appraisal requires that it be based on performance criteria—measurable standards to which performance is compared—that are comprehensive and actually reflect aspects of performance that are relevant to the program's work. In taking a traditional approach to performance appraisal, managers use the performance criteria as points of comparison while observing actual performance of participants.

Increasingly, however, a broader approach to performance appraisal is employed. This approach may involve combining a manager's appraisal of performance with a participant's self-appraisal. Self-appraisals can be especially useful in tailoring and guiding development efforts. One approach to appraisal in some programs is team-based appraisal, whereby the performance of a team or group, rather than that of a single participant, is appraised. The major benefit of this approach is that it encourages teamwork; it is especially appropriate when groups or teams of participants work toward achieving specific objectives, and when any one participant's performance is highly interdependent with that of other participants in the team or group.

Originally intended exclusively for development purposes, an ever more popular approach to performance appraisal is 360-degree appraisal, also known as multirater assessment or multisource feedback (Bracken, Timmreck, and Church 2001). In many settings, 360-degree appraisals are replacing the traditional performance appraisals of individual participants conducted by managers. The central concept of 360-degree appraisal (and the source of its name) is that an individual's performance can be usefully appraised from many perspectives. Picture a 360-degree circle of perspectives surrounding the individual.

The raters in this approach can include an individual's organizational superiors, subordinates, peers, and perhaps patients/customers, as well as other external stakeholders with whom he or she has contact. This type of appraisal can serve administrative or development purposes, although care should be exercised in tailoring appraisals for different uses (Toegel and Conger 2003). Because of the widespread popularity of this type of appraisal, commercial software for structuring 360-degree appraisals is readily available (see, for example, www.sumtotalsystems.com or www .halogensoftware.com), and books on the subject abound (Lepsinger and Lucia 2009).

Promotions, Transfers, Demotions, and Separations

The last step in the staffing process is the movement of participants within a program through promotions, demotions, or transfers, and eventually their separation from the program through resignation, layoff, discharge, or retirement. As the feedback loop in Figure 3.9 illustrates, these movements provide important information for human resource planning. Separation represents critical information because it may trigger a new round of recruitment.

Special Aspects of the Staffing Process

This overview of the staffing process is intended to show how the various steps in the process are interrelated. Each of these steps involves very complicated activities, and all aspects of staffing are conducted within a legal context that includes employment law, labor relations law, and equal employment opportunity law (Fried and Fottler 2011). It is advisable that every program manager use the skills and expertise of the human resource professionals in his or her organizational home, as well as legal counsel, in fulfilling his or her staffing responsibilities.

It is also advisable that managers pay special attention to diversity among the participants resulting from their staffing efforts. Demographic changes in the United States are creating a more culturally diverse labor pool, as well as a more culturally diverse patient/customer base for programs. Studies suggest that cultural diversity is associated with better performance in health services settings (Dansky et al. 2003), in part because of the relationship between greater diversity and increased cultural competence, which supports improved performance.

The U.S. Department of Health and Human Services, Office of Minority Health (2014) maintains a set of standards for culturally and linguistically appropriate health services. The standards, which managers should follow, are "intended to advance health equity, improve quality, and help eliminate health care disparities" (1). Among the recommended standards is one stating that all health services organizations—including health programs—should "recruit, promote, and support a culturally and linguistically diverse governance, leadership, and workforce that are responsive to the population in the service area" (1).

Summary

The organization designs of contemporary health programs are created through the application of a set of organization design concepts whose roots can be traced back to the ideas of general administrative theorists from early in the twentieth century. Their work established what are called the classical concepts of organization design.

This chapter includes a discussion of the important dimensions of the informal relationships that people establish within the formal organization design in which they work, and of how managers can tap into the potential of such informal aspects.

The classical concept of division of work—dividing the work of a program into specific positions or jobs that have specified activities—is discussed. For example, the job of a pharmacist is defined by the activities a person in this position is expected to accomplish. The same is true for nurses, counselors, and therapists. The corollary of division of work, specialization of the participants who perform the work, is also discussed.

Growing directly out of the division of work is a need to assign responsibility for and authority over the performance of work. This assignment occurs through the technical process of delegation, which results in scaling or grading the levels of authority and responsibility in an organization design.

A natural consequence of division and specialization of work is clustering or grouping (called departmentalization by the classical theorists) of positions under the authority of a manager. The bases used in clustering participants are examined: knowledge and skills, work processes or functions performed, timing, outputs, clients served, and place. The span of control concept is examined, with emphasis on the influence of span of control on the shape (tall or flat) of an organization design. A number of contingencies that help determine the proper span of control are discussed.

Coordination is described as a process intended to achieve unity of effort among the various parts of an organization design toward the accomplishment of a program's mission and objectives. An extensive menu of coordinating mechanisms available to managers is presented, including administrative systems and procedures; committees and teams; customs; direct supervision; feedback; hierarchy; mutual adjustment; planning; programming; standardization of work processes, work outputs, or worker skills; and voluntary action.

The design of logic models for programs is discussed. A logic model is defined as a schematic picture of the relationships among the resources available to a program, the work processes undertaken with the resources, and the results the program seeks to achieve.

Finally, a model of the staffing process, through which program managers fill the positions in an organization design, is presented (see Figure 3.9).

REVIEW QUESTIONS

1. Distinguish between the formal and informal aspects of organization designs.

2. Discuss the advantages and disadvantages of dividing work. What are the implications for managers of dividing work?

3. What is the relationship between authority and responsibility in organization designs? Discuss the sources of each.

4. Describe the important bases for clustering in the organization designs of health programs, and give an example of clustering using each basis.

5. What factors should be considered in determining an appropriate span of control for a program manager?

6. Discuss the menu of coordinating mechanisms available to managers as they seek to achieve coordination within a program.

7. Why do people form informal groups within formal organization designs?

8. What should managers do about informal groups in their programs?

9. Discuss the design of logic models for programs.

10. Model and describe the basic staffing process, and discuss the interdependence among the steps in the process.

KEY TERMS AND CONCEPTS

authority

clustering

coordinating mechanisms

coordination

departmentalization

designing

division of work

formal and informal organization designs

groups

human resource planning

integration

interdependence

interpersonal power

learning organization

logic model

matrix organization design

organization designs

responsibility

span of control

specialization

staffing

References

Bracken, David W., Carol W. Timmreck, and Allan H. Church. *The Handbook of Multisource Feedback*. San Francisco: Jossey-Bass, 2001.

Dansky, Kathryn H., Robert Weech-Maldonado, Gita De Souza, and Janice L. Dreachslin. "Organizational Strategy and Diversity Management: Diversity-Sensitive Orientation as a Moderating Influence." *Health Care Management Review* 28, no. 3 (July-September 2003): 243–253.

Dyer, W. Gibb, Jr., Jeffrey H. Dyer, and William G. Dyer. *Team Building: Proven Strategies for Improving Team Performance*, 5th ed. San Francisco: Jossey-Bass, 2013.

Fallon, L. Fleming, Jr., James W. Begun, and William Riley. *Managing Health Organizations for Quality and Performance*. Burlington, MA: Jones & Bartlett Learning, 2013.

Fayol, Henri. *General and Industrial Management*. Translated by Constance Storrs. London: Sir Isaac Pitman and Sons, 1949.

French, John R. P., and Bertram H. Raven. "The Basis of Social Power." In *Studies of Social Power*, edited by Dorwin Cartwright, 150–167. Ann Arbor, MI: Institute for Social Research, 1959.

Fried, Bruce J., and Myron D. Fottler. *Fundamentals of Human Resources in Healthcare*. Chicago: Health Administration Press, 2011.

Fried, Bruce J., Sharon Topping, and Amy C. Edmondson. "Teams and Team Effectiveness in Health Services Organizations." In *Shortell and Kaluzny's Health Care Management: Organization Design and Behavior*, edited by Lawton Robert Burns, Elizabeth H. Bradley, and Bryan J. Weiner, 6th ed., 121–162. Clifton Park, NY: Delmar, Cengage Learning, 2012.

Gulick, Luther, and Lyndall Urwick, eds. *Papers on the Science of Administration*. New York: Institute of Public Administration, 1937.

Hage, Jerald. *Theories of Organizations: Forms, Processes, and Transformations*. Hoboken, NJ: Wiley, 1980.

Harvard Business Review. Harvard Business Review on Building Better Teams. Boston: Harvard Business School, 2011.

Lepsinger, Richard, and Anntoinette D. Lucia. *The Art and Science of 360 Degree Feedback*, 2nd ed. San Francisco: Jossey-Bass, 2009.

Litterer, Joseph A. *The Analysis of Organizations*. Hoboken, NJ: Wiley, 1965.

Mintzberg, Henry. *The Structuring of Organizations*. Upper Saddle River, NJ: Prentice Hall, 1979.

Mintzberg, Henry. *Structure in Fives: Designing Effective Organizations*. Upper Saddle River, NJ: Prentice Hall, 1992.

Mondy, R. Wayne. *Human Resource Management*, 13th ed. Upper Saddle River: NJ: Prentice Hall, 2013.

Mooney, James D., and Alan C. Reiley. *Onward Industry! The Principles of Organization and Their Significance to Modern Industry*. New York: Harper & Brothers, 1931.

Pynes, Joan E. *Human Resources Management for Public and Nonprofit Organizations*, 4th ed. San Francisco: Jossey-Bass, 2013.

Schermerhorn, John R., Jr. *Management*, 12th ed. Hoboken, NJ: Wiley, 2013.

Schmitt, Neal. *The Oxford Handbook of Personnel Assessment and Selection*. New York: Oxford University Press, 2014.

Smith, Adam. *The Wealth of Nations*. Blacksburg, VA: Thrifty Books, 2009. First published 1776.

Smith, Mark, Robert Sanders, Leigh Stuckhardt, and J. Michael McGinnis, eds. *Best Care at Lower Cost: The Path to Continuously Learning Health Care in America*. Washington, DC: National Academies Press, 2012.

Thompson, James D. *Organizations in Action*. New York: McGraw-Hill, 1967.

Toegel, Ginka, and Jay A. Conger. "360-Degree Assessment: Time for Reinvention." *Academy of Management Learning and Education* 2, no. 3 (September 2003): 297–311.

U.S. Department of Health and Human Services, Office of Minority Health. *National Standards for Culturally and Linguistically Appropriate Services (CLAS) in Health and Health Care*. Washington, DC: U.S. Department of Health and Human Services, Office of Minority Health. Accessed May 11, 2014. http://www.thinkculturalhealth.hhs.gov/pdfs/EnhancedNationalCLASStandards.pdf.

Weber, Max. *The Theory of Social and Economic Organization*. Translated by A. M. Henderson and Talcott Parsons. New York: Free Press, 1947.

Wholey, Joseph S., Harry P. Hatry, and Kathryn E. Newcomer. *Handbook of Practical Program Evaluation*, 3rd ed. San Francisco: Jossey-Bass, 2010.

CHAPTER 4

LEADING TO ACCOMPLISH DESIRED RESULTS

As we discussed in Chapter 1, managers engage in three highly interrelated core activities as they perform management work: developing/strategizing, designing, and leading (see Figure 1.3). Developing/strategizing and designing are discussed in Chapters 2 and 3, respectively. This chapter discusses the third core activity of management work: leading.

It has been firmly established through extensive research that there are positive associations between, on the one hand, how well managers perform their leading activities and, on the other hand, "follower attitudes, such as trust, job satisfaction, and organizational commitment, and behaviors, such as job performance at the individual, group, and organizational levels" (Bono and Judge 2003, 554). This quote embodies a key point about leadership—its relationship to followership.

Followers, in the context of a program, are those participants who share with the leader a common view of the desired results established for the program, believe in what the program is trying to accomplish, and want both the leader and the program to succeed (Banaszak-Holl et al. 2012; Riggio, Chaleff, and Lipman-Blumen 2008). Leadership and followership are interdependent. Neither can exist without the other.

What managers do when leading is complex and multidimensional, although its essence is one person influencing other people. In his seminal study of leadership, for which he won a Pulitzer Prize, political scientist James M. Burns (1978) identified the central function of leadership: to achieve a collective purpose. This chapter focuses on ways in which managers can influence other participants' contributions to the accomplishment of the mission and objectives (the collective purpose) of a program. Thus, in

LEARNING OBJECTIVES

After reading this chapter, you should be able to:

- Define leading, and understand the relationships between influence and leading and between interpersonal power and influence

- Define motivation, and model the motivation process

- Distinguish between the content and process perspectives on motivation, and understand the implications of both perspectives for leading

- Understand the main approaches to studies of leading, including the traits, behaviors, and situational or contingency approaches

this chapter we will consider some basic concepts having to do with influence, as background for our discussion of leading.

A key aspect of managers' ability to influence participants' contributions is their ability to affect participants' motivation to contribute. Attention is therefore also given to motivation in this chapter, because skill at motivation is required for managers to be effective at leading.

Leading Defined

Adapting well-known definitions (Robbins and Judge 2012; Yukl 2012b), I define *leading* by a manager in a program as influencing others to understand and agree about what needs to be done to achieve the desired results established for the program, and facilitating the individual and collective contributions of others to the achievement of the desired results. Influencing is the most critical element of leading. Influence is the means by which leaders successfully persuade others to follow them.

In his classic study of leadership noted previously, Burns (1978) established that leading in organizations is of two distinct types: transactional and transformational. *Transactional leading* occurs as leaders—managers engaging in leading activities—enter into transactions with followers through which each receives something of value. In essence, if the followers perform their work in ways that contribute to accomplishing the mission and objectives of the program, the manager rewards them in some way. These transactions are ubiquitous in management work throughout all organizations. Effective transactional leading permits managers to facilitate better performance from participants, helping participants plan and coordinate their work and learn new skills.

In the second type of leading identified by Burns (1978), *transformational leading*, the leader's purpose is to effect significant change in the status quo. Transformational leadership means causing or helping bring about major changes in organizations. In practicing transformational leadership, managers focus on changes that involve an entire program and relate to such things as mission and objectives and modifying the level of support for the program from internal and external stakeholders. Unlike with the transactional leading process that occurs between managers and other participants, a transformational leader must have a vision for the entire program and must influence followers both inside and outside that program if the vision is to be realized.

The definition of leading given previously applies equally well to both transactional and transformational leading. Both are processes through which managers influence other internal and external stakeholders to contribute to a program's success. Important aspects of influencing are discussed in the next section.

Influence and Leading; Interpersonal Power and Influence

Because the essence of leading is the ability to *influence* others, one must fully understand influencing to understand leading. To understand the influence a manager can have over other participants in a program, however, one must first understand interpersonal power, which refers to the potential to exert influence over others.

Managers are able to exert influence in the workplace because they have interpersonal power. To a great extent, managers have interpersonal power in work settings because they are managers. It may be useful to review the discussion of authority in Chapter 3, where it is noted that the most important source of a manager's interpersonal power is the formal position he or she holds in a program's organization design. Formal power or authority is assigned to a manager in an organization design to support his or her ability to manage effectively.

All program managers have some degree of interpersonal power or authority based on their position, although managers at different hierarchical levels within organization designs have different amounts of positional interpersonal power. Positional interpersonal power permits managers to exert influence via control over a number of variables. They have, for example:

- The ability to reward or coerce participants' behaviors.

- Control over certain aspects of the physical environment in which work occurs.

- The ability to shape elements of a program's logic model, including determination of mission and objectives, work processes used, and resources available (see Figure 2.1).

- A key role in establishing the organization design for a program. When managers design work flow arrangements, for example, they can determine which participants interact with others, or who initiates a linked series of actions. Similarly, their ability to cluster certain individual positions into units, to assign reporting relationships, or to design an information system is a positional source of interpersonal power.

Control over information is a source of interpersonal power in any organizational setting. Managers have access to certain information because of their position in an organization design. To have interpersonal power derived from control over information, a manager must actively cultivate a network of information sources.

Another aspect of a manager's interpersonal power is that he or she can acquire such power through possession and use of political skills. Interpersonal power can derive from control over key decisions, the ability to form coalitions, the ability to co-opt or diffuse and weaken the influence of rivals, and the ability to interpret events in a manner that one deems favorable (Yukl 2012b). Position can help a manager use political skills, but those skills are inherent in the manager who possesses them. This serves as an example of another important source of interpersonal power, the characteristics and attributes of the person who possesses it.

Scholars have recognized for many years the existence of interpersonal power in work settings that is based on what an individual knows or is able to do. In their classic work on the subject, French and Raven (1959) called this type of interpersonal power "expert power," which is power held by a person who possesses knowledge that is valued by a program, or by the larger organization in which the program is embedded. Thus, expert power is different from positional interpersonal power, which, as noted previously, is primarily determined by a manager's position in the organization design. Any participant in a program can possess expert power. For example, physicians or nurses whose expertise is vital to the success of a program possess such power.

Another source of interpersonal power, sometimes called charismatic power or referent power, results when one individual engenders admiration, loyalty, and emulation to the extent that it permits him or her to influence others. As with power based on expertise, referent power cannot be assigned to a person based on his or her position in an organization design. Referent power is typically developed only over a long period of close interaction in which a person, who may or may not be a manager, demonstrates friendliness, concern for the needs and feelings of others, and fairness toward them. It is rare for a leader to gain sufficient power to heavily influence followers simply from referent or charismatic power, although this source of power can play a role.

Managers in all programs have multiple sources of interpersonal power, although they will have different levels of power because they will have different mixes of sources of power available to them. For example, one manager may have interpersonal power because of formal positional authority over a program and its participants. This manager may have some degree of control over resources, rewards, punishments, and information, and may have more relevant expertise in the work of the program than others. Yet this manager may possess little power based on political skill.

Another manager may derive interpersonal power from the same menu of sources, but in a different mix. For example, this manager may possess an exceptional level of political power by virtue of having the authority to control decision-making processes, the ability to form coalitions of key internal and external stakeholders, or the ability to co-opt opponents. Still another manager may have considerable charisma, extremely loyal followers in a program, and personal friendships with key leaders of the organization in which the program is embedded, all of which provide him or her with considerable interpersonal power.

Certainly, possessing interpersonal power derived from some mix of the sources noted previously is an important precursor to exerting influence over others or leading them effectively. But interpersonal power alone does not fully explain influence or leading. Another key aspect of leading is motivation, which is discussed in the next section to provide further background on leading.

Motivation as a Basis for Leading Effectively

To be effective at leading the participants involved in a program, managers must help create and maintain conditions under which the participants can and do contribute to accomplishing the program's established mission and objectives. Participants must be induced or motivated to contribute. Possessing knowledge of how motivation occurs is a means of understanding why people behave in particular ways—an understanding that is necessary for success in leading.

Managers need participants to exhibit a diverse set of contributory behaviors for a program to be successful. At the most basic level, they want participants they have selected for employment to attend work regularly, punctually, and predictably. These behaviors do not happen by chance; they are motivated behaviors. Managers also want participants to perform the direct or support work assigned to them, and they want this work to be performed at acceptable levels of quantity and quality. Finally, managers want participants to exhibit good citizenship behaviors, including such specific behaviors as cooperating, demonstrating altruism, protecting fellow workers and property, and generally going above and beyond the call of duty. High levels of good citizenship behaviors among the participants in a program invariably contribute directly to attaining the program's mission and objectives. How can managers create and maintain the conditions that evoke such desirable behaviors? Part of the answer lies in motivating participants to practice them.

Motivation is at once simple and complex. Motivation is simple because human behavior is goal directed, and because it is induced by increasingly well-understood factors, some of which are internal to the individual, and some of which are external. Motivation is complex because mechanisms that induce behavior rely on very complicated and individualized needs, wants, and desires that are satisfied in different ways for different people. Before exploring the key theories and models that have been developed to explain human motivation in the workplace, it is first necessary to define motivation and model the basic motivation process.

Motivation Defined and Modeled

Why does one participant in a program work harder than another? Why is one more cooperative than another? A partial answer lies in the fact that people have various needs and behave differently in attempting to fulfill them. Needs are, in effect, deficiencies that cause people to undertake patterns of behavior intended to remedy them. For example, at a very simple level, human needs are physiological. A hungry person needs food; is driven by hunger; and is motivated to satisfy the need for food (in other words, to overcome the deficiency). Other needs are more complex. Some needs are psychological (for example, the need for self-esteem); others are sociological (for example, the need for social interaction). In short, needs in human beings trigger and energize behaviors intended to satisfy those needs. This fact is the basis for a needs-based model of how motivation occurs. The needs-based perspective on motivation is very important to managers. If managers can identify the needs of a program's participants and design their work in ways that allow participants to satisfy or fulfill some of their needs, then motivation can occur, which in turn stimulates behaviors among participants that contribute to achieving the program's mission and objectives.

As shown in Figure 4.1, the motivation process is cyclical. It begins with unmet needs and cycles through the individual's assessment of the results of efforts to satisfy those needs. This assessment may confirm the continuation of unmet needs and permit the identification of new needs. Throughout this process, the person searches for ways to satisfy each need, chooses a course of action, and exhibits behaviors intended to satisfy the unmet need. The model is oversimplified, but contains the essential elements of the process by which human motivation occurs:

• Motivation is driven by unsatisfied or unmet needs.

• Motivation results in behaviors intended to satisfy the unmet needs.

• Motivation can be influenced by factors that are internal or external to the individual.

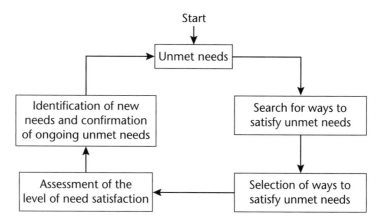

Figure 4.1   The Motivation Process for an Individual

This model also suggests a definition of ***motivation*** as an internal drive that stimulates behavior intended to satisfy an unmet need. It is "a state of feeling or thinking in which one is energized or aroused to perform a task or engage in a particular behavior" (D'Aunno and Gilmartin 2012, 93). It is important to note that the direction, intensity, and duration of this state can be influenced by outside factors, including the ability of a manager to contribute to or impede the satisfaction of an individual's needs.

Motivation is a key determinant of individual participant performance in work situations and is of obvious importance in accomplishing the missions and objectives established for health programs. Motivation alone, however, does not fully explain individuals' performance. Physical and mental ability and the nature of the work environment also affect performance. Knowing how to perform work and having the physical ability to perform it, good equipment, and pleasant surroundings facilitate performance. The variables affecting performance can be conceptualized as follows:

Performance = Physical and mental ability × Environment × Motivation

This equation shows that performance is a function of an interaction of several variables (Colquitt, LePine, and Wesson 2012). Without motivation, no amount of ability and no environmental conditions can produce acceptable performance. Although motivation alone will not result in a satisfactory level of performance, it is central to performance.

How Motivation Occurs

Because understanding motivation and applying knowledge of how it occurs are so critical to effectively leading others, a great deal of attention has been given to determining the mechanisms of human motivation. To motivate participants, managers need to know the answers to such questions as: What energizes or arouses participants to behave in contributory ways? What variables help direct their energy into particular behaviors? Can the state of arousal be intensified or made to last longer?

It is important to note at the outset that in seeking answers to questions about motivation, researchers have not established an undisputed and comprehensive theory about motivation, or about how managers affect motivation in the workplace. Instead, many competing theories have been posited to explain motivation. These varied approaches to motivation can be divided into two broad categories: the ***content perspective*** and the ***process perspective*** (see Figure 4.2). Each of the perspectives contributes something to an understanding of motivation and has implications for the core management activity of leading.

The content perspective on motivation focuses on identifying the internal needs and desires of individuals that cause them to initiate and sustain behaviors intended to satisfy the needs and desires, and that eventually cause individuals to terminate behaviors when the needs and desires are satisfied. The focus is on *what* motivates. In contrast, the process perspective seeks to explain *how* behavior is initiated, sustained, and terminated. Combined, these perspectives on motivation define variables that explain much about motivated behavior and show how the variables interact and influence each other to produce certain behavior patterns. Key theories and models that underpin contemporary thought about human motivation in the workplace are noted in Figure 4.2 and are briefly described in the following subsections, beginning with four theories that fall within the content perspective. Much of the literature on motivation is decades old. But as with our discussion of the designing activity in Chapter 3, do not be concerned that this information is out of date. It is as relevant today as it was when the theories and models were first developed.

Maslow's Hierarchy of Needs

Perhaps the most widely recognized model of what motivates human behavior—certainly the one with the most enduring impact—was advanced by Abraham Maslow in the 1940s. A psychologist, Maslow (1943) formulated a theory of motivation that stressed two fundamental premises. First, he argued that human beings have a variety of needs, and that unmet needs influence behavior; an adequately fulfilled need is not a motivator. His second premise was that people's needs are arranged in a hierarchy, with "higher" needs becoming dominant only after "lower" needs are satisfied.

Content Perspective

Focus:

> Identifying factors within individuals that initiate, sustain, and terminate behaviors

Key studies:

> Maslow's five levels of human needs in hierarchy
>
> Alderfer's three levels of human needs in hierarchy
>
> Herzberg's two sets of factors
>
> McClelland's three learned needs

Implication for managers in leading:

> Managers must pay attention to the unique and varied needs, desires, and goals of participants.

Process Perspective

Focus:

> Explaining how behaviors are initiated, sustained, and terminated

Key studies:

> Vroom's expectancy theory of choices
>
> Adams's equity theory
>
> Locke's goal-setting theory

Implication for managers in leading:

> Managers must understand how the unique and varied needs, desires, and goals of participants interact with their preferences and with rewards and accomplishments to affect their behavioral choices.

Figure 4.2   Comparison of the Content and Process Perspectives on Motivation

Figure 4.3 illustrates ***Maslow's hierarchy of needs,*** with examples showing how needs in each category can be fulfilled in the context of working in a health program.

From lowest to highest order, the five categories of needs in Maslow's hierarchy begin with basic physiological needs, such as air, water, food, shelter, and sex, which are necessary for survival. Participants can satisfy many of these needs through the resources that their paychecks provide.

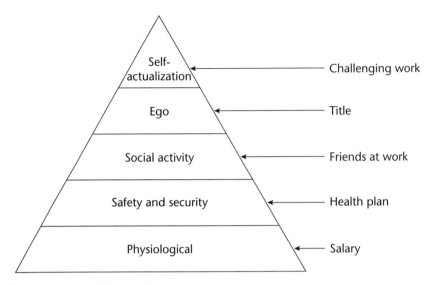

Figure 4.3   Maslow's Hierarchy of Needs

After basic physiological needs, safety and security needs come next. Once basic survival needs are met, participants can turn their attention to ensuring continued survival by protecting themselves against physical harm and deprivation. Participants seek to meet their safety and security needs through ensuring job security, having adequate health insurance, and other benefits. The third level of needs pertains to social activity, which relates to people's social and gregarious nature and includes their need for belonging, friendship, affection, and love. The ability to have friendships with other participants and to engage in social activity in the workplace helps satisfy these needs.

It is important to note that the third-level needs are something of a breaking point in the hierarchy, moving away from the physical or quasi-physical needs of the first two levels. This level reflects people's need for association or companionship, belonging to groups, and giving and receiving friendship and affection.

The fourth level, ego needs, includes two different types of needs, the need for a positive self-image and for self-respect and the need for recognition and respect from others. Examples of ego needs are the need for independence, achievement, recognition from others, self-esteem, and status. Opportunities for advancement within a program, or within the larger host organization, can help participants fulfill these needs.

The top level of Maslow's hierarchy includes self-actualization needs. These fifth-level needs have to do with realizing one's potential for continued growth and development. In effect, this level represents a person's need to become everything he or she is capable of being. Self-actualization needs are evidenced in people by their need to be creative and to have opportunities for self-expression and self-fulfillment. A challenging and satisfying job is a primary pathway to satisfying such needs in contemporary society.

In part because of its great intuitive appeal, Maslow's conceptualization of what motivates human behavior has been widely adopted. In a remarkable bit of candor, however, he once wrote of his concern that the theory was "being swallowed whole by all sorts of enthusiastic people, who really should be a little more tentative" (Maslow 1965, 56). Although Maslow's view of what motivates human behavior has limitations, it contains the valid point that people have numerous needs, which they seek to fulfill, and his theory accounts for how unmet needs influence need-fulfilling behaviors. Finally, Maslow's views on motivation provided a conceptual framework that was used to build and test more sophisticated theories about needs and how they affect human behavior, which are described in the following subsections.

Alderfer's ERG Theory

In another classic theory of what motivates human behavior, Clayton Alderfer (1969, 1972) advanced the idea that the hierarchy of needs is more accurately conceptualized as having only three distinct categories, not five as in Maslow's formulation described earlier. This theory is known as ERG theory because of the three categories of needs: **e**xistence, **r**elatedness, and **g**rowth. Existence needs include material and physical needs that can be satisfied by such things as air, water, money, and working conditions. Relatedness needs include all needs that involve other people. Relatedness needs are satisfied by meaningful social and interpersonal relationships. Growth needs, in Alderfer's scheme, include all needs involving creative efforts. Individuals satisfy these needs through making creative and productive contributions to achieving the mission and objectives in their workplace.

Alderfer's ERG theory is obviously similar to Maslow's theory. His existence needs are similar to Maslow's physiological and safety needs; his relatedness needs are similar to Maslow's social activity needs; and his growth needs are similar to Maslow's ego and self-actualization needs. The theories differ, however, in regard to how needs predominate in influencing behavior.

Maslow (1943) theorized that unfulfilled lower-level needs are predominant, and that needs at the next-higher level are not activated until the predominant (unmet lower-level) needs are satisfied. He called this the "satisfaction-progression" process. In contrast, Alderfer (1969, 1972) argued that three categories of needs form a hierarchy only in the sense of increasing abstractness, or decreasing concreteness: as an individual moves from existence to relatedness to growth needs, the means to satisfy the needs become less and less concrete.

In Alderfer's theory, people focus first on needs that are satisfied in relatively concrete ways; then they focus on needs that are satisfied more abstractly. This is similar to Maslow's idea of satisfaction-progression. Alderfer proposed, however, that what he called a "frustration-regression" process is also present in determining which category of needs predominates at any given time. By this he meant that someone frustrated in efforts to satisfy growth needs may regress and focus on satisfying more concrete relatedness needs or even more concrete existence needs. In Alderfer's view, the coexistence of the satisfaction-progression and frustration-regression processes leads to a cycling between categories of needs. A case example from a health program will help clarify Alderfer's concept of cycling:

Consider the case of Jennifer Smith, a thirty-two-year-old registered nurse who is a participant in a women's health program sponsored by a major hospital. Ms. Smith, a single parent of two children, is appropriately concerned about the security of her position and her pay and benefits, although she finds the social interactions with coworkers rewarding. Professionally, she is an excellent nurse who enjoys her work.

When a vacancy occurs in a nurse manager position in the program, Ms. Smith considers the opportunities this presents for professional growth and development, as well as for a higher salary. She applies for the position and looks forward to the challenges she will face if selected.

But a more experienced and equally qualified nurse is promoted. Ms. Smith's disappointment shows, and she also becomes quite concerned about her future in the program. Several other participants in the program notice her reaction and make special efforts to ease her disappointment. They tell her that other opportunities will arise, and that with more experience, she will be promoted.

The newly promoted nurse manager is sensitive to this situation and makes a point of telling Ms. Smith what valuable contributions she is making to the success of the program. After a few weeks, Ms. Smith returns to the same level of work enjoyment she felt before this episode.

In terms of needs, Ms. Smith cycled from having existence and relatedness needs predominate to focusing on growth needs represented by the promotion, and then returned to relatedness needs—all in a few weeks. In other words, Ms. Smith experienced both a satisfaction-progression process and a frustration-regression process.

Another important part of Alderfer's ERG theory, and another way in which it differs from Maslow's formulation, is Alderfer's view that when individuals satisfy their existence and relatedness needs, these needs become less important. The opposite is true for growth needs, however. In Alderfer's view, as growth needs are satisfied, they become increasingly important. As people become more creative and productive, they raise their growth goals and are dissatisfied until the new goals are reached. In the case of Ms. Smith, this means that when she becomes a nurse manager, she will probably raise her goals to include increased levels of responsibility and perhaps promotions to higher management positions, anticipating further growth and development in her career.

Herzberg's Two-Factor Theory

Frederich Herzberg took another approach to the study of what motivates human behavior in the workplace. His work advanced Maslow's needs theory by asking questions about what leads people to feel satisfied or dissatisfied at work, assuming that the answers would contribute to an understanding of what motivates people (Herzberg 1987; Herzberg, Mausner, and Snyderman 1959).

Herzberg and his associates (1959) found that one set of factors was associated with satisfaction and high levels of motivation, whereas another different set of factors was associated with dissatisfaction and low motivation. *Herzberg's two-factor theory* of motivation argues that one set of factors, called satisfiers or motivators, results in satisfaction and high motivation when the factors are present at adequate levels. These factors are achievement, recognition, advancement, satisfying aspects of the work itself, the possibility of growth, and the possibility of increased responsibility. The other set of factors, called dissatisfiers or hygiene factors, causes dissatisfaction and low motivation when the factors are not present at adequate levels. These factors include appropriate organizational policies, quality supervision, pleasant interpersonal relations, and positive working conditions.

The most important contribution of Hertzberg's formulation is that it has caused managers to think more carefully about the factors that contribute to motivation, and about what they can do to enhance opportunities for people to achieve intrinsic satisfaction from their work. If managers are to help participants be motivated, they must be concerned with one set of factors to minimize dissatisfaction and another to help them achieve satisfaction and be motivated in their work.

McClelland's Learned Needs Theory

Another important contributor to the content perspective on motivation was David McClelland (1961, 1983), who developed *McClelland's learned needs theory*. Extending Maslow's needs theory discussed earlier, he posited that people learn some of their needs through life experiences; they are not born with the needs. For example, children learn the need to achieve through encouragement and reinforcement of autonomy and self-reliance by adults who influence their early years. The learned needs theory builds on Maslow's (1943) theory and the even earlier work of Murray (1938), who theorized that people acquire an individual profile of needs by interacting with their environment. McClelland was also influenced by the work of Atkinson (1961) and Atkinson and Raynor (1974).

Both McClelland and Atkinson argued that people have three distinct sets of needs: (1) achievement needs, including the need to excel, achieve in relation to standards, accomplish complex tasks, and resolve problems; (2) power needs, including the need to control or influence how others behave and to exercise authority over others; and (3) affiliation needs, including the need to associate with others, form and sustain friendly and close interpersonal relationships, and avoid conflict.

McClelland posited not only that everyone has these three sets of needs but also that one predominates and most strongly affects each individual's behaviors. This point is important because it relates to how well people fit with particular work situations. In fact, the most useful aspect of McClelland's formulation is the idea of the importance of matching a person's dominant needs with his or her work situation. If this matching is done carefully in the context of a program, participants will be more motivated, which will be reflected in their performance.

The content perspective on motivation, as reflected in the four theories or models discussed previously, has significant implications for managers. These theories emphasize that human motivation originates from the needs of people and their search to satisfy those needs. The common thread running through the theories or models of motivation in the content perspective is their focus on needs that motivate human behavior. Each theory defines human needs differently, but all support the concept that managers can help motivate participants in a program by helping them identify their specific needs and assisting them in at least partially meeting those needs in the workplace.

These are extraordinarily complex tasks, considering the fact that each person has a unique and constantly changing set of needs. Managers can help participants identify and meet their needs by empathizing with them. Combining empathy with effective two-way communication, as discussed in Chapter 6, usually results in progress toward identifying and fulfilling needs.

The content theories or models of motivation, with their singular focus on what motivates behavior, provide managers with many useful insights. Other theories and models are needed, however, to shed light on the process of motivation—that is, to explain the mechanisms through which motivation occurs. The process perspective focuses on how individuals' expectations and preferences for outcomes that are associated with or that result from their performance actually influence performance. A central element in the process perspective on motivation is that people are decision makers who weigh the personal advantages and disadvantages of their behaviors. Continuing to follow the outline presented in Figure 4.2, three theories that fall within the process perspective on motivation are briefly presented next: Vroom's expectancy theory, Adams's equity theory, and Locke's goal-setting theory.

Vroom's Expectancy Theory

Victor Vroom's (1964) formulation of how motivation occurs is based on the idea that although people are driven by their unmet needs, they make decisions about how they will and will not behave in attempting to fulfill their needs. Their decisions, according to Vroom, are affected by three conditions: (1) people must believe that their effort to perform affects their level of performance; (2) people must believe that achieving the desired level of performance will lead to concrete outcomes or rewards; and (3) people must value the possible outcomes. Figure 4.4 models the three central components and the relationships in the expectancy theory model.

In **Vroom's expectancy theory**, expectancy is what individuals perceive to be the probability that their effort will lead to the desired level of

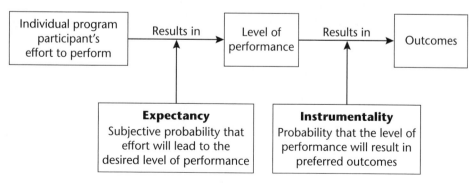

Figure 4.4   Basic Model of Expectancy Theory

performance. If a person believes that more effort will lead to improved performance, expectancy will be high. If, in a different situation, the same person believes that trying harder will not improve performance, expectancy will be low.

Instrumentality in Figure 4.4 is the probability perceived by individuals that their performance will lead to desired outcomes or rewards. If a person believes that better performance will be rewarded, the instrumentality of performance in relation to rewards will be high. Conversely, if the person believes that improved performance will not be rewarded, the instrumentality of improved performance will be low.

Outcomes are listed only once in Figure 4.4, but they play two important roles in expectancy theory. The level of performance (in the center of the figure) actually represents an outcome of the "individual program participant's effort to perform" component of the figure. Vroom called this a first-order outcome. Examples of first-order outcomes include productivity, creativity, absenteeism, and quality work resulting from an individual's effort to perform. The outcomes component shown on the right side of Figure 4.4 represents second-order outcomes that result from attainment of first-order outcomes. That is, these outcomes are the rewards (or punishments) associated with performance. Examples include merit pay increases, the esteem of coworkers, approval by the program's manager, promotions, and flexible work schedules.

Crucial to Vroom's expectancy theory is the concept that people have preferences for outcomes. Vroom referred to the value an individual attaches to a particular outcome as its valence. When an individual has a strong preference for a particular outcome, it receives a high valence; conversely, a weaker preference for an outcome yields a lower valence. People have valences for both first- and second-order outcomes. For example, a participant in a program might prefer (have a high valence for) a merit pay increase to a flexible work schedule, whereas another participant might prefer the flexibility (second-order outcomes). Or a participant might prefer to produce quality work (a first-order outcome) because he or she believes this will lead to a merit pay increase (a second-order outcome).

Expectancy, instrumentality, and valence for outcomes can be combined into an equation to express the motivation to work as follows:

$$\text{Motivation} = \text{Expectancy} \times \text{Instrumentality} \times \text{Valence}$$

or

$$M = E \times I \times V$$

It is important to note that because the equation is multiplicative, a low value assigned to any variable will yield a low result. For example, if a person is certain that effort will lead to performance, an expectancy value of 1.0 is assigned). If a person is certain that performance will lead to reward, an instrumentality value of 1.0 is assigned. And if a person does not have a very high valence or preference for the reward involved, a lower valence of 0.5 might be assigned. When multiplied ($1.0 \times 1.0 \times 0.5 = 0.5$), the result is low, indicating that motivation is low. For motivation to be high, expectancy, instrumentality, and valences all must be high.

Implications for Managers For managers of programs, expectancy theory explains a great deal about motivated behavior. By applying expectancy theory, managers focus on leverage points that help them influence the motivation of other participants. Managers who know what participants prefer in terms of second-order outcomes resulting from their efforts and performance have an advantage in developing effective approaches to their motivation. It is important to remember that implicit in Vroom's model is the fact that individuals have different preferences when it comes to outcomes. The design of approaches to motivation must reflect this fact; the approaches must be flexible enough to address differences in individual preferences concerning the rewards of work.

Bateman and Snell (2013) identified three crucial implications for management work inherent in expectancy theory. First, they argued that managers should take steps to increase expectancy. This means providing a work environment that facilitates work performance and establishing realistic performance objectives. It also means providing training, support, and encouragement in ways that permit participants to be confident that they can perform their work as they are expected to.

Second, Bateman and Snell (2013) urged managers to identify positive outcomes for participants they seek to motivate. This means thinking about what it is that jobs offer those who occupy them, as well as what is not provided by these jobs, but could be. Managers must think about how and why different participants assign different valences to outcomes and what this means for motivating behavior. In considering outcomes with high valences for participants, managers must think about the needs participants seek to fulfill through work.

Third, Bateman and Snell (2013) emphasized that managers should make good performance instrumental to positive outcomes for participants. Managers can do this, for example, by making certain that good performance is followed by such positive results as praise and recognition, favorable performance reviews, or pay increases. Conversely, managers should make certain that poor performance has more negative outcomes compared to good performance.

Adams's Equity Theory

An important extension of expectancy theory arose from the realization that, in addition to having preferences as to the outcomes or rewards associated with performance, individuals also assess the degree to which potential rewards will be equitably distributed. J. Stacy Adams (1963, 1965) recognized this phenomenon, which is reflected in **Adams's equity theory**. This theory posits that people calculate the ratio of their efforts to the rewards they receive and compare it to the ratios they believe exist for others in similar situations. They do this because they have a strong desire to be treated fairly. Adams argued that a person judges equity with the following equation:

$$\frac{O_p}{I_p} = \frac{O_o}{I_o}$$

where

O_p is the person's perception of the outcomes received

I_p is the person's perception of personal inputs

O_o is the person's perception of the outcomes that a comparison person (or comparison other) received

I_o is the person's perception of the inputs of the comparison person (or comparison other)

This formula suggests that participants believe equity exists when they perceive the ratio of inputs (such as experience, time, effort, dedication, intelligence, and the like) to outcomes (such as pay, promotions, status, esteem, monotony, fatigue, danger, and the like) received is equivalent to that of some comparison other or referent. Conversely, inequity exists when the ratios are not equivalent.

It is noteworthy that perception, not reality, is considered in this equation. Furthermore, the comparison other or referent in the equation could be any of the following (among other possibilities):

- A person in similar circumstances (a coworker or someone whose circumstances are thought to be similar)

- A group of people in similar circumstances (for example, all registered nurses working in a particular health program)

- The perceiving person under different circumstances (for example, earlier in the person's present position or when he or she previously occupied another position)

The choice of referent is a function of available information about the options for comparison as well as perceived relevance of the options to a particular situation. It is also important to note that in the equation there may be many different inputs and outcomes. Inputs are what people believe they contribute to their job; outcomes are what they believe they get from their job.

Equity theory recognizes that people are concerned both with the absolute rewards they receive for their efforts and with the relationship between these rewards and what others receive. In effect, equity theory recognizes that people are interested in distributive fairness—that is, in getting what they believe they deserve for their work. Extensive research (Gill 2011) supports the fact that people consider equity regularly in regard to how they are treated at work.

When faced with situations they perceive to be inequitable, people seek to restore equity in a number of different ways. Using pay as an example, people who feel an inequity (such as that their pay is too low or that they work harder than others with the same pay) can decrease their input by reducing effort to compensate for this perceived inequity. Alternatively, they could seek to change their total compensation package as a way to reduce the perceived pay inequity. Or they could seek to modify their comparisons or referents. For example, they might try to persuade low performers who are receiving equal pay to increase their effort, or they might try to discourage high performers from exerting so much effort.

Others who feel an inequity in their pay might, perhaps in desperation, distort reality and rationalize that the perceived inequity is somehow justified. As a last resort, people might even choose to leave an inequitable situation. This action usually occurs only when people conclude that the inequity will not be resolved. In summary, participants in a program can attempt to restore equity by changing the reality or their perception of the inputs and outcomes in the equity equation.

Implications for Managers   Equity theory shows that motivation is significantly influenced by both absolute and relative rewards. It also shows that if people perceive inequity, they act to reduce it. It is therefore important that managers minimize inequity—real and perceived—in their programs. This means helping participants understand the differences among jobs and the associated rewards, and making certain that reward differences actually reflect different performance requirements across jobs.

The bottom-line implication of equity theory for managers is that people who feel equitably treated in the workplace are more satisfied than those who feel inequitably treated. Although satisfaction alone does not ensure a high level of work performance, dissatisfaction, especially when many participants feel it in a work situation, has very negative consequences, including the following:

- Higher absenteeism and turnover rates
- Fewer good citizenship behaviors
- More grievances and lawsuits related to the work situation
- Stealing, sabotage, and vandalism
- More job stress
- Other costly, negative consequences for a health program and the participants in it

Above all, equity theory emphasizes the importance of managers' treating participants in a program fairly and ensuring that participants perceive themselves as being treated equitably.

Locke's Goal-Setting Theory

A third important model within the process perspective on motivation derives from the work of Edwin Locke (1987). Building on the idea that human behavior is largely goal directed, Locke viewed goal setting as a cognitive process through which conscious goals, as well as intentions about pursuing them, are developed and become primary determinants of behavior (Latham and Locke 2006; Locke and Latham 2004). In *Locke's goal-setting theory*, a goal is defined as something that an individual consciously attempts to attain (Latham and Locke 1987, 2006). The central premise here is that people focus their attention on the concrete tasks that are related to attaining their goals, and persist in the tasks until the goals are achieved.

In general, studies affirm the importance of goals in motivation (Petri and Govern 2013; Pinder 2012). Locke's theory includes the facts that goal specificity (the degree of quantitative precision of the goal) and goal difficulty (the level of performance required to reach the goal) are important to motivation; both facts have been affirmed by other studies (Latham 2007). It is also well established that goals that are specific lead to improvement in an individual's performance, because he or she has a better understanding of what is to be done. Finally, knowledge about the role of goals in motivation has been enhanced by research that shows the positive relationship between goals' being accepted as appropriate by a person and his or her performance.

Other studies (Petri and Govern 2013) show that people are more likely to accept goals, especially difficult goals set for them at work, when they participate in establishing them.

Implications for Managers   Goals that can effectively motivate desirable behaviors in the workplace have certain characteristics that managers should keep in mind as they set goals for participants in a program, collaboratively establish goals with participants, or encourage participants to set goals for themselves. For goals to have the greatest ability to motivate, they should be acceptable to participants. Acceptability is greater when work-related goals do not conflict with personal values, and when people have clear reasons to pursue them. Goals should also be challenging but attainable, and they should be specific, quantifiable, and measurable (Bateman and Snell 2013). It is also important for managers to provide participants with timely and specific feedback on their progress toward achieving established goals.

Many of the most significant challenges of leading and of helping participants be motivated in the workplace arise because managers do not clearly define and specify the desired results (mission and objectives) toward which they want participants to contribute. When participants know and understand a program's mission and objectives, it is easier for them to formulate or accept specific goals that contribute to the achievement of the mission and objectives. Effective leaders clearly state desired results, which all participants can then link to the work-related goals that they establish for themselves or that have been established for them or in consultation with them. Clear statements of a program's mission and objectives are especially useful in promoting desired behaviors and in leading in general when those who will be influenced by the statements have participated in formulating them and agree with what they say.

The Ongoing Search to Understand Effective Leading

From the previous discussion, we now know that greater understanding of influence and motivation supports a manager's core activity of leading, because leading effectively means influencing participants to make contributions that help accomplish the mission and objectives established for a program. That being said, neither influencing nor motivating a program's participants—nor a combination of these two actions—fully explains effective leadership by managers. The search for such an explanation is an ongoing and evolutionary process from which a better understanding of leading is emerging. This continuing search is considered in this section.

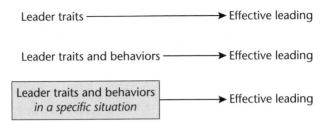

Figure 4.5   Comparing Three Approaches to Understanding Effective Leading

In seeking for many decades to understand how effective leading is accomplished in work settings, researchers have taken three general approaches. The ***traits approach*** is based on the proposition that traits—encompassing skills, abilities, or characteristics—inherent in some people explain why they are more effective at leading than others. The ***behaviors approach***, which grew directly out of the realization that traits cannot fully explain effective leading, is based on the assumption that particular behaviors or sets of behaviors that make up a style of leading might be associated with success in leading. A third approach, called the ***situational approach***, integrates the traits and behaviors approaches by arguing that traits and behaviors must be combined with particular situations to explain effective leading (see Figure 4.5 for the evolutionary progression of these approaches). Key insights drawn from studies conducted within each approach are described in the following subsections.

Leader Traits

The earliest studies of leading were based on the idea that particular physical or personality traits distinguish effective leaders. In attempting to prove the so-called trait theory of leadership, researchers sought to find traits that *all* effective leaders possess. Many different traits were studied, including physical characteristics, such as height, weight, and appearance, and personality traits, such as alertness, originality, integrity, and self-confidence, as well as intelligence or cleverness. Although the search for universal leader traits was not fruitful (Bass and Bass 2008), researchers have identified traits and patterns of traits that tend to be associated with effective leaders (Ledlow and Coppola 2014). For example, Kirkpatrick and Locke (1991, 48) concluded that "although research shows that the possession of certain traits alone does not guarantee leadership success, there is evidence that effective leaders are different from other people in certain key respects. Key leader traits include: drive (a broad term which includes achievement, motivation, ambition, energy, tenacity, and initiative); leadership motivation (the desire to lead but not to seek power as an end in itself); honesty and integrity; self-confidence (which is associated with emotional stability); cognitive ability; and knowledge. There is less clear evidence for traits such as charisma, creativity, and flexibility."

Goleman (2011) found an association between what he termed a leader's *emotional intelligence* and his or her effectiveness at leading. He identified five components of emotional intelligence: self-awareness, self-regulation, motivation, empathy, and social skill. Self-awareness is the ability to recognize one's own moods, emotions, and drives as well as to determine their effect on others. Self-regulation refers to the ability to control or redirect negative or disruptive moods or emotions. Motivation, in Goleman's view, reflects a strong drive to achieve and to pursue desired results with energy and persistence. Empathy means the ability to under-stand other people. Social skill refers to being proficient in building relationships and being persuasive. Goleman (1998, 94) argued that without emotional intelligence, "a person can have the best training in the world, an incisive, analytical mind, and an endless supply of smart ideas, but still won't make a great leader."

As research expanded the perspectives on the role of leader traits in effectiveness at leading, traits began to be seen as predispositions to behaviors. This viewpoint has been expressed as, "A particular trait, or set of them, tends to predispose (although does not cause) an individual to engage in certain behaviors that may or may not result in leadership effectiveness" (Pointer 2006, 132). This research led to an appreciation that traits have an impact on effectiveness at leading, but not in the way imagined in the earlier search for universal traits of leaders: "What seems to be most important is not traits but rather how they are expressed in the behavior of the leader" (Van Fleet and Yukl 1989, 67); also important is how they are expressed in a leader's style, which is a broader concept.

Leader Behaviors and Styles of Leading

Studies of the relationships between the behaviors and styles of leading exhibited by leaders and effectiveness were premised on the exciting possibility that, if especially successful behaviors or styles could be identi-fied, people could be taught how to be leaders (Pinder 2012; Yukl 2012a). Leaders would not have to be born with certain traits or attributes. The studies focused on describing leader behaviors, developing concepts and models of styles of leading (with styles being thought of as combinations of behaviors), and examining the relationships between different styles and effectiveness in leading.

One of the contributions of the studies of leader behaviors and styles has been the identification and definition of specific leader behaviors. Currently there is widespread agreement about what behaviors exhibited by leaders are related to success at leading. According to Yukl (2012a, 84–85), these behaviors are

- **Planning:** develops short-term plans for the work; determines how to schedule and coordinate activities to use people and resources efficiently; determines the action steps and resources needed to accomplish a project or activity.

- **Clarifying:** clearly explains task assignments and member responsibilities; sets specific goals and deadlines for important aspects of the work; explains priorities for different objectives; explains rules, policies, and standard procedures.

- **Monitoring:** checks on the progress and quality of the work; examines relevant sources of information to determine how well important tasks are being performed; evaluates the performance of members in a systematic way.

- **Problem Solving:** identifies work-related problems that can disrupt operations, makes a systematic but rapid diagnosis, and takes action to resolve the problems in a decisive and confident way.

- **Supporting:** shows concern for the needs and feelings of individual members; provides support and encouragement when there is a difficult or stressful task, and expresses confidence members can successfully complete it.

- **Recognizing:** praises effective performance by members; provides recognition for member achievements and contributions to the organization; recommends appropriate rewards for members with high performance.

- **Developing:** provides helpful feedback and coaching for members who need it; provides helpful career advice; encourages members to take advantage of opportunities for skill development.

- **Empowering:** involves members in making important work-related decisions and considers their suggestions and concerns; delegates responsibility and authority to members for important tasks and allows them to resolve work-related problems without prior approval.

- **Advocating Change:** explains an emerging threat or opportunity; explains why a policy or procedure is no longer appropriate and should be changed; proposes desirable changes; takes personal risks to push for approval of essential but difficult changes.

- **Envisioning Change:** communicates a clear, appealing vision of what could be accomplished; links the vision to member values and ideals; describes a proposed change or new initiative with enthusiasm and optimism.

- **Encouraging Innovation:** talks about the importance of innovation and flexibility; encourages innovative thinking and new approaches for solving problems; encourages and supports efforts to develop innovative new products, services, or processes.

- **Facilitating Collective Learning:** uses systematic procedures for learning how to improve work unit performance; helps members understand causes of work unit performance; encourages members to share new knowledge with each other.

- **Networking:** attends meetings or events; joins professional associations or social clubs; uses social networks to build and maintain favorable relationships with peers, superiors, and outsiders who can provide useful information or assistance.

- **External Monitoring:** analyzes information about events, trends, and changes in the external environment to identify threats, opportunities, and other implications for the work unit.

- **Representing:** lobbies for essential funding or resources; promotes and defends the reputation of the work unit or organization; negotiates agreements and coordinates related activities with other parts of the organization or with outsiders.

Studies of leader behavior have added an important dimension to the understanding of leading and new insights into effectiveness in leading. It should be noted, however, that as with the studies of traits, leader behavior studies have not fully explained successful leadership. As Yukl (2012a, 66) concluded, "Extensive research on leadership behavior during the past half century has yielded many different behavior taxonomies and a lack of clear results about effective behaviors." Even so, we will review the evolution of leader behavior studies because they add to our understanding of leading.

Early Studies of Leader Behavior

The most important early studies of leader behavior were conducted in the late 1940s at the Ohio State University and at the University of Michigan. In fact, most studies of leader behavior are based, at least in part, on this pioneering work. The ***Ohio State University leader behavior studies*** identified two separate dimensions of leader behavior: consideration and initiating structure (Ledlow and Coppola 2014; Stogdill and Coons 1957) Consideration refers to the degree to which a leader acts in a friendly and supportive manner, shows concern for followers, and looks out for their welfare. Initiating structure refers to the degree to which a leader defines and structures the work to be done by followers and the extent to which followers focus their attention on achieving desired results established by the leader.

Other researchers conducting the ***University of Michigan leader behavior studies*** did work that paralleled the studies at the Ohio State University. Based on extensive interviews of leaders and followers in a variety of organizations, Likert and his colleagues at the University of Michigan identified two distinct styles of leader behavior: job centered and employee centered (Likert 1961, 1977). Among the leaders these researchers studied, those who were employee centered emphasized interpersonal relations, took a personal interest in the needs of their followers, and readily accepted differences among work group members. These leaders were considerate, supportive, and helpful with followers. In contrast, job-centered leaders emphasized technical or task aspects of the job, were more concerned with participants' accomplishing their tasks than anything else, and regarded participants primarily as a means of getting work accomplished. These leaders spent their time planning, scheduling, coordinating, and closely supervising the work of participants.

Studies conducted in a variety of settings have found that effective leaders are employee centered and focus on the needs of participants. These studies have also demonstrated that effective leaders establish high performance objectives for participants, but permit them to participate in establishing the objectives (Katz and Kahn 1978).

Likert (1977), who was especially influenced by the findings on employee-centered behaviors, came to believe that a key element in effective leadership is the degree to which a leader allows followers to influence his or her decisions. He believed that follower participation in decision making encourages acceptance of decisions and commitment to them, both of which contribute directly to productivity and to follower satisfaction. His views on the benefits of participative leadership stimulated substantial research on its effects. Miller and Monge (1986) provided a good meta-analytic review of studies of the value of participative leadership. The relevance of these studies to managing health programs can be summarized as follows:

- Participation encourages those who work in a program to identify more closely with it. This enhances motivation, especially in regard to such contributory behaviors as cooperation, protecting fellow participants and property, avoiding waste, and generally going beyond the call of duty. If people have a voice in their work, they tend to be more enthusiastic in performing that work.

- Participation can be a means of overcoming resistance to change. Those who participate in making decisions about change will have a better understanding of the need for change and be less likely to resist it.

- Participation enhances followers' personal growth and development. By participating in decision making, they gain experience and become more proficient in decision making.

- Participation enables a wider range of ideas and experiences to be brought to bear on a problem or opportunity. Often participants who are closer to a situation and more familiar with it can develop ideas as to how to solve problems or take advantage of opportunities more readily than can managers.

- Participation increases the flexibility and adaptability of those who work in a program and improves how the program's organization design (see Figure 3.4) and logic model (see Figure 2.1) accomplish their purposes as participants gain a wider range of experience with how a program's various components fit together.

Studies of Leader Styles

The behavior studies provided the intellectual foundation for subsequent efforts to identify effective **leader styles** by identifying the optimal mix of leader behaviors for achieving effectiveness. (Remember that styles of leading mean particular combinations of behaviors.) One such effort that has been useful in its depiction of variations in leader styles was undertaken by Blake and Mouton (1985) and subsequently expanded by Blake and McCanse (1991). Their model of leader styles uses two variables: concern for people and concern for production.

The concern for people orientation focuses on the leader's relationships with followers. The concern for production orientation focuses on tasks and objectives in relation to performing work. The two orientations can be used as the axes on a diagram to help visualize the variation in possible styles of leading. For example, using a scale from 1 (minimum concern) to 10 (maximum concern), a style characterized by minimum concern for both people and production would be located at the bottom left of the diagram.

Similarly, a style characterized by maximum concern for people and for production would be located at the top right of the diagram. Different levels of concern for these two variables permit plotting of various styles of leading.

Slevin and Pinto (2007) developed another leader style model as a means of clarifying how leaders achieve consensus with followers in decision making. This model of leader styles is based on two dimensions: information input and decisional authority. Information input is determined by the degree of information inputted by followers into a decision-making situation. The decisional authority dimension is determined by whether leaders either make decisions by themselves or share the decision making with followers. These two dimensions form a grid, called the Bonoma-Slevin Leadership Model, with decisional authority on the x-axis, scaled from 0 to 100, and information input on the y-axis, also scaled from 0 to 100. The four extreme leader styles formed by this grid are as follows:

- *Autocrat* (100 on x-axis, 0 on y-axis), a style in which leaders seek little or no input from followers and make the decisions by themselves.

- *Consultative autocrat* (100 on x-axis, 100 on y-axis), a style in which leaders seek extensive input from followers, but keep substantive decisional authority for themselves.

- *Consensus leader* (0 on x-axis, 100 on y-axis), a style in which leaders seek maximum input from followers and allow for full participation in the decision-making process.

- *Stakeholder leader* (0 on x-axis, 0 on y-axis), a style in which leaders delegate ultimate authority for decision making to followers, but without obtaining any input from them. In effect, this style represents weak or failed leadership.

Turning Point in the Study of Leader Behaviors and Styles

Tannenbaum and Schmidt (1973) developed a model in which several possible styles of leading are arrayed as a continuum. This model shows alternative styles based on how much participation leaders afford other participants in their decision making. The resulting styles of leading, with the labels used in ***Tannenbaum and Schmidt's continuum of leader styles model***, can be described as follows:

- *Autocratic leaders* make decisions and announce them to other participants. The role of other participants is to carry out orders without an opportunity to materially alter decisions already made by a manager.

- *Consultative leaders* convince other participants of the correctness of a decision by carefully explaining the rationale for the decision and its effect on the other participants and on the program. A second consultative style is practiced when managers permit slightly more involvement by other participants. For example, a manager might present decisions to other participants and also invite questions to enhance understanding and acceptance.

- *Participative leaders* present tentative decisions that will be changed if other participants can make a convincing case for different decisions. A second participative style is practiced when a manager presents a problem to participants, seeks their advice and suggestions, but then makes the decision. This style of leading makes greater use of participation and less use of authority than do autocratic and consultative styles.

- *Democratic leaders* define the limits of the situation and problem to be solved and permit other participants to make the decision.

- *Laissez-faire leaders* permit other participants to have great discretion in decision making. The manager participates in decision making with no more influence than other participants. Leaders' and other participants' roles in decision making are indistinguishable in this style.

The importance of Tannenbaum and Schmidt's (1973) model to understanding leading lies in their conclusion that the best style of leading depends on the circumstances present in a particular situation. In their view, the choice of a style should be based on three sets of factors:

- Factors within managers, such as their value system, confidence in other participants, and tolerance for ambiguity and uncertainty

- Factors within the other participants in a situation, such as their expectations, need for independence, ability, knowledge, and experience

- Factors in a particular situation, such as the organization design, the logic model, the nature of the problem to be solved or the work to be done, and time pressure

Tannenbaum and Schmidt (1973) made a significant leap forward in understanding leading by arguing that no single style of leading is correct all of the time or in all situations. Leaders must adapt and change styles to fit different situations. An autocratic style might be appropriate in certain clinical situations in programs where work frequently involves a high degree of urgency. But this style could be disastrous in other situations, such as when a manager must decide how to offer a new service in a program or improve communication with participants. Tannenbaum and Schmidt's model, which couples a set of relatively discrete styles of leading with the concept that certain factors dictate choosing one style over the others, provides a bridge between the early traits and behaviors approaches to understanding leading and contemporary (and much more sophisticated) situational or contingency models of leading, which are described next.

Situational or Contingency Models of Leading

When it was found that leading effectiveness could not be fully explained by traits, behaviors, or styles, and especially when it was found that behaviors and styles appropriate and effective in one situation produce failure in others, researchers turned their attention to incorporating situational influences, or contingencies, into models of leading. Described briefly here are three from among the many resulting models that seek to explain how situational variables help determine the relative effectiveness of leader styles. The path-goal model developed by House and Mitchell (1974) is given the most attention because it is the most useful of the situational models.

Fiedler's Contingency Model

Fred Fiedler (1967, 1978) sought to identify situations in which certain leader traits are especially effective. His hypothesis was that effective leading is contingent on whether the elements in a particular leading situation fit specific traits of the leader. Complex theories have ample room for criticism, and *Fiedler's contingency model* is no exception. Considerable research, however, supports the model (Bass and Bass 2008).

Fiedler's work is important because it represents the first comprehensive attempt to incorporate situational variables, or contingencies, directly into a model of leading. The contingency model has utility in management practice, especially in suggesting to managers the importance of systematically assessing whether their relationships with the participants in a program are supportive. The contingency model also considers how the organization design and processes being used fit a manager's leader style and, in turn, how this affects his or her effectiveness as a leader.

Hershey and Blanchard's Situational Model

Paul Hershey and Kenneth Blanchard (2012) developed a model of leading that attempts to explain leading effectiveness in terms of the interplay among (1) the manager's relationship behavior, defined as the extent to which he or she maintains personal relationships with other participants through open communication and by exhibiting supportive behaviors and actions toward them; (2) the manager's task behavior, which is the extent to which he or she organizes and defines the roles of participants and guides and directs them; and (3) the participants' readiness levels, by which Hershey and Blanchard meant their readiness to perform a task or function or to pursue a particular objective.

Hershey and Blanchard's situational model identifies the participants a manager is attempting to lead as the most important situational variable, specifically focusing on participants' readiness to perform. The central premise is that the appropriate leader style depends on the readiness levels of the people the manager is seeking to influence. In this model, readiness is assessed according to two factors: ability and willingness. Ability refers to the knowledge, experience, and skills that an individual or group possesses. Willingness is the extent to which an individual or group has the commitment and motivation needed to accomplish a specific task.

This model, widely used by managers, suggests that managers engaged in leading must be concerned about other participants' readiness to be led, and must recognize their ability to affect the readiness levels of other participants. This model also reminds managers that it is important to treat all participants in a program as individuals, with real differences among them. Moreover, the model reminds managers to treat the same participant differently over time, as his or her readiness level changes (Bateman and Snell 2013).

House and Mitchell's Path-Goal Model

Like the other situational or contingency models of leading just described, *House and Mitchell's path-goal model* attempts to predict which leader behaviors will be most effective in particular situations. This model is perhaps the most generally useful situational model of leading effectiveness. Its name is derived from its focus on how leaders influence participants' perceptions of their work goals and the paths they follow toward attaining these goals. Robert House (1971), in originally conceiving this model, posited that a leader's functions are to increase the personal payoffs to followers for attaining their work-related goals, and to make the path to these payoffs smoother. House and Terence Mitchell (1974, 81), who helped develop the theory further, argued that "leaders are effective because of their impact on subordinates' motivation, ability to perform effectively, and satisfaction." The path-goal model incorporates the concept that leader behaviors are motivating or satisfying to the degree that they clarify the paths to and thereby increase participants' goal attainment.

This model of leading draws on the results of the Ohio State University (Ledlow and Coppola 2014; Stogdill and Coons 1957) and University of Michigan leadership studies from the 1940s (Likert 1961, 1977), and on the previously described expectancy theory of motivation (Vroom 1964). As already noted, expectancy theory describes the relationships between expectancy, instrumentality, and valence, where expectancy is the perceived probability that effort will affect performance, instrumentality is the perceived probability that performance will lead to outcomes, and valence is the value attached to an outcome by a person. The path-goal model of leading focuses on the factors that affect expectancy, instrumentality, and valence. Leaders can increase the valences associated with work-goal attainment, the instrumentality of work-goal attainment, and the expectancy that efforts will result in work-goal attainment.

The path-goal model is considered to be situational because its basic premise is that the effect of leader behavior on follower performance and satisfaction depends on the situation, specifically on follower characteristics and characteristics of the work to be performed (Polston-Murdoch 2013). According to House and Mitchell (1974), there are four categories of leader behavior, each of which might be best suited to a particular situation:

- *Directive leading* describes the behavior of the leader who tells followers what they must do, tells them how to do it, requires that they follow rules and procedures, and schedules and coordinates the work.

- *Supportive leading* describes the behavior of the leader who is friendly and approachable and exhibits consideration for the well-being and needs of followers.

- *Participative leading* describes the behavior of the leader who consults with followers, asks for opinions and suggestions, and considers what he or she hears.

- *Achievement-oriented leading* describes the behavior of the leader who establishes challenging goals for followers, expects excellent performance, and exhibits confidence that they will meet expectations.

House and Mitchell (1974) argued that all four styles of leader behavior can and should be used by leaders as the situation dictates, and that effective leaders match styles to situations. Situations can vary along two dimensions. One dimension is the nature of the people being led. Followers may or may not have the ability to do the job. They differ, too, as to the perceived degree of control they have over their work. The second dimension is the nature of the task, which may be routine and one with which followers have prior experience, or which may be new and ambiguous, meaning that followers require help if the task is to be performed well.

In using the path-goal model, effective leaders would diagnose the situation at hand and match behaviors to it. For example, directive leading could be used when followers are not well trained for their work and the work they are doing is partly routine and partly ambiguous. Supportive or participative leading might be most appropriate if followers are doing highly routine work and have experience with such work. Achievement-oriented leading would be effective if followers are doing highly innovative and ambiguous work, and if they have high levels of work-related knowledge and skill—conditions often found in health programs.

The path-goal model of leading, in essence, suggests that program managers improve leading effectiveness by (1) making the paths to achieving work goals smoother by providing participants with coaching and direction when needed, (2) removing or minimizing frustrating barriers that interfere with participants' ability to achieve work goals, and (3) increasing the payoffs for participants when they achieve work goals.

House and Mitchell's path-goal model is a useful construct because it merges concepts and knowledge of motivating and leading. The model also provides a pragmatic framework that is valuable to managers as they attempt to match their leader behaviors to characteristics of the participants they seek to lead, as well as to characteristics of a given work situation.

Toward an Integrative Approach to Effective Leading in Health Programs

Clearly, managers' effectiveness at leading contributes to the performance of individual participants, teams and work groups, and entire programs. Among the core activities of managers, effective leading is as important as effective developing/strategizing and designing.

Three approaches to understanding leading—traits, behaviors, and situational or contingency approaches (again, see Figure 4.5)—have been presented in this chapter. These different approaches have yielded numerous models over the years, each seeking to explain the phenomenon of effective leading. Individually, however, none of the models fully explains how a leader is effective. Levey (1990, 479) suggested, "We will probably never be able to achieve a truly elegant and rigorous general theory of leadership." This prescient view reflects the complexity and variety of variables involved in the dynamic process of leading. Even with this limitation, however, it is possible to integrate many of the findings from this research and the different models of effective leading described in this chapter into a useful, if incomplete, overall approach to considering effective leading in programs.

To reiterate some of the key points made in the chapter, we know that leading effectiveness results from interactions among such variables as leader traits and behaviors selected to fit situations, all of which are mediated or influenced by intervening variables, such as participants' efforts and abilities, organization design features, and the availability of appropriate resources. In health programs, participative styles of leading work best most of the time.

We also know that, above all else in regard to effective leading, it is important for managers to realize that because leading is a matter of influencing participants to contribute to achieving the mission and objectives established for a program, they must help participants be motivated to make their contributions. Motivation is a means to the end of leading participants to make contributions that help accomplish a program's desired results.

In terms of using motivation in the leading activity, the simplest and perhaps best advice is to select motivated participants to fill the positions in an organization design. People who have demonstrated appropriate levels of performance in the past are motivated to perform, and will in all likelihood continue to perform well under favorable conditions. Leading such participants to contribute to accomplishment of desired results is rather straightforward. This aside, however, some of the most significant challenges of leading and helping participants be motivated in the workplace arise because managers do not clearly define and specify the desired results (the mission and objectives) toward which they want participants to contribute. Being an effective leader, and using motivation to support the leading activity, begins with clear statements of desired results. These statements are especially useful when those who will be influenced by them have participated in their formulation and agree with them.

The models of how motivation occurs discussed in this chapter show us the powerful and direct connections among participants' efforts, performance, and rewards. A critical step in motivating people is choosing appropriate ways to reward desired performance, remembering that rewards can be intrinsically derived from the work itself, or extrinsically provided by managers. A contemporary approach to the issue of rewarding performance is what is termed pay-for-performance, or P4P. This approach to rewarding the performance of individuals or teams links the payment of bonuses to outstanding performance. The approach works at the level of health programs and is now being scaled up to apply to entire hospitals and physician practices. The reason for increased attention to P4P, especially at the level of entire organizations, is straightforward: "Payers, consumers, and other stakeholders believe that health care organizations are not providing services at a satisfactory level of quality or cost, and that strengthening the link between performance and financial rewards will produce better results" (D'Aunno and Gilmartin 2012, 109).

Also considering theories and models reviewed in this chapter, it is important to remember that people have different valences or preferences concerning rewards, making reward selection difficult at times. Some participants would rather have more challenging assignments or more vacation time than more money. For others, the reverse may be true. The point for managers to remember is that rewards must be important to the person receiving them if they are to be effective motivators. Prefer-ences often can be determined simply by discussing with participants what they want from work. Viewed broadly, managers' responsibility to provide suitable rewards can lead them into such areas as job redesign and job enrichment, cause them to change their leader styles, and induce them to change the degree to which they permit others to participate in decision making, which takes them well beyond the more traditional view of rewards as pay levels and benefits.

Selecting rewards that are appropriate is only part of the process of using rewards to motivate. Managers must link rewards to suitable job performance; that is, rewards must be made contingent on performance, and the linkage must be explicit. The more a participant knows about the relationship between performance (with clearly established expectations for performance) and rewards, the more likely it is that the rewards will help motivate the desired level of performance. The performance-reward linkage is strengthened by having rewards follow as soon as possible after desirable performance, and by providing participants with extensive feedback on performance. Finally, it is important to remember that people have a strong preference for being treated fairly or equitably. Their perceptions about the connection between performance and rewards at work are fundamental to their sense of fairness. Managers must pay careful attention to the equity implications of their use of rewards.

Reflecting on another important lesson from the work on motivation reviewed in this chapter, we know that motivation alone does not fully account for participants' performance or for their contributions to accomplishing the mission and objectives established for a program. A participant's performance is also determined, in part, by his or her abilities and by constraints in the work situation, such as uncoordinated work flow or an inadequate budget for technology or training. This means that it is important for managers to remove or minimize barriers to performance, which can be addressed in many ways, including through such actions as increased education and training, and in some cases by more careful matching of people with positions. Situational constraints, such as inadequate resources or an organization design that impedes performance, also can be addressed—once they are identified as constraints.

Managers' capacity to lead effectively, including using motivation to support leading, is greatly enhanced in work situations in which there is concern for the overall quality of work life (QWL). A program, and the larger organizations in which it is embedded, can approach QWL from several specific dimensions or foci of attention, such as the following (adapted from Bateman and Snell 2013):

- Adequate and fair compensation

- A safe and healthy work environment

- Commitment to the full development of participants

- A social environment that fosters freedom from prejudice and a sense of community

- Careful attention to the right of participants to personal privacy, dissent, and due process

- Work roles that minimize infringement on personal leisure and family needs

- Commitment to socially responsible organizational actions

Summary

In leading, program managers seek to influence other participants to understand and agree about what needs to be done to achieve the mission and objectives established for a program, and they facilitate the individual and collective contributions of others to achieve those results. To lead effectively, managers must help create and maintain conditions under which the other participants in a program can and do make their best contributions. An understanding of human motivation and of how to apply what is known about the process through which it occurs is therefore necessary for success in leading.

Motivation is defined as an internal drive that is a stimulus for behaviors intended to satisfy an unsatisfied need that an individual feels. Motivation thus stimulates goal-directed behavior. The basic process of motivation is modeled in Figure 4.1. An overview of the primary content and process perspectives of motivation is presented in Figure 4.2.

Models within the content perspective focus on the internal needs and desires that initiate, sustain, and eventually terminate behaviors. They focus on what motivates people. Four content theories of motivation are presented: Maslow's hierarchy of needs theory, Alderfer's ERG theory, Herzberg's two-factor theory, and McClelland's learned needs theory. Three process theories of motivation are also presented: Vroom's expectancy theory, Adams's equity theory, and Locke's goal-setting theory.

Motivation is a means to an end, a tool that a manager can use in leading participants to make contributions that help accomplish the mission and objectives established for a program. But there is more to leading than motivating program participants. Broader models of leading, based on leader traits, leader behaviors, and the application of traits and behaviors in various situations, are described (see Figure 4.5).

Models of leading based on leader traits, including intelligence, personality, and ability, are reviewed. Pioneering research about leader behavior conducted at the Ohio State University and the University of Michigan is presented as a prelude to reviewing the leader behavior models of leading developed by Likert, Blake and McCanse, and Tannenbaum and Schmidt. It is noted that Tannenbaum and Schmidt's (1973) model represented a significant advance in understanding how managers lead by recognizing that no single style of leading works best all of the time or in all situations.

Three key situational or contingency models of leading are reviewed: Fiedler's contingency model, Hershey and Blanchard's situational model, and House and Mitchell's path-goal model of leading. The House and Mitchell (1974) model is emphasized because of its widespread usefulness for managers, in that it shows that the effect of leader behavior on follower performance and satisfaction depends heavily on the situation in which leading is taking place.

This chapter describes how these theories and models of motivation and leading build on and complement one another. In the final section, this chapter integrates what is known from the reviewed theories and models and applies it to how managers can carry out the leading activity in health programs.

REVIEW QUESTIONS

1.   Define leading, and discuss its relationship to management work.

2.   Define motivation, and model the basic motivation process.

3.   Compare the content theories of motivation developed by Maslow, Alderfer, Herzberg, and McClelland.

4.   Compare the process theories of motivation developed by Vroom, Adams, and Locke.

5.   Describe the relationships between influence and leading and between interpersonal power and influence.

6.   Describe the sources of interpersonal power available to managers in health programs, and give an example of each.

7.   Discuss the evolution of approaches to understanding leading effectiveness.

8.   Why is Tannenbaum and Schmidt's model particularly important to understanding leading?

KEY TERMS AND CONCEPTS

Adams's equity theory

Alderfer's ERG theory

behaviors approach

content perspective

emotional intelligence

Fiedler's contingency model

Hershey and Blanchard's situational model

Herzberg's two-factor theory

House and Mitchell's path-goal model

influence

leader styles

leading

Locke's goal-setting theory

Maslow's hierarchy of needs

McClelland's learned needs theory

motivation

Ohio State University leader behavior studies

process perspective

situational approach

Tannenbaum and Schmidt's continuum of leader styles model

traits approach

transactional leading

transformational leading

University of Michigan leader behavior studies

Vroom's expectancy theory

References

Adams, J. Stacy. "Toward an Understanding of Inequity." *Journal of Abnormal and Social Psychology* 67 (November 1963): 422–436.

Adams, J. Stacy. "Inequity in Social Exchanges." In *Advances in Experimental Social Psychology*, edited by Leonard Berkowitz, vol. 2, 267–299. New York: Academic Press, 1965.

Alderfer, Clayton P. "A New Theory of Human Needs." *Organizational Behavior and Human Performance* 4 (May 1969): 142–175.

Alderfer, Clayton P. *Existence, Relatedness, and Growth: Human Needs in Organizational Settings.* New York: Free Press, 1972.

Atkinson, John W. *An Introduction to Motivation.* New York: Van Nostrand, 1961.

Atkinson, John W., and Joel O. Raynor. *Motivation and Achievement.* Washington, DC: Winston, 1974.

Banaszak-Holl, Jane, Ingrid Nembhard, Lauren Taylor, and Elizabeth H. Bradley. "Leadership and Management: A Framework for Action." In *Shortell and Kaluzny's Health Care Management: Organization Design and Behavior*, edited by Lawton Robert Burns, Elizabeth H. Bradley, and Bryan J. Weiner, 6th ed., 33–62. Clifton Park, NY: Delmar, Cengage Learning, 2012.

Bass, Bernard M., and Ruth Bass. *The Bass Handbook of Leadership: Theory, Research, and Managerial Applications*, 4th ed. New York: Free Press, 2008.

Bateman, Thomas S., and Scott A. Snell. *Management: Leading and Collaborating in a Competitive World*, 10th ed. New York: McGraw-Hill/Irwin, 2013.

Blake, Robert R., and Anne Adams McCanse. *Leadership Dilemmas—Grid Solutions.* Houston: Gulf, 1991.

Blake, Robert R., and Jane S. Mouton. *The Managerial Grid III: The Key to Leadership Excellence.* Houston: Gulf, 1985.

Bono, Joyce E., and Timothy A. Judge. "Self-Concordance at Work: Toward Understanding the Motivational Effects of Transformational Leaders." *Academy of Management Review* 46, no. 5 (October 2003): 554–571.

Burns, James M. *Leadership.* New York: Harper & Row, 1978.

Colquitt, Jason, Jeffrey LePine, and Michael Wesson. *Organizational Behavior: Improving Performance and Commitment in the Workplace*, 3rd ed. New York: McGraw-Hill/Irwin, 2012.

D'Aunno, Thomas A., and Mattia J. Gilmartin. "Motivating People." In *Shortell and Kaluzny's Health Care Management: Organization Design and Behavior*, edited by Lawton Robert Burns, Elizabeth H. Bradley, and Bryan J. Weiner, 6th ed., 91–120. Clifton Park, NY: Delmar, Cengage Learning, 2012.

Fiedler, Fred E. *A Theory of Leadership Effectiveness.* New York: McGraw-Hill, 1967.

Fiedler, Fred E. "The Contingency Model and the Dynamics of the Leadership Process." In *Advances in Experimental Social Psychology*, edited by Leonard Berkowitz, 59–112. New York: Academic Press, 1978.

French, John R. P., and Bertram H. Raven. "The Basis of Social Power." In *Studies of Social Power*, edited by Dorwin Cartwright, 150–167. Ann Arbor, MI: Institute for Social Research, 1959.

Gill, Roger. *Theory and Practice of Leadership*, 2nd ed. Thousand Oaks, CA: Sage, 2011.

Goleman, Daniel. "What Makes a Leader?" *Harvard Business Review* 76 (November-December 1998): 93–102.

Goleman, Daniel. *Leadership: The Power of Emotional Intelligence*. Northampton, MA: More Than Sound, 2011.

Hershey, Paul, Kenneth H. Blanchard, and Dewey E. Johnson. *Management of Organizational Behavior: Leading Human Resources*, 10th ed. Upper Saddle River, NJ: Prentice Hall, 2012.

Herzberg, Frederick. "One More Time: How Do You Motivate Employees?" *Harvard Business Review* 87 (September-October 1987): 109–117.

Herzberg, Frederick, Bernard Mausner, and Barbara Snyderman. *The Motivation to Work*. Hoboken, NJ: Wiley, 1959.

House, Robert J. "A Path-Goal Theory of Leader Effectiveness." *Administrative Science Quarterly* 16 (September 1971): 321–339.

House, Robert J., and Terence R. Mitchell. "Path-Goal Theory of Leadership." *Journal of Contemporary Business* 3 (Autumn 1974): 81–98.

Katz, Daniel, and Robert L. Kahn. *The Social Psychology of Organizations*. Hoboken, NJ: Wiley, 1978.

Kirkpatrick, Shelly A., and Edwin A. Locke. "Leadership: Do Traits Matter?" *Executive* 5 (May 1991): 48–60.

Latham, Gary P. *Work Motivation: History, Theory, Research, and Practice*. Thousand Oaks, CA: Sage, 2007.

Latham, Gary P., and Edwin A. Locke. "Goal-Setting—A Motivational Technique That Works." In *Motivation and Work Behavior*, edited by Richard M. Steers and Lyman W. Porter, 4th ed., 120–134. New York: McGraw-Hill, 1987.

Latham, Gary P., and Edwin A. Locke. "Enhancing the Benefits and Overcoming the Pitfalls of Goal Setting." *Organizational Dynamics* 34, no. 5 (2006): 332–340.

Ledlow, Gerald R., and M. Nicholas Coppola. *Leadership for Health Professionals: Theory, Skills, and Applications*, 2nd ed. Burlington, MA: Jones & Bartlett Learning, 2014.

Levey, Samuel. "The Leadership Mystique." *Hospital & Health Services Administration* 35 (Winter 1990): 479–480.

Likert, Rensis. *New Patterns of Management*. New York: McGraw-Hill, 1961.

Likert, Rensis. *Past and Future Perspectives on System 4*. Ann Arbor, MI: Rensis Likert Associates, 1977.

Locke, Edwin A. "The Ubiquity of the Technique of Goal Setting in Theories of and Approaches to Employee Motivation." In *Motivation and Work Behavior*, edited by Richard M. Steers and Lyman W. Porter, 4th ed., 111–120. New York: McGraw-Hill, 1987.

Locke, Edwin A., and Gary P. Latham. "What Should We Do about Motivation Theory? Six Recommendations for the Twenty-First Century." *Academy of Management Review* 29, no. 3 (July 2004): 388–403.

Maslow, Abraham H. "A Theory of Human Motivation." *Psychological Review* 50 (July 1943): 370–396.

Maslow, Abraham H. *Eupsychian Management.* Homewood, IL: Dorsey-Irwin, 1965.

McClelland, David C. *The Achieving Society.* Princeton, NJ: Van Nostrand, 1961.

McClelland, David C. *Human Motivation.* Glenview, IL: Scott Foresman, 1983.

Miller, Katherine I., and Peter R. Monge. "Participation, Satisfaction, and Productivity: A Meta-Analytic Review." *Academy of Management Journal* 29 (December 1986): 727–753.

Murray, Henry A. *Explorations in Personality.* New York: Oxford University Press, 1938.

Petri, Herbert L., and John M. Govern. *Motivation: Theory, Research and Application*, 6th ed. Belmont, CA: Wadsworth, Cengage Learning, 2013.

Pinder, Craig C. *Work Motivation in Organizational Behavior*, 2nd ed. New York: Psychology Press, 2012.

Pointer, Dennis D. "Leadership: A Framework for Thinking and Acting." In *Healthcare Management: Organization Design and Behavior*, edited by Stephen M. Shortell and Arnold D. Kaluzny, 5th ed., 125–147. Clifton Park, NY: Thomson Delmar Learning, 2006.

Polston-Murdoch, Leana. "An Investigation of Path-Goal Theory, Relationship of Leadership Style, Supervisor-Related Commitment, and Gender." *Emerging Leadership Journeys* 6, no. 1 (2013): 13–44.

Riggio, Ronald E., Ira Chaleff, and Jean Lipman-Blumen. *The Art of Followership: How Great Followers Create Great Leaders and Organizations.* San Francisco: Jossey-Bass, 2008.

Robbins, Stephen P., and Timothy A. Judge. *Organizational Behavior*, 15th ed. Upper Saddle River, NJ: Prentice Hall, 2012.

Slevin, Dennis P., and Jeffrey K. Pinto. "An Overview of Behavioral Issues in Project Management." In *The Wiley Guide to Project Organization and Project Management Competencies*, edited by Peter W. G. Morris and Jeffrey K. Pinto, 1–20. Hoboken, NJ: Wiley, 2007.

Stogdill, Ralph M., and Alvin E. Coons, eds. *Leadership Behavior: Its Description and Measurement.* Research Monograph No. 88. Columbus: Ohio State University, Bureau of Business Research, 1957.

Tannenbaum, Robert, and Warren H. Schmidt. "How to Choose a Leadership Pattern." *Harvard Business Review* 51 (May-June 1973): 162–180.

Van Fleet, David D., and Gary A. Yukl. "A Century of Leadership Research." In *Contemporary Issues in Leadership*, edited by William E. Rosenbach and Robert L. Taylor, 3rd ed., 65–90. Boulder, CO: Westview Press, 1989.

Vroom, Victor H. *Work and Motivation.* Hoboken, NJ: Wiley, 1964.

Yukl, Gary. "Effective Leadership Behavior: What We Know and What Questions Need More Attention." *Academy of Management Perspectives* 26, no. 4 (November 2012a): 66–85.

Yukl, Gary A. *Leadership in Organizations*, 8th ed. Upper Saddle River, NJ: Prentice Hall, 2012b.

CHAPTER 5

MAKING GOOD MANAGEMENT DECISIONS

This chapter focuses on decision making as a pervasive facilitative activity in management work. Managers of health programs constantly make decisions. This vital facilitative activity permeates the core activities of developing/strategizing, designing, and leading and the other facilitative activities (see Figure 1.4).

Examples of the decisions managers make in performing each of the core activities of their work illustrate the breadth of their decision-making activity. In developing/strategizing the future, managers, often with the involvement of other participants, decide what a program's desired results will be, expressed in terms of its mission and objectives. When managers establish a new program, they must decide what goes into the business plan. Further, they must make numerous decisions about how to conduct external and internal situational analyses, and they must decide whether acceptable progress is being made toward achieving the desired future state they have envisioned for the program.

In addition to making decisions about what a program is to accomplish, managers also decide how desired results will be achieved. In the designing activity, managers make myriad decisions as they establish the initial organization design and logic model of a program and subsequently reshape them as circumstances change. They must decide both what resources are needed and how to acquire them. They must decide what work processes will be used to achieve the desired results established through developing/strategizing. Other decisions are required when managers establish the intentional patterns of relationships among human and other resources within a program as they shape the program's organization design, the creation of which then stimulates other decisions in regard to staffing.

In leading, managers must decide how to encourage other participants in a program to contribute to

LEARNING OBJECTIVES
After reading this chapter, you should be able to:

- Define decision making and understand some of the important characteristics of management decisions in programs

- Understand and model the sequential steps in the decision-making process

- Identify some of the most popular quantitative models that support decision making, including decision grids, payoff tables, decision trees, cost-benefit analysis, the program evaluation and review technique, and decision support systems

- Understand the implementation and evaluation of management decisions as important steps in the decision-making process

accomplishing the program's mission and objectives, and they must decide how to facilitate those contributions. Managers decide what means of influencing other participants will work effectively, and how they will be applied. As leaders, managers focus on the various decisions that affect the entire undertaking, including those intended to ensure the program's survival and overall well-being. Because leading effectively means motivating participants to contribute to the program's performance, managers must decide how to motivate diverse participants, each of whom has a unique set of needs that can be partially met in the workplace.

Indeed, how managers conduct their decision making has a great deal to do with success in all the other activities of management work. We will begin our consideration of decision making with a definition.

Decision Making Defined

At its most basic level, ***decision making*** is simply making a choice between two or more alternatives (Adair 2013; McLaughlin and Olson 2012). Thinking of decision making in this way focuses attention on its essential element: making a choice. However, decision making by managers involves a process with a series of steps, which is described in detail in this chapter. The quality of managers' decisions is determined by how well they carry out all the steps in the decision-making process.

The many decisions program managers face can be divided into different types of decisions, but all of them involve choosing from among alternatives. One way of dividing decisions into categories is to consider programmed and nonprogrammed decisions (DuBrin 2011). Programmed decisions, on the one hand, are well defined, recurring, and more or less routine. Examples include decisions pertaining to scheduling, staffing, inventory, and selecting protocols to use with patients/customers. Nonprogrammed decisions, on the other hand, are not well defined; are not routine or recurring; and may involve consideration of new and complex alternatives, choosing among which is difficult. Examples include decisions about changes in a program's organization design, extending a program into new markets, selecting a new project director, or selecting a new information system.

An even more useful way to divide decisions into two types is to consider decisions as ***problem-solving decisions*** or ***opportunistic decisions.*** As the name implies, problem-solving decisions are made to solve existing or anticipated problems. Opportunistic decisions can be made when opportunities to advance accomplishment of a program's desired results arise, often by changing some element—perhaps a very small element—in the logic model or organization design. Such a decision might be called for, for example, when there is an opportunity to purchase some needed equipment or supplies at favorable prices, or an opportunity to recruit an especially skilled clinician for a program. Health program managers routinely make both problem-solving and opportunistic decisions in their work.

Although all management decisions are the responsibility of managers, managers can choose to involve other participants in the decision-making process to varying degrees. Answering the question of who makes decisions in programs is an important aspect of making good management decisions. In general, as discussed in this chapter, decision making is improved with more involvement of the participants in a program.

Involving Other Program Participants in Decision Making

Much of the literature on how managers make their decisions describes the process as one in which decisions are made by managers acting alone or by managers working with others (Adair 2013). Whether managers are making decisions alone or with others, the process is often described as taking place in an orderly, rational manner. In reality, decision making is more likely to be characterized by disorder and emotionality than by rationality and order (Yukl 2012). This is certainly the case when groups make decisions, as often happens in programs.

An important model that considers involving other program partic-ipants in decision making was developed by Victor Vroom (1973) and extended by Vroom and Yetton (1973), and subsequently revised by Vroom and Jago (1988). In this classic model, the approach managers take to involving other participants in decision making is shown to affect the resulting decisions in two important ways. First, it affects the *quality* of the decisions made. Second, it affects the level of *acceptance* of the decisions by those who must implement or those who will be affected by them.

As originally developed, Vroom's (1973) model features a flowchart of the various alternatives in a decision-making situation and a set of questions to guide users. The model assumes that managers can take any of five different approaches to including other participants in decision making. The approaches are defined and labeled as follows:

- Two types of *autocratic* decision-making approaches (AI and AII),

- Two types of *consultative* decision-making approaches (CI and CII),

- One approach that represents joint decision making by managers and other participants as a *group* (GII). (There is a GI approach, but it is not relevant to this discussion.)

Each of these five decision-making approaches is briefly described as follows:

AI   Managers make decisions alone, using information available to them at the time.

AII   Managers obtain the necessary information from other participants, and then decide themselves. Other participants merely provide managers with information, and play no part in generating or assessing alternatives in the decision-making process.

CI   Managers share information about the problem or opportunity requiring a decision with other relevant participants individually, obtaining their ideas and suggestions, but without bringing them together as a group. Then managers make the decision, which may or may not reflect the influence of the other participants.

CII   Managers share information about the problem or opportunity requiring a decision with other relevant participants as a group, obtaining their collective ideas and suggestions. Managers then make the decision, which may or may not reflect the influence of the other participants.

GII   Managers share the information about the problem or opportunity requiring a decision with other relevant participants as a group. In the GII approach, managers and the other participants involved generate and assess alternatives and attempt to reach agreement (consensus) on an alternative. The manager's role in this approach is much like that of the chairperson of a committee. Managers do not try to influence the group to adopt their preferred alternative, and they are willing to accept and implement solutions that the group prefers.

Figure 5.1 shows Vroom's decision model, which a manager can work through from left to right by answering seven questions to conclude which of the five decision-making approaches (AI, AII, CI, CII, or GII) is most appropriate in a given situation. The questions, which correspond to the letters *A* through *G*, are shown across the top of the model.

The Vroom decision model has practical value for managers because it demonstrates that they can effectively vary their approach to involving other participants in decision making to fit attributes of particular situations. When managers do seek the involvement of other participants in decision making, they can facilitate participation in several ways (Yukl 2012):

- Encouraging participants to express their ideas about alternatives in a decision-making situation and to express their concerns about other ideas being suggested

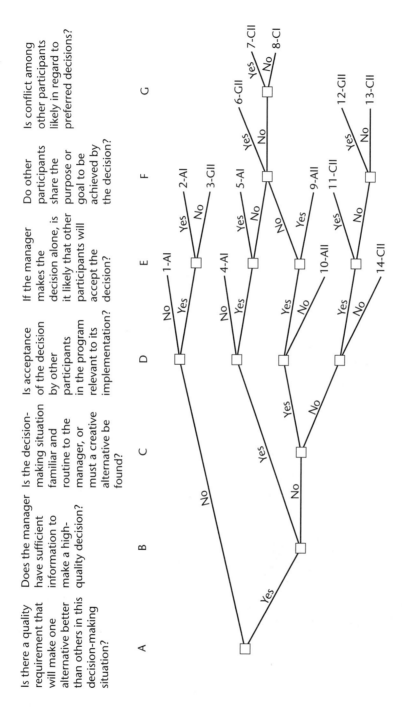

A. Is there a quality requirement that will make one alternative better than others in this decision-making situation?

B. Does the manager have sufficient information to make a high-quality decision?

C. Is the decision-making situation familiar and routine to the manager, or must a creative alternative be found?

D. Is acceptance of the decision by other participants in the program relevant to its implementation?

E. If the manager makes the decision alone, is it likely that other participants will accept the decision?

F. Do other participants share the purpose or goal to be achieved by the decision?

G. Is conflict among other participants likely in regard to preferred decisions?

By answering the questions in the sequence A through G, the manager reaches endpoints 1 through 14, each representing an autocratic, consultative, or group approach to decision making of the form AI, AII, CI, CII, or GII that is appropriate to a particular decision-making situation.

Figure 5.1 Vroom's Decision Model

Source: Adapted from Vroom, Victor. "A New Look at Managerial Decision Making." *Organizational Dynamics* 1, no. 4 (1973): 66–80. Adapted with permission from Elsevier.

- Describing alternatives as tentative and encouraging participants to try to improve them

- Recording ideas and suggestions as a way of demonstrating that they are important and not to be ignored

- Looking for ways to build on participants' ideas and suggestions by focusing on their positive attributes rather than on their negative attributes

- Being tactful in expressing concerns about ideas and suggestions and encouraging other participants to be tactful in how they express their concerns

- Listening to dissenting views or criticisms without getting defensive

- Actively seeking to use ideas and suggestions and to address concerns being expressed

- Demonstrating appreciation for the ideas and suggestions of other participants, especially giving credit to those who generate useful ideas and suggestions and explaining why other ideas and suggestions are not included in the decision

Even when managers correctly determine the appropriate degree of involvement in decision making by other participants in a program, many other variables affect the decision-making process. For example, some decisions made by managers must be based on imperfect information about available alternatives and their consequences and implications. Further, making decisions frequently involves risk, uncertainty, and conflict. These characteristics of management decisions and decision making, as described more fully in the next section, complicate the decision-making process, rendering it one of managers' most challenging activities.

Key Characteristics of Management Decisions and Decision Making in Programs

One of the most challenging characteristics of decision making for managers is that it often cannot be done in a completely rational manner. The underlying assumptions necessary for making completely rational decisions would require decision makers to know all the alternatives available in a given situation as well as all of the consequences of selecting each alternative, and would require that decision makers always act rationally so as to maximize a desired value, such as revenue or participant satisfaction, or minimize an undesired value, such as cost.

Because it usually is not possible to meet all of the assumptions required for complete rationality, managers make decisions using a more limited form of rationality, called bounded rationality (Simon 1982). Professor Herbert Simon won a Nobel Prize in Economics for this conceptualization of how managers make decisions.

The assumptions of bounded rationality are (1) that managers rarely have enough information and knowledge to maximize or minimize any result of their decision making; (2) that they face vaguely defined problems or opportunities about which decisions are to be made; and (3) that they have human limitations in regard to memory, reasoning power, and objectivity. These bounds on rationality mean that managers are forced to "satisfice," a word created by Simon (1956, 129) from the words *satisfy* and *suffice.* That is, in their decision making, managers typically choose alternatives that appear adequate and acceptable, rather than those that will completely maximize or minimize some result of their decision making (Liebler and McConnell 2012). The satisficer considers possible alternatives until a satisfactory one is found. Satisficing is a fact of life in making management decisions.

Another characteristic of decision making by managers in programs is that decisions must often be made under conditions of uncertainty. Just as managers are forced to rely on bounded rationality and are not able to make perfectly rational decisions, so too must they typically make their decisions under conditions of uncertainty. This means that in making decisions, managers must accept some degree of risk. Risk exists because managers cannot know with certainty the probability that their decisions will lead to positive results.

Under conditions of certainty, a manager would fully understand the problem to be solved or opportunity requiring a decision, would know all of the available alternative choices, and would be able to predict accurately the results of selecting each alternative. Uncertainty can be reduced by acquiring more information, but in complex decision-making situations it cannot be completely removed. Sometimes managers are required to make intuitive decisions that are based on nothing more than instincts, feelings, and personal experience with similar situations. In contrast to decisions that are guided by large amounts of relevant information, intuitive decisions tend to involve a high degree of uncertainty and risk.

Another important characteristic of management decisions is that they are often influenced by significant conflicting demands and expectations. The appropriate decision, from the standpoint of what contributes most to achieving the desired results established for a program, might have painful consequences for some participants—for example, a decision to downsize a program or to merge a project into a larger set of projects. Most managers faced with decisions like these experience significant internal conflict.

In addition to creating personal conflict for the decision maker, many decisions generate conflict between individuals or between groups within a program or even within the program's larger organizational home. A decision to emphasize one of a program's services automatically deemphasizes others. A decision to allocate space to one group involved in a project automatically means that others cannot use that space.

Finally, as noted earlier, management decisions are also characterized by the fact that they can be programmed or nonprogrammed. Nonprogrammed decisions are made when problems or opportunities demand decisions but there are no existing models or formulae to call on for guidance. This is in contrast to programmed decisions, for which previously made decisions, operating policies, or standard practices provide guidance. For example, the amount of money paid to a new employee is programmed by human resource policies that dictate pay ranges and by salaries paid to others with similar qualifications occupying similar positions. Nonprogrammed decisions are usually more difficult to make than programmed decisions. Managers, however, must make both types of decisions.

The Decision-Making Process

Although decision making was defined earlier as making a choice from among alternatives, the full *decision-making process* includes several sequential steps that precede the actual choice. Once the choice is made, the process includes additional steps to implement and evaluate the decision. In reality, managers rarely go through all the steps in sequence. Frequently, under constant pressure to make decisions, managers skip or combine steps. As Figure 5.2 and the following subsections illustrate, however, decision makers can go through a process that comprises seven separate steps and a feedback loop.

Becoming Aware That a Problem or Opportunity Exists

Effective decision makers must be sensitive to situations that represent problems or opportunities for a program. This sensitivity, termed perceptual skill, enables managers to collect and interpret cues from their surroundings. The initial step in the decision-making process is being aware that problems or opportunities requiring decisions exist. Managers with limited perceptual skill may remain oblivious to potential problems until the problems blossom into full-blown crises, or until they discover too

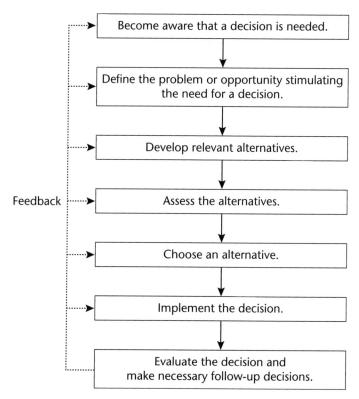

Figure 5.2   The Decision-Making Process

late that they did not seize a potential opportunity. It is difficult to gain perceptual skill except through experience. The development of such skill is one of the reasons why managers usually become more effective with experience.

One way for managers to increase their awareness of instances in which problem-solving and opportunistic decisions are called for is to acknowledge their ubiquity. Many decisions are required simply to respond to the performance gaps in programs that managers routinely identify in their efforts to determine whether ongoing performance is acceptable and whether appropriate progress is being made toward achievement of a program's mission and objectives. Remember from the discussion in Chapter 2 that a key part of a manager's developing/strategizing activity is an ongoing assessment of performance and progress. The discussion of program evaluation in Chapter 9 is also highly relevant to this topic. Managers must make adjustments and corrections if they detect inadequacies. All such changes require decisions.

In addition to the decisions managers must make in the interest of closing ongoing performance gaps in a program, other decisions are imposed on them from outside their domain of responsibility. In some instances, pressure comes from inside the organizational home of the program. For example, a decision to merge one hospital with another, when both operate hospice programs, will necessitate many decisions in both programs, such as decisions about who will manage the merged program or where it will be physically located.

The changes that continuously occur in the dynamic external environments in which most health programs exist force decisions within those programs. For example, a growing, declining, or aging population in the community served by a health program, as well as the plans and actions of competitors, have significant implications for the program. Such environmental changes trigger numerous decisions by the affected program as its manager seeks to adapt and adjust the program to fit the new environmental conditions.

Changes in public policies and regulations that apply to a program, such as changes in Medicare or Medicaid reimbursement policies, frequently necessitate decision making. Similarly, National Labor Relations Board rulings can instantly change how programs relate to unionized employees, again requiring decisions. Because health programs are so often dependent on particular technologies, advances in these technologies also stimulate change. For example, telemedicine programs have evolved concurrent with changes in the technologies on which they are based, with each step in the evolution requiring decisions about how programs will adjust to new technologies.

Perceptive managers in complex and dynamic environments should be aware of the constant need both to solve problems and to make opportunistic decisions. Knowing that decisions are needed and knowing how to precisely define the problem or opportunity at hand, however, are two different things. This leads to the second step in the decision-making process described in Figure 5.2.

Defining the Problem or Opportunity

Defining the real problem or opportunity in a given situation is not always a clear-cut task. What appears to be the problem may only be a symptom. For example, an apparent problem of conflicting personalities when two participants in a program cannot work together well might in fact be only a symptom of such real problems as poorly coordinated work, conflicting schedules, inadequate training, or ill-defined work expectations. Few things are more frustrating in decision making than finding the right solution to the wrong problem—except perhaps the effort wasted in responding to a perceived opportunity that does not really exist.

A simple but effective way to move past the symptom to get at the underlying problem or opportunity is to ask, Why? Answers to this question can be used to trace back from symptoms to underlying root causes, and thus to real problems (Andersen, Fagerhaug, and Beltz 2012). Similarly, the answer to a question about why some event, trend, or situation appears to be an opportunity for a program can also lead to a clearer delineation of the opportunity. Two useful tools available to managers to help with defining problems and opportunities are described in the next subsections.

Cause-and-Effect (Fishbone) Diagram

A device useful in getting to the root cause or causes of a problem is a cause-and-effect diagram, or, as it is frequently called because of its shape, a fishbone diagram. Figure 5.3 is a *fishbone diagram* drawn by the manager of a specialized surgical program embedded in an acute care hospital. The problem of concern to this manager is a higher-than-expected rate of nosocomial pneumonia among patients in the program. In the diagram, pneumonia is the effect, and as the diagram shows, this effect has many possible causes. The manager is interested in what is causing pneumonia, because the underlying root cause or causes of the high rate of nosocomial pneumonia must be addressed through decisions and subsequent actions.

In using a fishbone, or cause-and-effect, diagram to organize ideas about what might be causing the nosocomial pneumonia among the program's patients, the manager begins by identifying categories of possible causes. Common causes of nosocomial infections have to do with equipment, interventions or procedures, participants, and patients. The manager organizes the diagram around these potential categories of causes, which form the larger bones in the diagram. Within each category, specific ideas about the causes are developed, and are shown as the smaller bones in the diagram. The diagram does not identify the causes, but it organizes the manager's thinking, and perhaps the ideas of other participants involved in making this determination about the possible causes of the high rate of nosocomial pneumonia. More information will be needed to determine the causes of the nosocomial pneumonia, but identifying the possible causes is the first step in determining causation.

Pareto Chart

Another tool useful for this manager in determining and addressing the causes of the pneumonia is a *Pareto chart,* which is a bar graph showing the relative importance of several causes of a problem. Charts or graphs of this

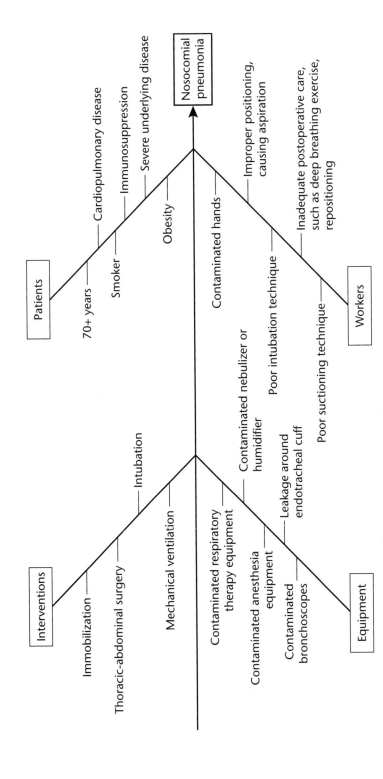

Figure 5.3 Fishbone Diagram of Possible Causes of Nosocomial Pneumonia

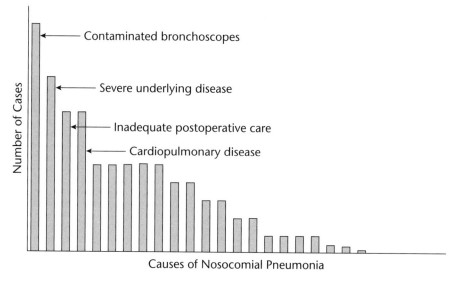

Figure 5.4   Pareto Chart of Causes of Nosocomial Pneumonia

nature can help managers determine where to focus their attention. Figure 5.4 is a Pareto chart showing the relative importance of the several causes of nosocomial pneumonia identified by the manager in this example; it directs the manager's attention to the most important causes that require decisions.

As can be seen in the Pareto chart, the largest number of cases of nosocomial pneumonia in the analysis resulted from contaminated bronchoscopes. The next largest number of cases resulted from severe underlying disease in patients. Inadequate postoperative care and cardiopulmonary disease are tied for the third-largest number of cases. Based on the information assembled in the Pareto chart, the manager will focus initial efforts to address the problem on contaminated bronchoscopes and inadequate postoperative care, variables concerning which the manager can intervene. Unless the program's patient mix changes, the manager cannot do anything about the fact that some patients have severe underlying disease or have cardiopulmonary disease.

To completely diagnose problems or define opportunities, decision makers analyze a great deal of information. Judgment is required to determine what information should be used in decision making, and decision makers must endeavor to be as comprehensive, fair, and objective as possible in gathering and examining information. The most difficult pieces of information to deal with are often intangible factors, which can play a significant role in defining problems and opportunities. Intangible factors include such things as reputation, morale, satisfaction, and personal biases. It is difficult to be as specific about these subjective factors as one can be about those more readily subject to physical measurement. Nevertheless, such information must be considered in fully defining problems or opportunities, which is an important step in the decision-making process.

No matter which tools a manager might use, defining problems or opportunities is much easier when they fall within the scope of the manager's experience. Problems and opportunities that look familiar are easier to diagnose and understand. Experience sharpens a manager's ability to define and specify problems or opportunities, just as it allows him or her to hone perceptual skill, as noted previously.

The degree of success in the definition step of the decision-making process is almost always directly proportional to the amount and quality of relevant information gathered and analyzed in relation to a problem or opportunity. Of course, good judgment is required in determining whether enough information is in hand to make an accurate diagnosis of that problem or opportunity. In general, more information is better, but some decision makers paralyze themselves by continuing to gather information about a problem or opportunity long after they should have moved on to the next step in the decision-making process.

Developing Relevant Alternatives

Once problems or opportunities that require decisions are fully diagnosed and understood, decision makers can search for and develop alternatives for consideration. One simple rule should guide decision makers in this step: the greater the number of alternatives considered, the greater the likelihood of eventually selecting a satisfactory alternative. Alternatives can be categorized as ready made or custom made.

Ready-made alternatives are based on approaches or solutions that decision makers have tried before, or on recommendations of others who have faced similar problems or opportunities. Custom-made alternatives are designed specifically for a particular decision-making situation. Developing them generally involves greater expenditure of time and effort, and thus they are less likely to be considered than the familiar, ready-made alternatives.

In considering alternatives, decision makers should not think in terms of one best alternative. Most problems have several solutions with both positive and negative characteristics, and for many opportunities there is a continuum of responses that would be appropriate. The task in developing relevant alternatives is to develop as many potentially satisfactory alternatives as is reasonably possible.

It is during this step in the decision-making process that creative and innovative alternatives can be developed, if decision makers are not inappropriately wedded to the idea of considering only ready-made alternatives. Essentially, creativity is the art and science of making new things or generating new ideas. Some decision makers focus on ready-made alternatives because they doubt their own ability to develop truly creative, custom-made alternatives.

Logic and experience play important roles in idea generation, as does imagination. The use of imagination and creative thinking in this step of the process is important in establishing the fullest possible set of relevant alternatives. Creative thinking is "a way of looking at problems or situations from a fresh perspective that suggests unorthodox solutions" (BusinessDictionary 2014a). It is useful to remember that creativity is latent within all people. Ordinary people working in an atmosphere of freedom, trust, and security can create new alternatives to address both problems and opportunities. It is therefore important for managers to encourage and foster the creative process, which is described next.

The Creative Process

Embedded within the decision-making process, the *creative process* itself can be viewed as a series of interconnected steps, including: (1) feeling a personal need to be creative, (2) preparing by acquiring information, (3) incubating both the problem or opportunity and possible alternatives by considering them as fully as possible, and (4) verifying by making certain the problem or opportunity is understood and that appropriate alternatives have been identified and reviewed. The concept of a personal need to think creatively emphasizes that a motivating force must initiate the creative process. Such motivation can come in the form of a serious problem or a rich opportunity.

Creative, custom-made alternatives usually emerge after a period of intensive preparation during which the decision maker becomes saturated with information and makes a concerted effort to perceive new and meaningful relationships among the factors at hand. To a large extent, the originality of ideas depends on the number of avenues the decision maker explores and the extent to which he or she considers all possibilities. The preparation step represents much of the work of engaging in the creative process.

It is certainly possible for an original alternative to be developed quickly as the result of a brief period of analysis. Sometimes this is necessary when a decision, for which there is no ready-made alternative, is urgently required.

For example, a manager whose program faces termination may have to respond quickly and creatively if the program is to be preserved. When circumstances permit, however, a period of incubation that allows the decision maker to mull over the problem or opportunity and possible alternatives is valuable.

The value of an incubation period lies in the fact that a more fully developed idea for a custom-made alternative may result. It is useful to set a deadline for the incubation period so that problems do not go unsolved for unduly long periods, and so that opportunities do not pass by while the decision maker mulls over various alternatives. But some period of incubation tends to be necessary if original alternatives are to be developed.

The final step in the creative process is verification. When the decision maker first envisions a custom-made alternative, it is rarely in a polished and final form. The verification step in the creative process is a period of refining an idea, changing it, and improving it. In effect, this step often represents the difference between an interesting idea and a truly innovative and creative alternative.

Sometimes the creative process is facilitated by having a group of program participants work on the development of relevant alternatives in a decision-making situation. Groups of people usually bring more experience and information, and therefore more ideas for alternatives, to the task than do individuals acting alone. A group, through its interactions, can stimulate each individual group member's creative abilities as well. Brainstorming is a standard method by which groups develop alternatives (Miller 2012). In a brainstorming session, participants are asked to produce ideas (without fear of censorship or control by the group) through free association of their ideas and those of others. In this way, one idea can stimulate a chain reaction of additional ideas.

Another approach to having a group establish alternatives is the nominal group technique, in which participants are asked to generate possible alternatives independently (that is, without group interaction), and then to have the ideas reviewed and prioritized by the group (Levi 2014). Unlike with the free association of brainstorming, ideas are discussed within the group only after those ideas have been independently developed and then presented by each participant. Following a round of discussion, during which initial ideas can be reworked, each participant privately rates the alternatives from first to last. The tabulated ranking of the group's alternatives are then openly discussed again, after which point there is a final, private ranking. The tabulated results of this vote are considered the nominal group's prioritized list of the alternatives. Both brainstorming and nominal groups generate a set of alternatives, which must then be assessed by the decision maker before one is chosen.

Stimulating and Supporting Creativity in Decision Making

Managers who want a program to benefit from the development of creative and innovative alternatives in decision making must stimulate and support creativity and innovative thinking. These characteristics can be fostered among participants by managers who make it a specific and important aspect of managing a program, and who establish and maintain a culture in which creativity and innovation are valued. Managers can also facilitate these characteristics by placing a high priority on creativity in making at least some of their staffing decisions. Workplace climates in which creativity and innovation are stimulated and facilitated share a number of characteristics (Robbins and Coulter 2013):

- Risk-taking is tolerated, even encouraged. Participants are pushed to take risks, and mistakes are treated as learning opportunities.

- Rules, procedures, policies, and similar formally imposed controls are kept to a minimum.

- Cross-training and participation in diverse and multiple teams and groups are encouraged. Managers recognize that narrowly defined jobs create myopia, whereas diverse job activities and experiences give participants a broader perspective.

- Tolerance for ambiguity is widespread in the program. Participants are given opportunities to express their respective identities through work as individuals and as members of teams and groups.

- A healthy degree of conflict is permitted. Differences in opinions about how to do things are recognized as a means of increasing creativity. Harmony and agreement between individuals and teams and groups is not seen as necessary for good performance.

- There is a high degree of tolerance for the impractical. Participants who offer improbable or even foolish answers to "what if" questions are not penalized or ridiculed. There is recognition of and appreciation for the fact that what seems impractical at first might turn out to be a great alternative in a decision-making situation.

- The focus is on the ends more than on the means. If participants are encouraged to consider alternative routes toward the accomplishment of the program's mission and objectives, innovation may result.

- Communication flows freely. Communication flows horizontally as well as vertically and diagonally, facilitating the cross-fertilization of ideas.

There are also certain characteristics and behaviors that managers who wish to stimulate creativity and innovation should avoid, minimize, or change. Managers often reduce the chance of developing innovations and creative ideas when they are isolated from the other participants in a program, when they focus on short-term performance, and when they maintain an incentive and reward system that does not support innovation.

Assessing the Alternatives

Managers who successfully rely on their own insights and experiences, the insights and experiences of others, and the creative processes available to them will develop a robust set of alternatives to consider—and each alternative must be assessed against the others (see Figure 5.2).

In this step in the decision-making process, quantitative models can be very helpful in structuring a careful assessment of the alternatives. Five useful quantitative techniques that are widely used in decision making are described in the paragraphs that follow: decision grids, payoff tables, decision trees, cost-benefit analysis, and the program evaluation and review technique. In addition, the use of decision support systems, which combine many decision-making models with a database to support decision making, is discussed. Many other quantitative decision-making techniques and tools for managers exist, but these are outside the scope of this book (see, for example, Anderson et al. 2012; Ozcan 2009).

Decision Grids

The most basic and in many ways the most useful decision-making tool is the *decision grid.* This is nothing more than a display of the possible alternatives in making a decision, along with the various elements that will affect the decision. Figure 5.5 illustrates a decision grid involving a program's decision to open and operate a satellite clinic. The four alternatives are listed in the first column, with the elements affecting the decision forming the rest of the grid. The grid's main advantage is that a large amount of pertinent information can be displayed in a convenient and understandable manner. This becomes especially important in making complex decisions and when multiple program participants are involved in the decision making and need to discuss and consider various alternatives.

Alternatives	Patients/ Customer's Preferences	Program Participants' Preferences	Financial Impact	Relative Feasibility	Decision
1. Maintain the status quo	Unacceptable	Mixed	Negative	Feasible, but undesirable	Not recommended
2. Purchase a new site for the clinic	Acceptable	Mixed	Positive over a 5-year period	Feasible, but expensive	Not recommended
3. Lease a new site for the clinic	Acceptable	Mixed	Positive in 2 to 3 years	Readily feasible	2nd priority
4. Enter into an agreement to use a community-based organization's existing facilities for the clinic, rent-free for 10 years	Highly acceptable	Mixed	Positive within the first year of operation	High feasible	1st priority

Figure 5.5   Decision Grid for the Possible Addition of a Satellite Clinic in a Program

The preferences of the program's participants are mixed for all alternatives, thus neutralizing the impact of this factor. Patients/customers have a preference for the fourth alternative, although they find any alternative acceptable except maintaining the status quo. The key factor in this decision is the financial impact of the alternative selected. The fourth alternative is the most attractive because the financial impact is positive and almost immediate, and none of the other factors in the decision preclude selecting this alternative.

Payoff Tables

If probabilities can be determined for the various possible outcomes of each alternative being assessed in a decision-making situation, a *payoff table* can be created. For example, suppose the manager of a clinical program must decide how many disposable syringes should be ordered and stocked each week.

Based on past usage patterns, the manager determines that there is an 80 percent probability that 800 syringes will be needed per week, and a 20 percent probability that 1,000 syringes will be needed per week. The manager can also assign costs to each of these two alternatives. In this case, storage space is allocated at $10 per 1,000 syringes. In addition, if too few syringes are ordered and stocked, an extra cost of $20 will result

Events and Results

Alternatives	800 syringes needed (0.8)	1,000 syringes needed (0.2)
800 syringes stocked	1 $8.00	2 $28.00
1,000 syringes stocked	3 $10.00	4 $10.00

Figure 5.6 Payoff Table for Ordering Syringes

for special ordering and messenger pickup. Figure 5.6 illustrates the two alternatives (1,000 and 800 syringes) and the costs associated with each of the two outcomes.

For the first alternative, if 800 syringes are stocked and the usage during the week is 800, the costs will be $8 (see cell 1). If 800 syringes are stocked and 1,000 are needed that week, the costs will be $28 ($8 for storage and $20 for the special order [see cell 2]). For the second alternative, if 1,000 syringes are stocked and the usage during the week is 800, the costs will be $10 (see cell 3). Also, if 1,000 syringes are ordered and stocked and 1,000 are used, the costs will be $10.

If the clinic manager orders and stocks 800 syringes, then 80 percent of the time this decision will be correct, and only an $8 storage cost will be incurred; 20 percent of the time there will not be enough, and the $28 storage and reorder costs will be incurred. The expected cost can be determined for each alternative as follows:

Expected cost if 800 syringes are ordered: $8(0.8) + $28(0.2) = $12

Expected cost if 1,000 syringes are ordered: $10(0.8) + $10(0.2) = $10

Thus, to minimize cost, 1,000 syringes should be ordered and stocked, although this number will be needed only 20 percent of the time.

Although the savings is modest, if the technique is applied to many items, the cumulative savings could be quite substantial. The basic difficulty in using this technique is in determining probabilities. When possible, the preferred procedure is to use historical data or experimental samples so that the probabilities have a clear basis in fact. Where this is not possible, a best estimate may have to suffice.

Decision Trees

Decision grids and payoff tables are useful tools in assessing alternatives in a decision-making situation, although both suffer from a common limitation. In reality, decisions are seldom one-time occurrences. They are more often linked to other decisions in the sense that one decision tends to necessitate other decisions. A **decision tree** is quite helpful in assessing alternatives when decisions that must be made are linked together over time, each with various possible outcomes. It is especially useful when probabilities can be determined for the possible outcomes.

To illustrate this technique, suppose the manager in a program determines that there is a 60 percent probability that demand for a certain procedure will increase by 20 percent next year, and that there is a 40 percent probability that demand for the procedure will decrease by 10 percent. The decision is whether to buy a piece of automated equipment (at a cost of $50,000) or to pay existing employees overtime wages to do the increased work, should that be necessary. (The manager determined that it would cost less to pay overtime than to hire an additional worker.)

Because of the vital nature of the procedure, simply deciding not to do the increased work is not acceptable. Figure 5.7 illustrates a decision tree based on this decision-making situation. The decision tree assumes that quality is not an issue because it will be the same whether the procedure is done manually or on the automated equipment. The decision therefore hinges on making the wisest expenditure of money by choosing the lower-cost alternative.

Assume that revenue from this procedure is currently $100,000 per year. If the 60 percent probability of a 20 percent increase holds up, the revenue for the next year (and future years if everything stays the same) will increase to $120,000; if the 40 percent probability of a decrease in demand of 10 percent holds, then revenue will decrease to $90,000 in both cases (see column 3 of the figure).

The cost of the machine (with installation and the first year's operation included) is $50,000; the cost of overtime wages is figured at $10,000 if the increased work has to be done, and at $0 if it does not (see column 4). Net cash flow can be determined in all events by subtracting cost from revenue (see column 5). The expected value at the end of the first year can be obtained in all events by multiplying net cash flow (column 5) by the probability of the event. A 60 percent chance of increase times $70,000

(1) Alternative Actions	(2) Possible Events	(3) Revenue from Procedures	(4) 1st-Year Costs	(5) Net Cash Flow	(6) 1st-Year Expected Value	(7) 2nd-Year Costs	(8) Net Cash Flow	(9) 2nd-Year Expected Value
Automate	Increased demand (0.6)	$120,000	$50,000	$70,000	$42,000	$2,000	$118,000	$70,800
	Decreased demand (0.4)	$90,000	$50,000	$40,000	$16,000 / $58,000	$1,500	$88,500	$35,400 / $106,200
Pay overtime	Increased demand (0.6)	$120,000	$10,000	$110,000	$66,000	$10,000	$110,000	$66,000
	Decreased demand (0.4)	$90,000	-0-	$90,000	$36,000 / $102,000	-0-	$90,000	$36,000 / $102,000

Decision point

Figure 5.7 Decision Tree for Automation or Overtime Pay

equals an expected value of $42,000 (see column 6). At the end of the first year the expected value of automation is $58,000 ($42,000 + $16,000), and the expected value of paying overtime is $102,000 ($66,000 + $36,000). At that point in time the lower-cost alternative clearly would be to forego the machine and pay overtime. If the decision is projected out over additional years, however, this may not be the lower-cost decision.

At the end of the second year (see column 9), the expected value of the choice to automate is greater. Although the initial $50,000 outlay must still be overcome, it will not take many years to do this. By extending the computation, the number of years it would take to overcome the initial outlay could be determined, and when compared to the expected useful life of the machine, this information could form the basis of a complete assessment of the alternatives in this decision-making situation.

Cost-Benefit Analysis

A manager deciding among alternative additions to the service mix provided in a program will be interested in how the alternatives compare in terms of financial impact. A useful way to make relative comparisons of multiple alternatives is to calculate the cost-benefit ratio (Z) of each alternative. Although these ratios should only be one factor in a decision, comparing them can nevertheless assist the decision maker. Z is defined as the ratio of the present value of the benefits of an alternative to the present value of the alternative's costs:

$$Z = \frac{\text{Present value of benefits}}{\text{Present value of costs}}$$

It is usually relatively easy to determine the financial costs of an alternative. In health programs, however, the financial value of benefits is often much more difficult to determine. What is the value of a human life? What is the value of improved health? Is it better to spend money on making older people more comfortable in their declining years, or to spend the money on improving infant mortality rates? When such questions are at issue, this technique has limited use.

There are, however, many decision-making situations in which the costs and benefits of various alternatives can be determined rather straightfor-wardly. In such cases, *cost-benefit analysis* is a useful tool for assessing alternatives. For example, a manager might find a cost-benefit comparison very useful in assessing a choice between two competing models of a particular piece of imaging equipment.

Model A costs $80,000 (installed) and requires a person to operate it at an annual cost of $64,000, plus $12,000 in other operating costs. The total cost for a year is $156,000. Model A will produce revenues of $185,000 per year because of its rate of operation.

Model B of this equipment will have a total cost of $175,000, but will permit revenues of $205,000 because of its superior rate of operation. Which is the better alternative, assuming that they both produce equal-quality results and have the same useful life expectancy and salvage value?

$$\text{Model A} : Z = \frac{\$185,000}{\$156,000} = 1.186$$

$$\text{Model B} : Z = \frac{\$205,000}{\$175,000} = 1.171$$

All other factors being equal, the cost-benefit ratio here argues that the better alternative in this situation is to purchase Model A because of its better Z value. This analysis is limited to one year. The manager should make additional calculations for future years based on operating costs and expected revenues from each model to decide which is the better alternative over the life of each piece of equipment.

Program Evaluation and Review Technique

In some operational planning situations, the assessment of alternatives involves considering the timing of activities or the best sequence for a series of actions. In such situations the *program evaluation and review technique (PERT)* can be very useful. PERT is the title given to this technique by its developers (Fazar 1959). The basic concept used in this technique, which was created to guide development of the U.S. Navy's Polaris submarine, is the network, or flow plan (Kerzner 2013). The network is composed of a series of related events and activities. Events are defined as sequential, required accomplishment points in a program, a project, or some other complex undertaking. Activities are defined as the time-consuming elements of a program, project, or undertaking that connect the various events.

For example, suppose a hospital initiates a project to establish an open-heart surgery program. A number of events and activities will have to take place, including renovation of an existing operating room, installation of new equipment, hiring and training of an open-heart surgery team, and many others. As with other situations in which many events and activities are involved, PERT can be used here. One alternative in this project is to do everything in a single sequence. For example, the hospital can begin by renovating the operating room, then purchase and install equipment, and then hire and train the team. The flaw in this approach is that the events and activities will be strung out for an unnecessarily long time, thus delaying the project. PERT can eliminate this flaw by giving the manager of this project a better way to time and integrate events and activities in the sequence.

Figure 5.8 shows a PERT network for the development of an open-heart surgery program. Events are shown as boxes in the network, and arrows connecting the events represent activities. This example illustrates the three basic characteristics of a situation that make it amenable to using PERT. First, it must be possible to estimate how long it will take to accomplish each activity. Second, there must be definite starting and ending points for each activity. Without them, there can be no events, which are the beginnings or endings of activities. Finally, and this is the key to PERT's usefulness, there must be parallel activities. That is, several activities must be taking place simultaneously for PERT to be of any real use to a manager. The technique relies on finding the critical path, which is the longest path through the sequence of events to completion. This path is shown as a dashed line in the figure.

To make the network usable, the times between the various events (activity times) must be computed. Usually, these can only be estimates, and the standard approach involves coming up with three different time estimates for each activity. Experience with the timing of similar activities is often used in developing the time estimates. The first is an optimistic time estimate, representing the time if everything goes smoothly in completing the activity. The second is the most likely time estimate and represents the most accurate forecast based on normal or typical circumstances. If only one estimate were given, this would be it. The third is a pessimistic time estimate and is based on maximum potential difficulties. The assumption here is that whatever can go wrong will go wrong.

The pessimistic, most likely, and optimistic time estimates for developing the open-heart surgery program can be used to form a beta curve or probability distribution as illustrated in Figure 5.9. This probability distribution assumes that the most likely time estimate is four times more likely to occur than either the optimistic or the pessimistic time estimate.

Based on the probability distribution of the three time estimates involved in performing an activity, a formula can be used to calculate the estimated activity time to use in the PERT network as follows:

$$\text{Activity time} = \frac{O + 4M + P}{6}$$

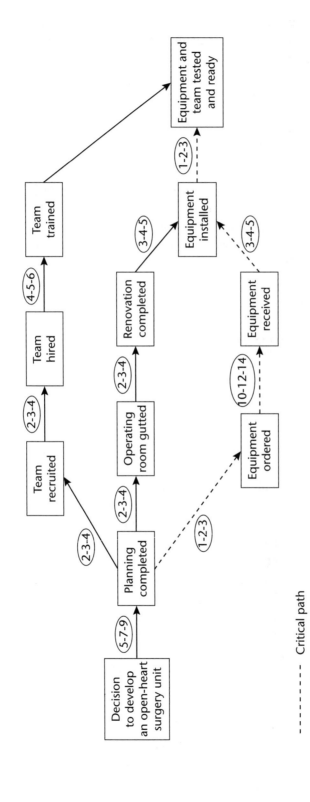

Figure 5.8 PERT Network for the Development of an Open-Heart Surgery Program

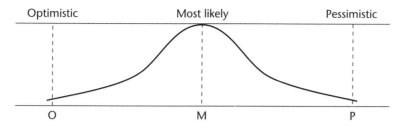

Figure 5.9   Beta Curve for Optimistic, Most Likely, and Pessimistic Time Estimates for Activities in Developing the Open-Heart Surgery Program

where O is the optimistic time estimate, M is the most likely time estimate, and P is the pessimistic time estimate.

Referring to Figure 5.8, it can be seen that the time estimates between the first two events, which are based on the manager's experience with the timing of similar activities, have been made as follows: $O = 5$ weeks, $M = 7$ weeks, and $P = 9$ weeks. The estimated activity time would then be

$$\text{Activity time} = \frac{5 + 4(7) + 9}{6} = 7 \text{ weeks}$$

Using the resulting value, one can be reasonably certain that the activity time between the first two events will be 7 weeks. The process of calculating estimated activity times must be completed for all activities in the network.

The next step in using PERT to help evaluate timing and sequencing of activities and events is to determine the critical path through the network. Among the several pathways of events and activities, the critical path (again, shown as the dashed line in Figure 5.8) is the one that takes the longest to complete. Inasmuch as the critical path takes the longest time to complete, it determines the completion time for developing this open-heart surgery program. Other activities and events that do not lie along the critical path are less important in terms of their timing because their completion will not shorten or lengthen the total completion time.

The time differential between the amount of time scheduled to complete these noncritical events and the amount of time that would actually alter the critical path through the project is the project's slack time. Slack time provides an opportunity for the manager to reassess whether certain resources should be transferred to activities along the critical path as a means of shortening the critical path and therefore the completion time for developing the open-heart surgery program. In the example represented in Figure 5.8, it would do no good to speed up recruitment, hiring, or training of the team or the renovation of the operating room in an effort to shorten the completion time. The only way to accomplish this is to shorten the time needed for equipment delivery and installation, because these activities form the critical path in this project.

PERT, and even more sophisticated time management and scheduling techniques (Project Management Institute 2013), can be used to great advantage by managers in making timing and sequencing decisions in many building or remodeling projects, in adding new equipment, in physically moving a unit, in preparing budgets, and in developing policy manuals or patient care protocols.

Managers may be supported in applying tools and techniques such as PERT by a formal planning department and professional planners in the larger organization in which a program is embedded. Most large health services organizations employ people with such expertise in their planning, marketing, government affairs, and finance departments—and perhaps in other departments as well. In addition, consultants can help managers assess alternatives.

Decision Support Systems

The intensified pressure to make good management decisions in health programs, combined with improved technology specifically designed to support the management decision-making process, may cause managers to consider using a ***decision support system (DSS).*** Such a system uses computer-based technology to provide decision makers with information that permits them to make better decisions (Burstein and Holsapple 2008; Glandon, Slovensky, and Smaltz 2013; Schuff et al. 2011). In essence, decision support systems incorporate data and models for analyzing this data to support decision makers in assessing their alternatives (Holsapple and Joshi 2001). They turn raw data into information. You should recall from the discussion in Chapter 2 that information is raw data that is "(1) accurate and timely, (2) specific and organized for a purpose, (3) presented within a context that gives it meaning and relevance, and (4) [possibly leading] to an increase in understanding and decrease in uncertainty" (BusinessDictionary 2014b).

A DSS can be constructed in various ways, although effective systems share the following characteristics:

• Interacting with the DSS is easy.

• Retrieving and displaying data are supported by the system.

• Modeling capabilities are built into the system.

• The system can produce clear and usable reports of the results of analyses.

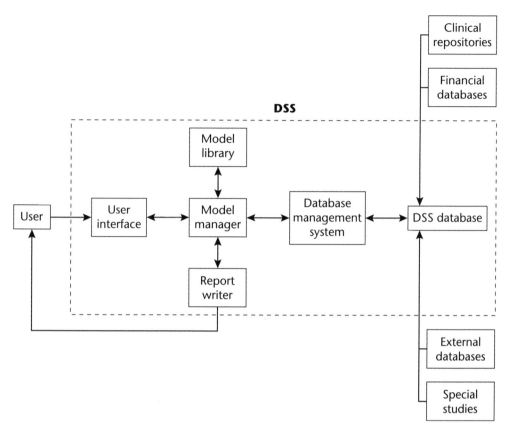

Figure 5.10   Conceptual Model of a Decision Support System

Figure 5.10 shows a conceptual model of the components of an effective DSS, each of which is described briefly in the following paragraphs.

The user engages the DSS through the user interface. The interface should have the ability to communicate with the DSS simply and intuitively.

An effective DSS contains a model library. The appropriate mix of models in a specific library depends on the requirements of decision makers who use the system. Typically, a DSS designed for use in a health program contains a mix of (1) statistical models (to summarize data, test hypotheses, make forecasts, and the like); (2) financial models (to predict cash flows, expenses, and revenues, as well as to perform break-even analyses or compute internal rates of return on investments that might be made in a program); and (3) "what if" models that can be used to determine the effect of changing one or more variables on a value of interest.

The model manager is software that links a DSS user's request to the appropriate model in the model library so that the desired analysis can be conducted. The models in an effective DSS can support decision making in clinical areas (such as patient scheduling and quality assessment) as well as in nonclinical areas (such as personnel scheduling, inventory control, and accounting).

A critical part of any DSS is the database from which the models can draw necessary information for analysis. Depending on the particular situation, a program's database could contain data from many sources, including clinical repositories, financial databases, special studies, and even commercially available external databases. Among the specific elements that might be found in a program's DSS database are the number of units of service provided, resources used in providing the services, data for assessing the quality of the services (see the broader discussion in Chapter 7), and data for evaluating results. A database can contain data relating to any of the components of a program's logic model (see Figure 2.1).

The final components of a DSS are a database management system, which is software that retrieves data at the request of a user or makes needed data available to the model manager for use in a particular decision-making model, and a report writer, which provides a user with a report of the analysis. Depending on the features of a given DSS, the reports produced may show comparisons of several alternatives, the consequences of a particular choice compared to alternatives, or a recommended choice.

Effective decision support systems are expensive. Even small ones cost tens of thousands of dollars and are not available to all programs. When affordable, however, these systems can greatly assist decision makers in assessing alternatives in decision-making situations.

Choosing an Alternative

After developing and assessing alternatives, decision makers must choose the alternative they think best in a given decision-making situation. If the other steps in the decision-making process (see Figure 5.2) have been carried out properly, the decision maker will typically be able to choose from among several relevant alternatives.

Of course, one alternative always available is to do nothing. This alternative must be considered most carefully of all. The decision maker should visualize the likely results of taking no action. If taking no action would result in the most desirable consequences, the decision maker should take no action. This alternative should never be taken lightly, however. After all, a problem or opportunity—or a potential problem or opportunity—triggered the decision-making process. Unless analysis reveals that there really is no problem or opportunity, the no-action alternative is usually inappropriate.

Making the choice from among alternatives in a decision-making situation—whether done based on experience, intuition, advice from others, experimentation, or analytical decision making—is rarely easy. Management decisions tend to be gray rather than black or white. They usually are made in the context of a constantly changing environment, which means that what is initially the most appropriate alternative may not remain the most desirable choice as circumstances change.

Aside from the difficulties encountered in collecting and properly analyzing enough information to fully inform a decision, problems can develop from the influence of the decision maker's personal prejudices and biases. These problems can interfere with the decision maker's effectiveness by forcing the selection of an alternative that fits some preconceived notion rather than the realities of the particular situation.

For some decision makers, the largest impediment to effectiveness is their own indecisiveness. But the opposite situation can exist and may be just as detrimental to the quality of decision making. Impulsiveness, or a tendency to jump headlong into a situation without considering all factors, is not uncommon among inexperienced decision makers as they make management decisions early in their career. If enough of their decisions turn out to be wrong, they may become indecisive.

To improve the quality of their decisions, managers should answer three questions concerning the alternatives in each decision-making situation. First, they should ask how each alternative contributes to the attainment of the program's desired results—that is, to its mission and objectives. This question is important because it reflects the fact that the alternatives in a decision-making situation are but means to an end—an end that has been clearly thought out and stated in the form of a mission and objectives. If an alternative under consideration does not improve the likelihood of achieving these desired results as well as or more than other alternatives, it should not be adopted.

Second, managers should ask whether alternatives under consideration represent a high degree of financial effectiveness. In other words, does an alternative make maximum use of available resources? There will be times, of course, when financial considerations should not unduly affect decision making, especially in a health program, where such considerations as need or quality may appropriately take precedence. Usually, however, financial aspects of a decision offer useful guidelines in selecting an alternative.

Third, managers should ask whether alternatives under consideration are feasible or capable of being implemented. In answering this question, the decision maker must think in very practical terms about how a particular alternative will be implemented within the context of the program's resources and organization design.

Answering these three questions does not guarantee that the best alternative—or even a good one—will be chosen. Doing so, however, increases the probability of an appropriate selection.

Implementing the Decision

The process of decision making does not end with the selection of an alternative. Managers are concerned about the effects of their decisions. Thus, implementing the decision is an important step in the overall decision-making process (see Figure 5.2). A well-chosen alternative, poorly implemented, can be useless or even harmful to a program. Successful implementation of a decision begins with carefully planning how the implementation will take place.

Planning for Implementation

Ideally, there are three interconnected components of good planning for implementation of a decision: (1) making a situational diagnosis, (2) choosing a general approach to implementing the decision, and (3) selecting a set of techniques to support the decision and its implementation and to reduce resistance from those affected by the decision. Each component is an important precursor to successful implementation.

Making a Situational Diagnosis   The process of making a situational diagnosis differs from the internal and external situational analyses discussed in Chapter 2 in that this diagnosis focuses specifically on the situation in which a particular decision is being implemented. The situational diagnosis that occurs as part of planning for implementation is a natural extension of the information-gathering effort that occurs in the second step of the decision-making process. During the second step, the decision maker explores the nature of the problem or opportunity he or she faces.

The situational diagnosis that precedes implementation of an alternative, however, goes well beyond the original gathering of the information needed to identify the nature of the problem or opportunity. It includes collecting information about resources available for implementing the chosen alternative as well as information on the views and attitudes of key participants (and perhaps others outside the program) concerning the choice that has been made. It is necessary to know about resource availability and constraints before the actual implementation begins, because this information can influence the selection of a general approach to implementation.

Choosing a General Approach to Implementation   In selecting a general approach to implementation, the decision maker can choose an approach from one of three broad categories: top-down, bottom-up, or participative approaches. In top-down approaches, which are also called power approaches, the decision maker simply announces to other participants in a program the decision that is to be implemented, and explains how it is to be implemented. The other participants are expected to accept the decision and take whatever part they are told to take in its implementation.

Power approaches are necessary and appropriate in some situations. For example, a change in the reimbursement policy of a major insurance carrier might require an immediate decision in a health program, leaving little time for anything but a top-down edict as a means of implementing the resulting decision. On the one hand, top-down approaches have the advantage of speed: decisions can be communicated quickly to affected participants in a program. On the other hand, a major drawback of top-down approaches is disruptiveness, particularly if those affected do not accept or understand the decision.

In bottom-up approaches to implementing decisions, participants in a program other than its manager are much more responsible for developing the details of how to implement the decision at hand. In this case the manager permits and encourages participants to decide how best to implement the chosen alternative. The primary advantage of bottom-up approaches to implementing decisions is that they foster widespread commitment to accomplishing the implementation task within a program.

In participative approaches to implementing decisions, participants responsible for implementation are involved in the entire decision-making process, along with the manager. Participation is formally sought through such devices as assigning participants to groups or teams specifically created to develop alternatives, to choose from among the alternatives, and to implement an appropriate alternative in response to a problem or opportunity. Participative implementation obviously differs from top-down edicts. It also differs from bottom-up approaches to implementation, which tend to focus on the details of implementation rather than on permitting participants to be involved fully in the entire decision-making process, as is characteristic of true participative approaches.

Developing Support for and Reducing Resistance to Decisions   The third component of good planning for implementation of a decision involves selecting techniques that help develop support for and reduce resistance to decisions and their implementation. In considering useful supportive techniques for use with program participants, and perhaps with other program stakeholders in certain situations, decision makers should remember that people respond to many types of change, including that resulting from decisions and their implementation, in predictable and often negative ways. Resistance may seem to managers like an inappropriate response, but it may seem to the resistant participants to be perfectly reasonable, especially if their past experiences with similar situations have been bad.

One of the underlying reasons why some participants view change negatively, and resist it, is their personal history, including their previous work and social experiences. For example, people who have experienced personal failures in their relationships with others or who have lost a previous job to downsizing or some other organizational change may be more concerned about changes than people who have experienced great success. A second cause can be the work environment itself. For example, if a program has been stable for a long time, participants may resist decisions that represent change. When participants have adjusted to the status quo and believe it is permanent, the introduction of even minor changes can be disruptive. Conversely, in a program with a history of continual change and in which change is seen as part of the culture, participants expect change and much more readily accept it.

There are many other reasons, which are discussed in the next paragraphs, for the resistance to change that is common among participants in programs, including the following:

- Feelings of insecurity
- Fears of potential social and economic losses, to say nothing of experience with actual losses
- Distaste for being inconvenienced
- Resentment that others are exerting control over them

Insecurity among affected participants is a major source of resistance to decisions that involve change. For many people, there is great comfort in the status quo, and any change is viewed as undesirable because it introduces a degree of uncertainty or unfamiliarity. Even a seemingly simple change can have far-reaching repercussions. For example, changing the schedule of meetings that a program's participants must attend may symbolize for some the manager's lack of concern for inconvenienced participants. To others it means interference with other aspects of their work schedule or routine. A third group may see it as more evidence of the autocracy of managers.

Participants also may fear or be concerned about social losses of various kinds that could result from implementation of a particular decision. Even the potential of such losses can cause people to resist a particular alternative in a decision-making situation. For example, modifications in the organiza-tion design of a program may mean that close friends have to work in separate rooms or are no longer able to interact during work. Complex informal relationships among participants are often affected by changes. Established status symbols may be destroyed in the process of reorganizing a program. Further, someone may jeopardize social acceptance by other participants if he or she supports an alternative that these coworkers have rejected. In such circumstances, a person may be forced to choose between cooperating with the manager or compromising friendships with and acceptance by other participants. Thus, what may seem a desirable and logical alternative in a decision-making situation can meet with heavy resistance because the price in terms of social relationships is too costly.

Possible social losses are not the only concerns participants may have about alternatives under consideration. Real or perceived economic losses may also be involved. In many situations new technology allows more work to be done by the same or even fewer people, and resistance by those affected is understandable. Even if they do not lose their job or have their earnings reduced, workers may find that changes in technology lead to a faster pace of work or to a redistribution of their workload.

Even when a decision does not cause significant economic or social losses, participants may be inconvenienced because of it. Any change causes some inconvenience, and extra effort is required to adjust to it. When old habits and routines must be replaced because of a decision, the inconvenience often stimulates resistance. If inconvenience is the only factor present, however, the degree of resistance may be minor.

Clearly there are many reasons for the often-encountered resistance to particular alternatives in a decision-making situation. People affected by a decision may resist for reasons ranging from little more than their dislike of being inconvenienced, to concerns about the decision's economic impact on them, to such complex factors as resentment of the manager's power to affect them so directly. Such factors often act in combination to strengthen their resolve to resist. There are a variety of techniques, however, that managers can use to help overcome resistance.

Key to any successful effort to reduce resistance to a decision or its implementation is informing and educating those affected by the decision about the decision itself and its implications for them before it is imple-mented. Effective communication about a change and education in regard to its implications can turn resistance into support.

Involving participants in the entire decision-making process, including determining how best to implement a given decision, can help overcome resistance by reducing uncertainty and misunderstandings about the decision and its implications. Participating in decision making gives participants an opportunity to gain a clearer picture of the changes that might occur as a result of the decision and enhances their commitment to successful implementation.

Supportive techniques that managers may find useful in helping participants accept decisions include offering training programs, granting requests for leave during a painful transition period, or even providing special counseling sessions for people adversely affected by a decision. It is sometimes possible to mitigate resistance by giving additional resources or promising to make a desired change at a later date, in exchange for participants' support of a decision.

Which support-enhancing and resistance-reducing techniques are used at any given time depends on how best to mollify the participants whose resistance must be overcome. Selecting and packaging the appropriate set of techniques to support the implementation of a decision and reduce resistance to it, as well as choosing a suitable general approach to implementing the decision, both of which should be based on a thorough situational diagnosis, are important precursors to actual implementation.

Actual Implementation

The actual implementation of a decision involves three distinct steps: (1) unfreezing the status quo; (2) changing to a new state; and (3) refreezing to make the new state permanent, at least until a future decision triggers a new round of implementation. This classic model of implementing changes, including those resulting from making and implementing decisions, traces back to the decades-old work of psychologist Kurt Lewin (1947). Figure 5.11 illustrates the steps in Lewin's model of implementing a decision. This three-step approach to change remains popular and provides contemporary managers with useful guidance.

Using the general approach selected to implement a decision, whether a top-down, bottom-up, or participative approach, the manager (or others responsible for the implementation) first unfreezes the status quo. This means making participants aware that a decision has been made and that the decision will necessitate changes. It may also involve steps to overcome resistance to the impending change as discussed earlier.

Once the status quo is unfrozen, change can occur. As shown in the figure, this means inserting different concepts, ideas, practices, or physical things into the situation. In a top-down approach, a simple announcement of a decision and plans for its implementation can unfreeze the status quo. Decisions and plans for their implementation reached through bottom-up

---

Step 1: Unfreezing

The manager's task is unfreezing the status quo and preparing those who will participate in or be affected by the decision and the resulting change.

This is done by

• Making participants aware of the decision and impending change
• Reducing or minimizing participants' resistance

Step 2: Changing

The manager's task is introducing the actual change necessitated by the decision.

This is done by

• Inserting different concepts or ideas, practices, or physical things into a situation

---

Step 3: Refreezing

The manager's task is refreezing the situation with the implemented decision and resulting change in place.

This is done by

• Restabilizing the situation
• Establishing conditions that will contribute to permanence

Figure 5.11   Lewin's Three Steps in Implementing Changes Resulting from a Decision

or more elaborate participative approaches can also be used to unfreeze the status quo and initiate change.

If the change is a physical thing, such as a new piece of equipment, it is put in place, and participants begin using it. If the change is a concept or practice, such as new reporting relationships in a revised organization design for a program, a new marketing strategy, or a modified accounting system, it is initiated, and participants begin using it.

The third step in implementing a decision involves incorporating the change into the routines of those carrying out the implementation. In effect, a new equilibrium is established as participants adapt and accept the decision as the norm. The situation is refrozen, until another decision requires more change and the cycle begins again.

There is no assurance that a decision can be implemented, no matter how appropriate a response to a problem or an opportunity it is, or how carefully its implementation is planned. That being said, managers can perform certain actions to increase the likelihood that their decisions will be successfully implemented. Most important is for managers to be certain that participants involved in implementing a decision understand the situation fully. Participants who understand the necessity and appropriateness of a particular decision are more likely to accept and adjust to it. Managers implementing a decision should provide information as far in advance as possible, and should include specifics pertaining to the reasons for the decision, its implications, the timing of its implementation, and the expected impact on the program as well as on participants.

Some decisions can be implemented on a trial basis. When feasible, managers should consider this option. Familiarity gained through experience with the implementation of a decision, along with assurances that the decision is not irrevocable, can reduce initial concern and increase the likelihood of acceptance. Allowing participants to assimilate changes that result from the implementation of a decision, which usually requires the passage of time, may also ultimately increase acceptance by those involved.

It is also useful when implementing decisions to minimize the impact on existing customs and informal relationships, where possible. Change almost invariably disrupts the culture in which it occurs. But participation in the entire decision-making process can help minimize such disturbance. Participants then feel less threatened by the resulting changes because, having helped plan those changes, they understand them better—and through their involvement in decision making they usually become more committed to the successful implementation of decisions.

Evaluating the Decision

The final step in the decision-making process outlined in Figure 5.2 is often given inadequate attention by managers; in fact, it may be overlooked altogether. Managers must evaluate their decisions, because they have a responsibility to optimally use resources entrusted to them. Almost all management decisions involve expending resources, such as money and time, that have alternative uses. Systematic evaluation determines whether the use of resources as a consequence of a decision yielded sufficient benefits, such as improved or enhanced quality, efficiency, satisfaction, adaptiveness, and survival potential, to justify the decision.

In addition, evaluation provides a basis for feedback, which can lead to adjustments to previously made decisions in the form of new or modified decisions. The evaluation of a decision requires collection and assessment of information on how well the decision is working; whether the decision has been effectively implemented; and, most important, whether the problem or opportunity that triggered the decision-making process has been either solved or successfully seized, respectively.

Information obtained in evaluating a decision may show that actual results do not match intended results, which provides feedback on the decision-making process. The manager may cycle back to the first step in the decision-making process after becoming aware that a problem or unmet opportunity still exists. The process then begins again, but this time the manager has more information, new insights into what might or might not work, and a bit more experience with the challenging process of making decisions in the context of a program. Alternatively, as shown by the feedback loop in Figure 5.2, the manager can cycle back to any prior step in the decision-making process, where he or she can make adjustments in the continuing effort to solve a problem or take advantage of an opportunity.

Summary

Decision making is defined as making a choice between two or more alternatives. It is critical to effectively performing the core developing/ strategizing, designing, and leading activities in management work and is discussed as a pervasive, facilitative activity in all management work. Figure 1.4 shows how decision making is intertwined with the core management activities and the other facilitative activities.

A seven-step process of decision making (see Figure 5.2) is presented in the chapter as follows:

1. Becoming aware that a problem or opportunity exists

2. Defining the problem or opportunity

3. Developing relevant alternatives

4. Assessing the alternatives

5. Choosing an alternative

6. Implementing the decision

7. Evaluating the decision

Several analytical tools that can be helpful in evaluating the alternatives in a decision-making situation are described. Most basic is the decision grid, which displays possible alternatives in a decision-making situation along with the various elements that will affect each. The payoff table is more useful than the decision grid in situations where probabilities can be assigned to various possible outcomes. The decision tree is a tool that can be helpful in evaluating decisions that are linked together over time, each with various possible outcomes. Cost-benefit analysis can be a useful tool, too, so long as decision makers recognize the difficulty in determining the true costs and benefits of various alternatives. The program evaluation and review technique, which can be very useful in considering the timing of activities or the best sequence for a series of actions, is discussed. The general structure of a decision support system is presented.

Many factors go into successful decision making by managers, including experience, intuition, advice from others, experimentation, and analysis. Effective decision makers take advantage of all these aids in carrying out their decision-making responsibilities, because decision making in programs is often fraught with uncertainty, risk, and conflict.

REVIEW QUESTIONS

1. Define decision making, and discuss the two types of management decisions.

2. Describe some of the most important characteristics of management decisions.

3. List the sequential steps in the decision-making process, and describe each briefly.

4. Discuss creative thinking as a component of developing alternatives in decision-making situations.

5. Describe some of the commonly used quantitative techniques available to help decision makers choose from among alternatives in decision-making situations.

6. What is a decision support system?

7. Discuss the three interconnected components of good planning for implementation of a decision.

8. Discuss the three steps involved in implementing a decision. What can managers do to improve the likelihood of successful implementation?

9. Why is it important for managers to evaluate their decisions?

KEY TERMS AND CONCEPTS

cost-benefit analysis

creative process

decision grid

decision making

decision-making process

decision support system (DSS)

decision tree

fishbone diagram

opportunistic decisions

Pareto chart

payoff table

problem-solving decisions

program evaluation and review technique (PERT)

References

Adair, John. *Decision Making and Problem Solving*. Philadelphia: Kogan Page, 2013.

Andersen, Bjorn, Tom Fagerhaug, and Marti Beltz. *Root Cause Analysis and Improvement in the Healthcare Sector: A Step-by-Step Guide*. Milwaukee, WI: ASQ Quality Press, 2012.

Anderson, David R., Dennis J. Sweeney, Thomas A. Williams, Jeffrey D. Camm, and R. Kipp Martin. *An Introduction to Management Science: Quantitative Approaches to Decision Making*, 13th ed. Mason, OH: South-Western, Cengage Learning, 2012.

Burstein, Frada, and Clyde W. Holsapple, eds., *Handbook on Decision Support Systems 1: Basic Themes*. New York: Springer, 2008.

BusinessDictionary. "Creative Thinking." Accessed May 17, 2014a. http://www.businessdictionary.com/definition/creative-thinking.html.

BusinessDictionary. "Information." Accessed May 30, 2014b. http://www.business-dictionary.com/definition/information.html.

DuBrin, Andrew J. *Essentials of Management*, 9th ed. Mason, OH: South-Western, Cengage Learning, 2011.

Fazar, Willard. "Program Evaluation and Review Technique." *The American Statistician* 13, no. 2 (April 1959): 10.

Glandon, Gerald L., Donna J. Slovensky, and Detlev H. Smaltz. *Information Systems for Healthcare Management*, 8th ed. Chicago: Health Administration Press, 2013.

Holsapple, Clyde W., and Kshiti D. Joshi. "Organizational Knowledge Resources." *Decision Support Systems* 31, no. 1 (May 2001): 39–54.

Kerzner, Harold. *Project Management: A Systems Approach to Planning, Scheduling, and Controlling*, 11th ed. Hoboken, NJ: Wiley, 2013.

Levi, Daniel. *Group Dynamics for Teams*, 4th ed. Thousand Oaks, CA: Sage, 2014.

Lewin, Kurt. "Frontiers in Group Dynamics: Concept, Method, and Reality in Social Science, Social Equilibria, and Social Change." *Human Relations* 1 (June 1947): 5–41.

Liebler, Joan Gratto, and Charles R. McConnell. *Management Principles for Health Professionals*, 6th ed. Burlington, MA: Jones & Bartlett Learning, 2012.

McLaughlin, Daniel B., and John R. Olson. *Healthcare Operations Management*, 2nd ed. Chicago: Health Administration Press, 2012.

Miller, Brian Cole. *Quick Brainstorming Activities for Busy Managers: 50 Exercises to Spark Your Team's Creativity and Get Results Fast*. New York: American Management Association, 2012.

Ozcan, Yasar A. *Quantitative Methods in Health Care Management: Techniques and Applications*. San Francisco: Jossey-Bass, 2009.

Project Management Institute. *The Standard for Program Management*, 3rd ed. Newton Square, PA: Project Management Institute, 2013.

Robbins, Stephen P., and Mary K. Coulter. *Management*, 12th ed. Upper Saddle River, NJ: Pearson, 2013.

Schuff, David, David Paradice, Frada Burstein, Daniel J. Power, and Ramesh Sharda. *Decision Support: An Examination of the DSS Discipline*. New York: Springer, 2011.

Simon, Herbert A. "Rational Choice and the Structure of the Environment." *Psychological Review* 63, no. 2 (1956): 129–138.

Simon, Herbert A. *Models of Bounded Rationality*. Cambridge, MA: MIT Press, 1982.

Vroom, Victor H. "A New Look at Managerial Decision Making." *Organizational Dynamics* 1, no. 4 (1973): 66–80.

Vroom, Victor H., and Arthur G. Jago. *The New Leadership: Managing Participation in Organizations*. Upper Saddle River, NJ: Prentice Hall, 1988.

Vroom, Victor H., and Philip W. Yetton. *Leadership and Decision Making*. Pittsburgh, PA: University of Pittsburgh Press, 1973.

Yukl, Gary A. *Leadership in Organizations*, 8th ed. Upper Saddle River, NJ: Prentice Hall, 2012.

CHAPTER 6

COMMUNICATING FOR UNDERSTANDING

This chapter focuses on communicating, a pervasive facilitative management activity that is both vital to the successful performance of management work and a challenge for managers (O'Rourke 2012). In essence, *communicating* is "a two-way process of reaching mutual understanding, in which participants not only exchange (encode-decode) information, news, ideas and feelings, but also create and share meaning" (BusinessDictionary 2014). Communicating involves senders (individuals, groups, or organizations) conveying ideas, intentions, and information to receivers (also individuals, groups, or organizations). Communication is effective when receivers understand ideas, intentions, and information as senders intend.

Like decision making, communicating is a ubiquitous facilitative activity that managers engage in as they perform their core activities of developing/strategizing, designing, and leading, as depicted in Figure 1.4. When managers interact with other participants in developing/strategizing the future of a program, they must communicate about the program's mission and objectives. They must also communicate about the means through which these desired results will be sought. When managers develop a business plan for a new program, they prepare a document to use in communicating their ideas to others. In the designing activity, managers communicate as they establish the intentional patterns of relationships among human and other resources within a program, staff the program's organization design, or develop or reshape its logic model. Finally, in leading, managers communicate extensively with other participants in a program as they encourage and facilitate their contributions to accomplishing the program's mission and objectives. Because leading effectively requires managers to help motivate participants

LEARNING OBJECTIVES

After reading this chapter, you should be able to:

- Define communicating, and model the basic communication process
- Appreciate the importance of communicating effectively with internal and external stakeholders
- Understand the contextual and personal barriers to communicating effectively and how to manage them
- Understand how communication flows within programs and how these flows are combined into communication networks
- Understand the importance and mechanisms of informal communication
- Understand the special challenges and importance of communicating with a program's external stakeholders

to contribute positively to the program's performance, managers must communicate with participants about their needs and how these can partially be met in the workplace.

Like making good decisions, communicating effectively greatly influences the degree of success managers achieve in their core activities and also in their other facilitative activities. For example, effective communication is vital to managing quality, as will be discussed in Chapter 7, and is crucial in marketing, as will be discussed in Chapter 8.

Communicating: Key to Effective Stakeholder Relations

Every program has a variety of stakeholders, the individuals, organizations, or groups with a stake or significant interest in the program (Freeman 2010; Freeman et al. 2010). Managers must communicate effectively with a program's internal stakeholders and ensure effective communication between the program and a wide variety of its external stakeholders, all in the interest of maintaining productive relationships with them. Managers must identify key stakeholders and ask themselves such questions as, "What do these stakeholders expect?" and "How satisfied are they with current performance?" (Kovner, McAlearney, and Neuhauser 2009, 5). Good communication is critical to good *stakeholder relations* (Dunn 2010).

Internal stakeholders are the participants in a program, whether employees or volunteers. External stakeholders include a program's existing and potential patients/customers, as well as accrediting agencies, competitors, government bodies (both payers and regulators), commercial insurance plans, the media, and suppliers, among many others. Figure 6.1 is a prototype external *stakeholder map* for health programs. Such a map can be uniquely drawn for any program.

Communicating with stakeholders provides managers with many opportunities to put into practice their commitment to ethical behavior. You may wish to review the section on ethically managing programs in Chapter 1. The guidelines for ethical behavior presented in that discussion boil down to the following simplification: "Generally speaking, behaving ethically means avoiding lying, cheating, and stealing, as well as cruelty, deception, and subterfuge" (Seglin 2002, 76). This is useful guidance for communicating with those who have a stake in a program.

Relationships with internal and external stakeholders fall along a continuum of positive to neutral to negative, with positive and negative relationships varying in intensity. Figure 6.2 depicts examples of the internal

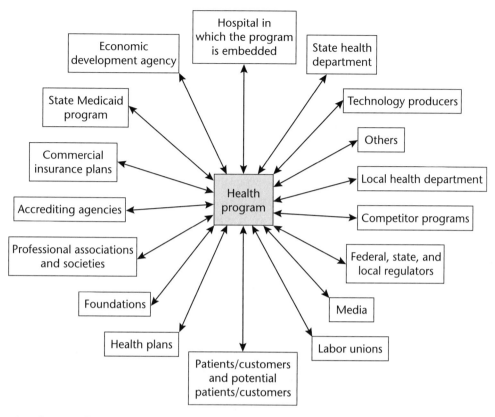

Figure 6.1   Prototype of an External Stakeholder Map for Health Programs

and external stakeholders a program might have, arrayed according to the typical—but by no means universal—nature of the relationships with these stakeholders. Although in Figure 6.2 stakeholders occupy typical patterns of relationships, patterns vary across programs, depending on each program's unique circumstances. It is important to note that managers can alter these

Typically positive relationships	Typically neutral relationships	Typically negative relationships
Participants Patients/customers Suppliers	Accrediting agencies Foundations Noncompeting programs	Competitors Regulators Media

Figure 6.2   Typical Relationships between a Program and Its Stakeholders

relationship patterns. It is possible, for example, to move a relationship with a stakeholder from negative to neutral or positive.

Managing Stakeholder Relationships

As might be expected, positive and neutral relationships with stakeholders provide better starting points for effective communication than do negative relationships. Managers thus improve the likelihood that they will communicate effectively with stakeholders by maximizing the proportion of stakeholders with whom a program enjoys positive relationships, and by minimizing the proportion of negative relationships. Because the intensity of positive and negative relationships varies, the manager's objective is to cultivate strongly positive relationships. Finally, because neutral relationships are better than negative relationships, but not as good as positive relationships, it is desirable to take steps to convert neutral stakeholders into positive ones.

It takes considerable, sustained effort to establish and maintain positive relationships with both internal and external stakeholders. In essence, as managers seek to establish and maintain good relationships with a program's stakeholders, they attempt to do the following:

- Achieve among internal and external stakeholders a widespread understanding and acceptance of the mission and objectives established for the program, and of its logic model and organization design

- Garner support for and secure contributions toward achievement of the mission and objectives

- Achieve and maintain a workable balance between the program's mission and objectives and the needs and preferences of its stakeholders

Relationships between programs and their stakeholders can be effectively managed in two ways, both of which are heavily dependent on communicating well. A manager can seek to establish and maintain good relationships with stakeholders by fitting a program's organization design, performance, and logic model (if there is one) to the preferences, requirements, and expectations of its stakeholders. Alternatively, a manager can seek a closer match between a program and its stakeholders by changing the stakeholders in some way.

Fitting Programs to Stakeholders

In trying to fit a program to the preferences, requirements, and expectations of its stakeholders, the manager at least partly uses knowledge of these preferences, requirements, and expectations to guide decisions that help mold the program into a form that facilitates positive stakeholder relationships. The manager gains this necessary knowledge by communicating with stakeholders.

Efforts to build positive internal stakeholder relationships by fitting a program to the preferences, requirements, and expectations of internal stakeholders are exemplified by the provision of more satisfying working conditions or better pay and benefits for participants. An example of working to build positive external stakeholder relationships is responding to the identified preferences of patients/customers. For example, patients/customers might be provided with child care while they receive services in response to their expressed preferences for such a service. Or a program might redesign its physical layout to appeal to and accommodate the preferences of an older clientele. In each case, the program is altering or reshaping itself in some manner to better fit the preferences, requirements, and expectations of some of its external stakeholders—efforts that are likely to improve stakeholder relations.

Altering Stakeholders

In the second approach to managing stakeholder relationships, managers can seek to alter stakeholders to achieve a closer match between the stakeholders' preferences, requirements, and expectations and what the program offers. This approach also depends on communicating with stakeholders.

Examples of efforts to build better relationships through changing internal stakeholders include providing participants with additional training and education to better equip them to contribute positively to accomplishing the program's mission and objectives, using participative decision-making processes to gain participants' commitment to implementing decisions, and adding new participants with needed expertise to the staff. When such efforts work, the internal stakeholders better fit the needs of the program, and relationships are improved.

Examples of efforts intended to cause desired changes in external stakeholders include marketing activities designed to educate and inform potential patients/customers about services, and communicating with regulators in the hope of providing them with useful information as they decide whether to approve a new technology. If these communication efforts succeed, better and more positive relationships will exist between the program and its external stakeholders.

A Model of the Communication Process

In communicating, as was noted previously, senders convey ideas, intentions, and information to receivers. The *communication process* is essentially an exchange process, as depicted in Figure 6.3. When the process works well, the receiver understands the idea, intention, or information. But conveyance of ideas, intentions, and information between senders and receivers is more readily and easily accomplished than achievement of understanding.

Components of the Communication Process

The communication process has a number of interrelated components that are identified here and given more attention later on. In regard to the components of the communication process depicted in Figure 6.3, *senders* want *receivers* to understand their *message; that is, senders want their message *decoded* exactly as they were *encoded.* Unfortunately, understanding can be difficult to achieve because of the many *contextual and interpersonal barriers* to effective communication. *Channels* are the mechanisms through which messages are conveyed, including face-to-face or telephone conversations, e-mails, facsimiles, letters, memoranda, policy statements, work schedules, reports, electronic message boards, videoconferences, newspapers, television and radio commercials, and written or intranet newsletters for external or internal distribution. Finally, communication exchanges ideally include a *feedback* loop. The likelihood of there being effective communication is improved if receivers give feedback to senders, who can then adjust a message if it is not received as intended. When a sender encodes and transmits a message to a receiver, and the receiver decodes the message and indicates understanding by giving feedback, effective two-way communication occurs.

Using the Communication Process Effectively

Explicit attention to each component in the communication process shown in Figure 6.3 and identified earlier is necessary for managers to communicate effectively. In addition, there are many other practical steps managers can take to improve communication. Some of the most important ones are briefly described here.

A first step for a sender wishing to improve communication is often for the sender to simply consider whether the receiver is better able to interpret information received verbally or in writing. The sender can also help the receiver by cueing him or her as to whether the purpose of a message is to

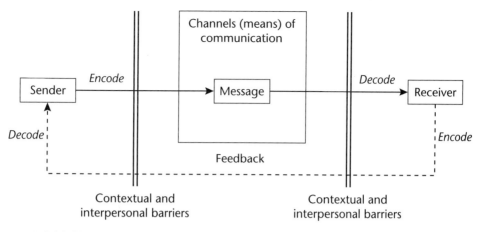

Figure 6.3 A Model of the Communication Process

provide information, elicit a response or reaction, or support a particular alternative in a decision-making situation.

Communication can also be improved if the sender carefully considers the content, importance, and complexity of a message in determining the channels through which the message is communicated. Similarly, the time frames associated with particular communication situations should be considered in choosing the channels through which messages are sent. That is, faster channels and more precise cues are needed with shorter time frames. Paper memoranda are too slow to use in effectively communicating emergency situations, for example.

In communicating, a sender uses words and symbols to encode an idea, an intention, or information into a message for a receiver. Because words can have different meanings for different people, care must be taken to communicate in words that are easily understood and that perhaps are augmented with other symbols. Communication is not restricted to words alone, because achieving understanding may require multiple channels, including both verbal and nonverbal means. Even silence conveys meaning and is thus a means of communicating.

In health programs, many symbols have a role in communication. These symbols can be physical things, pictures, or actions. For example, a particular uniform (physical thing) may permit quick identification of people in some health services settings. Everyone knows who wears a long, white coat.

Pictures or visual representations are another type of symbol that can be quite efficient and helpful in communicating, and they increase under-standing in many situations. Consider how many words, in lieu of a chart such as that in Figure 1.1, would be needed to explain the organization design of a large program. Or imagine the difficulty of using only words to communicate all the information in a sophisticated image of a patient's heart.

Finally, an action is a symbol that communicates. A smile or a congratulatory handshake has meaning. A promotion or pay increase conveys a great deal to the recipient, as well as to others. Lack of action can also have symbolic meaning. When managers fail to follow through on promises of new resources or promotions, or fail to acknowledge work that is done especially well, they are sending a clear message that they do not keep their word or that they do not value the work of participants.

Action or inaction that is inconsistent with words transmits a contradictory message. The manager who tells a participant, "I have confidence in your ability; your performance is excellent, and I want to expand your duties by delegating more to you," but then becomes angry when the participant makes a small technical error, is acting inconsistently. The receiver who says to the sender, "I am listening," but then looks at the clock impatiently or starts to walk away while a conversation is under way, sends a mixed message.

The selection of channels is an important part of the communication process. Communicating effectively often involves using multiple channels to convey a message. For example, a major revision in the mission of a program might be announced in a letter or memorandum from the manager to all participants; graphically illustrated by posters in key locations; and then reinforced in group meetings, where the manager might explain the change and respond to questions about it.

A decision to lobby the state legislature for more generous Medicaid reimbursement might result in messages conveyed through such channels as letters to individual legislators, direct contact between a program's manager and legislators, and newspaper advertisements stating the program's position. If other similar programs would benefit from the legislation, their managers might also participate—perhaps through an association—in producing and distributing television commercials or using other communication channels to boost support for increased Medicaid funding.

Those who receive a message must decode it, no matter what channels were used in conveying it. The surest way to determine if a message has been received as intended is through feedback. In the absence of feedback, communication is a one-way process. Feedback can be direct or indirect. Direct feedback is a receiver's response to a sender concerning a specific message. For example, in response to a sender's inarticulate and confusing message about a change in work schedules, the confused receiver might respond with, "I don't understand. Please explain the change further."

Indirect feedback is more subtle, involving consequences that result from a particular message. For example, indirect feedback on a message about changing a program's physical location might be expressed by higher levels of participant satisfaction if the change is liked, or increased turnover among participants if the change is disliked. Similarly, indirect feedback on communication intended to cause legislators to change Medicaid reimbursement levels might include an increase in rates if legislators agree with proponents of the increase, no action if they disagree, or even hostile action if they disagree with the message and are upset by the means used to communicate it.

No matter how carefully and skillfully a manager seeks to communicate, however, there are almost always barriers that must be overcome if communication is to be effective. These barriers apply whether a manager is communicating with internal or external stakeholders. It is so crucial to understand and overcome these barriers to effective communication that they receive special attention in the following section.

Barriers to Communicating Effectively

The *contextual and interpersonal barriers* depicted in Figure 6.3 are ubiquitous in the communication process for managers in health programs. Contextual (or environmental, as they are also called) barriers of several types arise in programs, including in the organizational homes in which programs are embedded. Interpersonal barriers arise from the nature of individuals and their interactions with others as they communicate. Contextual and interpersonal barriers can block, filter, or distort messages as they are encoded and sent, or as they are decoded and received. Overcoming these barriers is vital to communicating effectively, and understanding them is the first step in addressing them.

Contextual Barriers

There are a number of common contextual barriers found in programs, as in all busy work settings. These barriers include competition for the attention and time of both senders and receivers; complexity of the organization design of a program; the prevailing attitude about communication, which can affect senders and receivers alike; and characteristics of the messages.

Competition for Attention and Time

Multiple and simultaneous demands on a sender's time and attention may cause a message to be encoded inadequately; similar demands may also interfere with its receiver, causing the message to be incorrectly decoded. In such situations, a receiver may receive a message without comprehending it because the receiver is not giving the message sufficient attention. Similarly, time constraints may be a barrier to effective communication by giving a sender inadequate opportunities to think through and carefully structure a message to be conveyed, or by giving its receiver too little time to determine its meaning.

Organization Design Complexity

The complexity of the organization design of a program can be an important contextual barrier to effective communication. The existence of multiple layers in the organization design, as well as other organization design complexities, such as the program's size and diversity of activity, creates a barrier that tends to cause message distortion.

As messages are transmitted up or down through a hierarchy of layers in a program, and as participants at each level interpret the messages according to their personal frame of reference and vantage point, there are many opportunities for information to be filtered, dropped, or added, or for emphasis to be rearranged. As a result, messages sent through many layers are more likely to be distorted. Furthermore, there are more opportunities for messages to be blocked as they are transmitted along a chain of participants. A message sent from a manager to participants through several layers of a program may be received in a form that is quite different from what was originally sent. Or a report prepared for the manager that passes up through layers in the organization design may not reach its destination due to being blocked along the way by someone who disagrees with the message.

Prevailing Attitudes about Communication

In addition to the structural aspects of a program that can interfere with the communication process, the attitudes about communication in a particular context can either facilitate or serve as a barrier to communication for senders and receivers alike. A manager's attitude about communication can directly inhibit or promote effective communication. As a rule, managers who are not interested in promoting communication within a program will establish procedural and organizational blockages, which are serious contextual barriers to effective communication. Symptoms of an anticommunication attitude, which invariably retards communication, include requiring all communication to flow through formal channels; being inaccessible; showing a lack of interest in participants' frustrations, complaints, or feelings; and not allocating sufficient time to communicate.

Managers' attitudes about communication also have a significant impact on communication with external stakeholders. Differences in attitudes could lead two managers to act very differently in communicating with external stakeholders in a crisis. For example, knowledge that patients/customers might have been exposed to a dangerous infection while being served in a program could lead one manager to conceal this information, whereas another manager faced with the same situation would make wide use of the media in the hope that everyone who might have been exposed would come forth to be tested and treated as needed.

Characteristics of Messages

A final contextual barrier that may cause a breakdown in communication lies in the messages themselves. When messages contain specific terminology unfamiliar to the receiver, or when they are especially complex, these features can be barriers. Each profession has its own jargon. Managers of programs may use very different terminology (such terms as payoff tables or logic models, for example) from that used by participants who are responsible for direct or support work. Further, many of the participants in health programs routinely use terminology that is unfamiliar to external stakeholders.

Communication between people who use different terminology can be ineffective simply because people attribute different meanings to the same words. When a message both is complex and contains terminology that is unfamiliar to the receiver, it is particularly likely that misunderstanding will occur. This contextual barrier often inhibits communication not only within health programs but also between health programs and many of their external stakeholders.

Interpersonal Barriers

Interpersonal barriers are always possible in the communication process, because it involves people interacting with others. The interpersonal relationships that exist among participants within a program can promote effective communication, but they can also distort the encoding or decoding of messages or inhibit their conveyance. For example, a discordant relationship between a manager and another participant in a program can negatively influence the flow and content of information between them, and can certainly interfere with achieving understanding. There are other interpersonal barriers, as described in the following subsections.

Different Frames of Reference

When people encode and send messages or decode and receive them, they tend to do so according to their personal frame of reference, which shapes how messages are encoded and decoded, or even whether these individuals attempt to communicate. In some instances, for example, a participant's past experiences may inhibit communication because of his or her fear of reprisal, negative sanctions, or ridicule. On the one hand, it is not unusual to find participants in a program who are reluctant to communicate with the manager because of negative past experiences when communicating that something was wrong or communicating that they disagreed with a manager's idea or decision. On the other hand, good interpersonal relationships, especially those characterized by trust, generally support and facilitate communication.

An individual's socioeconomic background and previous experiences largely determine his or her frame of reference. For example, someone whose cultural background emphasizes not challenging authority may be inhibited in communicating with organizational superiors. Naive people tend to accept communication at face value without filtering out erroneous information or noticing gaps in the information they receive. Self-aggrandizing people may send distorted messages intended to provide them with some advantage or gain for themselves.

Furthermore, unless all those involved in communication exchanges have had similar experiences, it may be difficult for communicators to completely understand each other's messages. The wealthy may have difficulty understanding the concerns of people without health insurance. Those who have never had a serious illness or lost a loved one may be unable to fully understand messages about these experiences.

Different Values

Closely related to the different frames of reference of individuals are their different values, which can cause messages to be distorted in sending or receiving, and which can also cause messages to be blocked. People hold different values in regard to such issues as politics, ethics, religion, fairness in the workplace, race, gender, sexual orientation, and lifestyle, which filter and distort communication and are thus important interpersonal barriers to communicating effectively.

Selective Perception

Selective perception is another interpersonal barrier. People often screen out derogatory information and amplify words, actions, and meanings that flatter them; people tend to filter out the "bad" of a message and retain the "good." Selective perception can be conscious or unconscious. When it is conscious, often because one fears the consequences of the truth, intentional distortion results. For example, managers whose programs have a high rate of turnover among participants may fear that those they report to will notice it. They might argue that turnover is due to low wages over which they have no control (or responsibility), or delete, alter, or minimize the importance of this information in reports to their organizational superiors.

Sometimes jealousy, especially when coupled with selective perception, may result in conscious efforts to filter and distort incoming information, transmit misinformation, or both. For example, a manager with a superb assistant who routinely makes the manager look good may block or distort information that would reveal this fact to organizational superiors, preferring that they give the manager full credit. Sometimes nothing more than petty personality differences, the feeling of professional incompetence or inferiority, or greed can lead to jealousy and result in communication distortion.

Judgmental Attitudes

Another potential interpersonal barrier to communicating effectively arises because people receiving a message have a tendency to evaluate and judge the sender. They do this to decide whether to ignore the message or filter out or discount part of it. Participants who distrust a manager, for example, may ignore messages from him or her; or managers may ignore messages from program participants with whom they frequently disagree. Source evaluation may help communicators cope with the barrage of messages exchanged in a typical health program, but it also can mean that legitimate messages are misunderstood or disregarded.

Lack of Empathy

A final interpersonal barrier to effective communication is a lack of empathy on the part of communicators. Having empathy means being sensitive to the frames of reference or emotional states of other people in the communication situation. Such sensitivity promotes understanding. Empathy helps the sender decide how to encode a message for maximum understanding, and it helps the receiver interpret the message's meaning. For example, participants in a program who empathize with its manager may discount an angry message because they are aware that temporary, extreme pressure and frustration are causing such a message to be sent even though it is not warranted.

Similarly, a sender who is sensitive to the receiver's circumstances may, based on what he or she knows, decide how best to encode a message or decide that it is better left unsent. For example, if a participant is having a bad day, a reprimand may be interpreted more negatively than intended. If a participant has just emerged from a traumatic experience, such as family illness, the empathetic manager might decide to delay bad news until later. A manager who is empathetic with external stakeholders might delay announcing a generous across-the-board wage increase or a substantial price increase just after a major local employer has announced a plant closure in the community.

Minimizing Barriers to Communicating Effectively

Awareness that contextual and interpersonal barriers to effective communication exist is the first step in minimizing their impact. However, overt actions are needed to overcome them. Although the specific steps necessary to overcome the barriers depend on circumstances, several general guidelines can be suggested.

Reducing Contextual Barriers

Contextual barriers are reduced by establishing a culture within a program that encourages and facilitates communication. These barriers can also be reduced if receivers and senders pay attention to their messages and devote adequate time to sending and receiving messages.

Reducing the number of links (layers in the organizational hierarchy of a program, or steps between a program as a sender and its external stakeholders as receivers) through which messages pass reduces opportunities for distortion. For example, a flat organization design may mean that a message from a program manager can go to all participants simultaneously rather than moving through two or three layers (as would happen in a tall organization design). Similarly, an e-mail message sent directly to an external stakeholder—rather than a letter that passes through one or more assistants before being read by the intended receiver—may enhance understanding. Consciously tailoring words and symbols so that messages are understandable, and reinforcing words with actions, significantly improves communication among people with different positions. Finally, using multiple channels to reinforce complex messages decreases the likelihood of misunderstanding.

Reducing Interpersonal Barriers

Interpersonal barriers to effective communication are reduced by conscious efforts on the part of the sender and the receiver to understand each other's frame of reference. Recognizing that people engage in selective perception and are prone to jealousy and fear is a good place to begin eliminating, or at least diminishing, these barriers. Empathy with those to whom messages are directed is one of the surest ways to increase the likelihood that the messages will be received and understood as intended.

Both contextual and interpersonal barriers can be overcome or minimized by effective listening within the communication process. Rice (2003, 1) has suggested the following good listening habits:

- Clear away physical distractions, such as noise or interruptions.

- Express your interest in listening.

- Maintain your focus while listening.

- Ask questions as you listen.

- Listen with your mind as well as your ears.

- Take notes whether you need to or not.

- Listen early and often.

Communicating within Programs

Communication flows in programs in all directions: downward, upward, horizontally, and diagonally. These *communication flows* form directional patterns that are also found in the organizational home in which a program is embedded (see Figure 1.1). Each flow pattern has its appropriate uses and unique characteristics (see Figure 6.4). Typically, downward or upward flow is communication between organizational superiors and subordinates in a program; this flow is typical of communication between managers and other participants. Horizontal flow is between organizational equals, such as between managers of similar sections or subunits of a program, or between coworkers. Diagonal flow cuts across sections or subunits and layers.

Downward Flow

Downward communication primarily involves transmitting information from organizational superiors to subordinates. It commonly consists of information, orders, or instructions from organizational superiors to subordinates, and is often transmitted on a one-to-one basis. It also may include speeches to groups of participants in meetings. The myriad written means

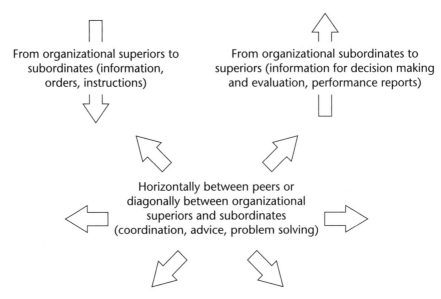

Figure 6.4   Communication Flows in a Program

of communicating—through such devices as handbooks, procedure manuals, newsletters, bulletin boards, and the ubiquitous memorandum—also are downward flows of communication. Computerized information systems contribute greatly to downward flow in many contemporary health programs.

Upward Flow

Upward communication primarily involves providing managers with information to be used in decision making, revealing problem areas, supplying data for performance evaluation, indicating the status of morale, and in general underscoring the thinking of the manager's organizational subordinates. Upward flow becomes more important with increasing size and complexity in the organization design of a program. Managers rely on effective upward communication, and they encourage it by establishing trust and respect as integral components of a program's culture (Robbins and Coulter 2013).

In addition to being directly useful to managers, upward communication flow helps other participants in a program fulfill personal needs. It permits them to feel a greater sense of participation and typically increases their level of satisfaction in the work setting. The hierarchical chain of command is the main channel for upward communication in most organizations, including in programs. Upward communication may be supported, however, with grievance procedures, open-door policies, counseling, questionnaires and surveys of participants, exit interviews, and participative decision-making techniques.

Horizontal and Diagonal Flows

No matter how smoothly downward and upward communication flows in a program, especially in one that is subject to abrupt demands for action and reaction, there must also be horizontal flow. For example, when the work of interdependent components of a program must be coordinated, horizontal communication flow may be necessary.

Diagonal communication flows can also be vital in a health program. For example, diagonal communication is necessary if a program's pharmacist is to alert a physician about a potential adverse reaction between two medications ordered for a patient. Diagonal flows violate the usual pattern of upward and downward communication by cutting across a program's sections or subunits, and these flows violate the usual pattern of horizontal communication in that the communicators are at different hierarchical levels.

In addition to diagonal flow that results when individuals take the initiative to communicate in this way, committees, groups, or teams comprising participants from different organizational layers of a program can serve as useful mechanisms of diagonal communication. In fact, the prevalence of committees, groups, and teams in health programs is largely attributable to a need for horizontal and diagonal communication flows.

Grouping permits participants from different components of a program, including those from different hierarchical levels, to overcome many of the contextual or personal barriers to effective communication as they discuss and clarify issues and common concerns, identify potential problems, solve problems face-to-face, and coordinate activities. It is important to remember, however, that groups have negative potential as well. As a group develops cohesion and commitment to common purposes, attitudes and norms within the group can either facilitate or impede group performance. Group decision making can be time consuming and expensive, and a group's decisions often are compromises. Fortunately, there is abundant guidance available in the literature on developing effective groups by taking advantage of their positive potential while avoiding the negative (Harris and Sherblom 2011).

Communication Networks

Downward, upward, horizontal, and diagonal communication flows can be combined into patterns called *communication networks* (Richmond,

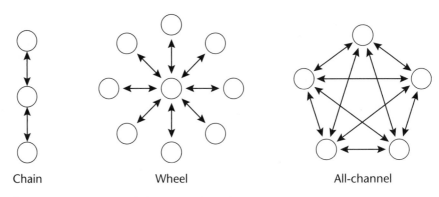

Chain   Wheel   All-channel

Figure 6.5   Common Types of Communication Networks in Programs

McCroskey, and Powell 2012). Three common types of communication networks—chain, wheel, and all-channel—are illustrated in Figure 6.5. The chain network is the standard pattern for communicating upward and downward between organizational superior and subordinate pairs of participants involved in a program. An example is a program in which a staff nurse (an organizational subordinate) reports to a nurse manager (an organizational superior of the staff nurse and an organizational subordinate of the program manager), who reports to the program manager (an organizational superior of both the staff nurse and the nurse manager).

The wheel pattern in the figure shows a situation where eight organizational subordinates report to one superior. This pattern can be expanded to include any number of subordinates reporting to a superior. For example, two social workers in a program can report to the director of the social work unit, as can a larger number of social workers. The all-channel network permits each communicator in the network to interact with every other communicator in the network.

Communication networks vary along several dimensions, and no one type of network is best in all situations. A wheel or all-channel network tends to be faster and more accurate than a chain network, but the chain pattern promotes clear-cut lines of authority and responsibility. An all-channel network enhances morale among those in it because everyone is equal in terms of how communication occurs; the drawback is that communication is relatively slow. Slow communication is a serious problem if an immediate decision is needed, or if an action must be taken quickly. Managers should choose types of networks to fit the various communication situations they face.

Informal Communication

Coexisting with the formal communication flows and networks that are established as part of the organization designs of health programs are informal communication flows, which have their own networks. Informal communication flows and networks result from the interpersonal relationships among participants. Informal communication flows are often referred to as the **grapevine,** a term that arose during the early wartime use of telegraph lines strung between trees, forming something similar to a grapevine. A communicator wishing to give credence to a rumor could claim that it came through the grapevine.

Informal communication flows are as natural as the patterns of social interaction that develop in all work situations. You may wish to review the discussion of informal aspects of organization designs in Chapter 3, because, just as informal designs coexist with formal designs, informal communication flows coexist with the formal patterns established by managers. There is no doubt that informal communication channels can be and routinely are misused in health programs, especially in transmitting rumors. Yet properly managed informal communication flows can be beneficial in ways that are discussed in the following paragraphs.

Downward flow of informal communication moves through the grapevine much faster than it does through formal channels. In many programs, much of the coordination among clusters of work groups occurs through the give-and-take in informal horizontal and diagonal flows. In the case of upward flow, informal communication can be a rich source of information about performance, ideas, feelings, and attitudes. Because of the potential usefulness and pervasiveness of informal communication flows, managers should try to understand them and use them to their advantage.

Similar to formal communication flows, informal communication flows follow certain predictable patterns and form identifiable networks. One pattern resembles a string in which participant A tells participant B, who tells C, who then tells D, and so on, until twenty participants later, X gets the information—late and inaccurate.

A more typical pattern for informal communication flow is one in which participant A tells several others (C, D, and F). Only one or two of these receivers pass the information forward, and they usually tell several other participants. As the information grows older and the proportion of those knowing it gets larger, spreading gradually ceases. This network is a cluster chain, because each link in the chain tends to inform a cluster of other people instead of only one person (as in the string pattern mentioned previously).

Informal communication flow is present in every health program and can either aid or inhibit the manager in his or her efforts to attain suitable levels of performance and results. Managers can take advantage of this flow by paying close attention to it (even inaccurate rumors may reflect certain aspects of participants' feelings and views) and by occasionally and selectively using informal communication channels, especially when speed is critical.

To summarize, the multidirectional communication flows and the networks they form within programs each have a purpose, and each is an important tool for managers. To the extent that these flows are planned and designed by managers, they are part of a program's formal organization design, and they represent formal communication channels and networks. To the extent that they result from the natural communication between people that arises within the formal organization design, they represent informal communication channels and networks. Understandable messages, whether they flow through formal channels or through the informal give-and-take among participants, are as crucial to the life of a health program as the circulation of blood is to human life.

Having discussed the formal and informal communication that occurs within programs, we now turn our attention to communication with a program's external stakeholders.

Communicating with External Stakeholders

In addition to communication that occurs within health programs, managers also communicate extensively with a program's external stakeholders. As noted earlier, these stakeholders include the people a program serves (such as its current and potential patients/customers), as well as others (such as those depicted in the stakeholder map in Figure 6.1). Effective communication between a program and each of its external stakeholders is necessary because programs are affected, sometimes quite dramatically, by what external stakeholders think and do.

Managers as Boundary Spanners

Boundary spanning is another name for the process through which managers of health programs communicate with external stakeholders. Although managers may have help with their boundary spanning efforts from the larger organizational home in which a program is embedded, they are the primary *boundary spanners.*

On the one hand, as boundary spanners, managers obtain information from external stakeholders that can be useful to a program. Obtaining demographic information about a service area for use in developing/ strategizing in regard to a program's future service mix is an example of this sort of boundary spanning. Obtaining information about possible changes in an important regulation affecting a program is another example.

On the other hand, boundary spanners also represent a program to its external stakeholders. Examples of this include activities undertaken in marketing or through public relations, patient/customer relations, government relations, or community relations efforts. Because information is the object of boundary-spanning activities—whether obtaining information from external stakeholders or providing them with information about the program—communicating is critical to successful boundary spanning.

The technical process of communicating with external stakeholders is no different from the process used within a program, as depicted in Figure 6.3. Furthermore, as is the case with communication flows occurring within a program, contextual and interpersonal barriers to effective communication affect communication between a program and its external stakeholders. But some specific aspects of communicating with external stakeholders deserve additional attention, beginning with knowing who the external stakeholders are.

Being a good communicator with external stakeholders requires a systematic approach to knowing who these stakeholders are and as much about their views, preferences, and positions on issues as possible. The process of acquiring and organizing important information about who a program's external stakeholders are is often a matter of judgment. An example of this is determining which state legislators are most important in policymaking so that their views can be observed and monitored. Such judgments can usually be improved by involving multiple people in making them through such mechanisms as ad hoc committees, task forces, or the use of outside consultants. One output of such an effort is an external stakeholder map, or a diagram showing the program at the center with its various external stakeholders radiating out like the spokes of a wheel (see Figure 6.1). Such a map increases the likelihood that the manager will know which external stakeholders he or she should communicate with.

Once stakeholders are clearly identified, their views, preferences, and positions on issues of relevance to a program can be monitored, providing a solid base for effectively communicating with them. For example, a program manager concerned about revenue from Medicaid-related services will be interested in what those who set Medicaid reimbursement rates are thinking for the next fiscal year. As part of an extension of their monitoring efforts, managers will benefit from forecasts of likely changes in stakeholders' thinking on relevant issues, giving managers time to factor this information into their decisions.

Identifying a program's external stakeholders and carefully monitoring their perspectives and opinions, and even accurately forecasting trends in this information, do not ensure that managers will communicate effectively with them. It does, however, mean that managers will have clearer ideas about what the subjects of communication should be. This will help them in both sending and receiving messages in exchanges with the external stakeholders.

Given the vital linkage between programs and such external stakeholders as current and potential patients/customers, payers, and regulators, it is unlikely that any program can succeed without an effective process through which a manager routinely communicates with external stakeholders.

Two of the most important types of communication with external stakeholders, discussed in the following subsections, are those associated with (1) marketing a program, and (2) communicating with the public sector, especially as managers advocate in support of a program or on behalf of patients/customers.

Communicating in Marketing

Marketing is discussed in depth in Chapter 8. Suffice it to say, the central purpose of marketing is to support the voluntary exchange of something of value between buyers and sellers (Pride and Ferrell 2014). Successful programs produce services or products that are of value to certain people, groups, or organizations (for example, individual patients/customers, health plans, or government agencies) and make the services or products available to them. In turn, individuals, groups, or organizations seek out the services or products and choose them. Communication is vital to how this process occurs; indeed, communicating effectively is necessary for the exchanges to occur at all.

Marketing can ensure that a program has patients/customers for its services or products, that the needs of patients/customers are identified and met, and that the program receives value in return (Berkowitz 2011). The major activities in commercial marketing include the following:

- Determining what groups of potential patients/customers (or markets) exist; determining the needs of potential patients/customers; and identifying which of these groups of potential patients/customers the program wishes to serve. In essence, these activities determine a program's target markets. If the program has competitors, it is also necessary to determine what they are doing or may do in regard to the target markets.

- Assessing the program's current service mix or product lines relative to the identified target markets' needs to determine what products or services the program can provide in response, or can develop and then provide.

- Deciding how to facilitate exchanges between the program and its target markets and implementing these decisions. Prerequisites to mutually satisfactory exchanges between a program and its target markets include responding to how and where patients/customers prefer to gain access to and use the products or services, as well as developing pricing structures that both attract patients/customers and provide the necessary financial resources to support the program. Both determining patient/customer preferences and providing information on pricing and other aspects of products or services require effective communication between a program and its target markets.

Carrying out all of the activities involved in commercial marketing depends on information's being exchanged through effective communication. Similarly, as can be seen in the discussion of the topic in Chapter 8, effective communication is also essential in the use of social marketing techniques in programs.

Communicating with the Public Sector

Health programs are affected by public policies, such as laws and regulations. For example, some public policies may determine reimbursement rates for a program or have a bearing on its grant funding. Other policies pertain to regulation of a program, regulation of technologies used by it, or licensure of the participants who work in it. There are also public policies that have an impact on the direct work of programs. Seat belt and motorcycle helmet laws are obviously of interest to programs focused on highway safety, and laws related to smoking in public places are of interest to programs focused on smoking cessation. The impact of public policies on health programs makes effectively communicating with the public sector important.

Managers have two categories of responsibilities in regard to communicating with the public sector. First, they are receivers of information from the public sector. They must acquire sufficient information to understand the consequences for their programs of events and forces in the public sector. In effect, they listen to the public sector by tracking and assessing decisions and actions in that sector.

In addition to receiving information from the public sector, managers also send information to this sector. They do this to influence the formulation of new policies, modification of existing policies, and implementation of policies in ways that support their programs. So long as these efforts to shape policies are made ethically and through appropriate means, such as advocacy, managers are acting responsibly. Managers have many available avenues through which to help influence public policies. For example, they can work with legislators to include relevant issues on the policy agenda and formulate new or revised laws. They can also participate in rule making by offering expert opinions as rules are developed or revised (Longest 2010).

Advocacy is a primary mechanism through which program managers can influence public policy, using various forms of communication. Figure 6.6 illustrates *advocacy* as a six-step process: analysis, strategy, mobilization, action, evaluation, and continuity. For more information about these steps, refer to www.jhuccp.org/sites/default/files/A%20Frame%20for%20 advocacy%20color.pdf.

Communicating When Something Goes Wrong

Figure 6.7 indicates the types of things that can go wrong in clinical settings. One of the verities of life for managers of health programs is that on occasion, even in well-managed programs, something will go wrong (Kohn, Corrigan, and Donaldson 2000; Smith et al. 2012). After all, many programs employ, under fallible human direction, dangerous drugs, devices, and procedures in their battles against disease and injury. The situation is complicated by the fact that these mechanisms are employed on behalf of people at vulnerable stages or moments in their lives, people who often have an inflated and unrealistic expectation of what can be done for them or their loved ones (Chuang, Ginsburg, and Berta 2007).

Clinical mishaps are not the only potential problems in health programs. Often a program is also an important economic entity in the organization in which it is embedded, and a larger program may even play an important economic role in its community. Programs employ people, buy goods and services, and generate costs for others who pay for their services. The finances and operations of programs present another set of things that can possibly go wrong. Financial problems in health programs not only affect internal stakeholders but also may have ramifications for external stakeholders. Indeed, health programs provide many opportunities for things to go wrong, and for there to be serious consequences when they do. It is on such untoward occasions that managers' actions may matter the most.

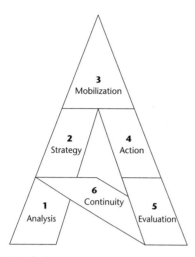

Analysis
Analysis is the step to effective advocacy, just as it is the first step to any effective action. Activities or advocacy efforts designed to have an impact on public policy start with accurate information and in-depth understanding of the problem, the people involved, the policies, the implementation or non-implementation of those policies, the organizations, and the channels of access to influential people and decision makers. The stronger the foundation of knowledge on these elements, the more persuasive the advocacy can be.

Strategy
Every advocacy effort needs a strategy. The strategy phase builds upon the analysis phase to direct, plan, and focus on specific goals and to position the advocacy effort with clear paths to achieve those goals and objectives.

Mobilization
Coalition-building strengthens advocacy. Events, activities, messages, and materials must be designed with our objectives, audiences, partnerships, and resources clearly in mind. They should have maximum positive impact on the policy-makers and maximum participation by all coalition members, while minimizing responses from the opposition.

Action
Keeping all partners together and persisting In making the case are both essential In carrying out advocacy. Repeating the message and using the credible materials developed over and over help to keep attention and concern on the Issue.

Evaluation
Advocacy efforts must be evaluated as carefully as any other communication campaign. Since advocacy often provides partial results, an advocacy team needs to measure regularly and objectively what has been accomplished and what more remains to be done. Process evaluation may be more important and more difficult than Impact evaluation.

Continuity
Advocacy, like communication. Is an ongoing process rather than a single policy or piece of legislation. Planning for continuity means articulating long-term goals, keeping functional coalitions together, and keeping data and arguments in tune with changing situations.

Figure 6.6   "A" Frame for Advocacy

Source: Adapted from Center for Communication Programs. *"A" Frame for Advocacy.* Baltimore, MD: Johns Hopkins University, Bloomberg School of Public Health, 1999. Adapted with permission.

Diagnostic

Error or delay in diagnosis
Failure to employ indicated test
Use of outmoded tests or therapy
Failure to act on results of
monitoring or testing

Preventative

Failure to provide prophylactic
treatment
Inadequate monitoring of
condition or progress or
inadequate follow-up treatment

Treatment

Error in the performance of an
operation, procedure, or test
Error in administering the
treatment
Error in the dose or method of
using a drug
Avoidable delay in treatment or
in responding to an abnormal test
Inappropriate (not indicated) care

Other

Failure of communication
Equipment failure
Other system failure

Figure 6.7   Types of Errors in Clinical Settings
Source: Adapted with permission from Leape, Lucian L., Ann G. Lawthers, Troyen A. Brennan, and William G. Johnson. "Preventing Medical Injury." *Quality Review Bulletin* 19, no. 5 (May 1993): 144–149.

Consequences When Something Goes Wrong

There are direct and indirect consequences when something goes wrong in a health program. Clinical mistakes can directly cause pain and suffering, even death. Downsizing, laying participants off, or terminating a program due to funding shortages is obviously felt directly by those who work in the affected program, but the effects may also ripple out into the surrounding community.

A health program often is an integral component of a habitable, stable community. People want a network of supportive institutions in their community. In addition to valuing jobs and economic security, people also tend to value good schools; comforting centers of religious life; responsive government entities; an effective public safety system; and accessible, high-quality health services. Anything that diminishes these vital signs of stability and well-being also diminishes the quality of life. If something goes seriously wrong in a visible health program, it will invariably have a disturbing effect on its internal and external stakeholders and intensify the need for effective communication.

What Managers Can Do When Things Go Wrong

The approaches managers can take to address the fact that things can go wrong in a program are conceptually similar to what clinicians do to ensure the safety of their patients. Both clinicians and managers focus on preventing things from going wrong. When something does go wrong, however, the focus shifts to containing and minimizing the damage. Finally, the focus centers on addressing the consequences of the negative event.

In seeking to prevent mishaps, to contain and minimize the resulting damage when they do occur, and to address their consequences, managers make important decisions and take specific actions. Throughout, communication is vital. The activities managers undertake to manage and communicate about mishaps are considered next.

Preventing Things from Going Wrong

In attempting to prevent the occurrence of negative events, managers are increasingly turning to integrated sets of activities aimed at making certain that the right things are done, that they are done correctly, and that they are done correctly the first time (White and Griffith 2010). As is discussed more fully in Chapter 7, these sets of activities go by various names. A popular one is continuous quality improvement (CQI), or simply quality improvement efforts (James and Savitz 2011). These integrated sets of activities are referred to in Chapter 7 in terms of a total quality (TQ) approach, which is discussed extensively. Each of these sets of activities relies heavily on communication.

Regardless of what they are called, these substantial and organized efforts focus on continuous improvement in performance (including preventing the occurrence of negative events) and provide a framework within which undesirable events, at least those under the control of managers, can be avoided or minimized. The framework works best in combination with activities designed to reduce risk and reap the benefits of organizational learning (Smith et al. 2012). Although there is no way to avoid all unwanted occurrences, concerted efforts can help reduce the frequency and severity of such events in health programs.

Containing and Minimizing the Damage

No matter how hard managers work to prevent it, and no matter what means they employ to this end, things will go wrong in health programs—at which point managers shift their focus to containing and minimizing the damage. In seeking to do this, managers engage in activities that are guided by concepts of and models for assessing and controlling performance. (You may wish to review the section on this topic in Chapter 2.)

In controlling, managers seek to ensure that the processes used in their domain of responsibility, as well as the results achieved in their domain, are continuously monitored; that the results are assessed; and, when necessary, that interventions are undertaken to contain the damage caused when something has gone wrong. In addition, the CQI or TQ programs and the risk management programs instituted to prevent problems also should include elements intended to help contain the damage when such events occur.

In exerting control, managers seek to regulate activities and events in accordance with preestablished plans and standards. When managers exercise control effectively, they quickly notice deviations from established standards and take corrective actions to curb the damage that might otherwise be done. Both the detection of deviations and the corrective responses rely on good communication between managers and other participants.

The reality is, however, that when prevention fails, regardless of how well the resulting damage has been contained, some damage will have been done. As noted previously, damage done in health programs often has significant direct and indirect consequences for both internal and external stakeholders. When things go wrong, the manager's focus eventually shifts to addressing the consequences.

Addressing the Consequences

Before anything constructive can be done to address the consequences of something's having gone wrong in a program, those who suffer the consequences must be identified. Sometimes this is easily done. Patients/customers who are harmed, their families, participants who are injured on the job or who are laid off, and their families, endure obvious consequences. Less obvious, perhaps, is that potential patients/customers and other participants who learn of such events and whose feelings about a program are subsequently less positive are also experiencing consequences.

Indeed, when something goes wrong in a health program, there may be consequences for many individuals, groups, and organizations. Collectively, those who might be harmed when things go wrong are the same as those who stand to benefit when things go right: the program's internal and external stakeholders. The best way for managers to fully understand and appreciate the consequences of events for stakeholders is through communicating with them, or at least with representative samples of them.

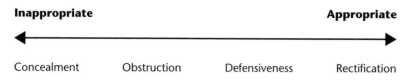

Figure 6.8   Continuum of Management Responses When Something Goes Wrong

Once those directly or indirectly affected have been identified, the ethically sound goal of fully addressing the consequences of a negative event requires restoring these stakeholders as closely as possible to positions and conditions extant before the event. Achieving this goal across the board may not be possible (some wrongs can never be righted), but it is the appropriate goal and should guide decisions and actions, including how the manager communicates with stakeholders.

Each instance in which something has gone wrong requires its own unique set of decisions and actions to appropriately manage the event's consequences. There are few hard-and-fast rules to guide managers in developing this set of decisions and actions, although their potential decisions and actions range along a rather clear-cut continuum of appropriateness, as illustrated in Figure 6.8.

Concealment   At one end of the continuum of responses managers can have in addressing the consequences of adverse events, the most inappropriate one is characterized by attempts to conceal the fact that something has gone wrong—by doing and communicating as little as possible about what has happened or, in the extreme, by telling lies and misleading others about what has happened.

Obstruction   Somewhat less extreme is to respond by acknowledging that something has gone wrong, but to deny wrongdoing, avoid or minimize responsibility, and take no action to address the consequences. A manager who is guided by a preference for this type of obstructive response will probably seek to communicate only minimally about a negative event.

Defensiveness   A third type of response when something has gone wrong is defensiveness. In this case, the manager (or another spokesperson) follows the letter of the law when taking action or communicating about what has gone wrong. This is a common response to serious negative events and reflects the intention to minimize legal liability. Decisions and actions based on this approach may be entirely legal, but they also can be far from the ethical high ground.

A defensive response to dealing with the consequences of a negative event partly reflects how costly taking responsibility can be. Addressing serious problems involving human health and life can be very expensive. But a defensive approach may be taken even when the problems have to do with layoffs, program service reductions or terminations, or other operational issues that affect internal or external stakeholders. Managers can find themselves conflicted in choosing between fully addressing the consequences of untoward events and upholding their responsibility to preserve a program's financial assets, good name, and reputation. But the defensive position, so often occupied when something goes wrong, falls short of being the most appropriate response.

Rectification   At the most appropriate end of the continuum of responses in Figure 6.8 is rectification. Rectification is characterized by accepting responsibility for what has gone wrong and undertaking aggressive actions to address the consequences for, and rectify the harm done to, all those who have been affected—a process that includes communicating extensively with them.

Managers who pursue a rectification response take a positive and proactive stance when it comes to addressing negative consequences. Their decisions and resultant actions reflect this stance. Communication is characterized by openness and candor about what went wrong, why, and the actions being taken to deal with the consequences.

The pattern of how a program manager responds to negative events builds on itself. Responses characterized by concealment, obstruction, and, to a large extent, defensiveness, once detected by stakeholders, increase distrust and invite intensified scrutiny of the immediate situation and of similar future situations. In contrast, a program with an established history of undertaking rectification responses when things go wrong builds trust among its stakeholders. In light of such a history, stakeholders waste little or no effort wondering whether they are being given all relevant information about a negative event or about the program manager's determination to fully address its consequences. The payoff for the program that behaves in this way includes an easier and faster return to equilibrium with its stakeholders after an unfortunate event.

Summary

Communicating is defined as a "two-way process of reaching mutual understanding, in which participants not only exchange (encode-decode) information, news, ideas and feelings, but also create and share meaning" (BusinessDictionary 2014). Communicating involves senders (individuals, groups, or organizations) conveying ideas, intentions, and information to receivers (also individuals, groups, or organizations). Communication is effective when receivers understand ideas, intentions, and information as senders intend.

Communication is not restricted to words; it includes all methods (verbal and nonverbal) through which meaning is conveyed. The technical process of communication is modeled in Figure 6.3. Particular attention is given to the contextual and interpersonal barriers to effective communication and to the means available to managers for overcoming those barriers.

Managers must be concerned with two basic types of communication: communication that is internal to a program, and communication with the program's external stakeholders. Communication within a program depends on formal channels and networks to transmit information and understanding in all directions as well as on widespread, effective use of these channels. Communication flows downward, upward, horizontally, and diagonally in programs. Flows in each direction have characteristics that make them useful for specific purposes. For example, as illustrated in Figure 6.4, downward flows facilitate organizational superiors' communication of information, orders, and instructions to organizational subordinates.

Coexisting with formal communication flows are informal communication flows, which consist of channels and networks (the grapevine) that arise naturally from the interpersonal relationships among the participants in programs.

Managers increasingly are concerning themselves with communication between programs and external stakeholders. Effective formal and informal communication flows to and from external stakeholders are important in successfully managing programs. Examples of important communication with external stakeholders include marketing a program's services, monitoring regulatory changes in government agencies that might affect a program, or lobbying for more favorable reimbursement rates for services provided by a program.

As discussed in this chapter, the best way to manage negative events in health programs is to prevent their occurrence. Carefully orchestrated continuous quality improvement or total quality efforts can be beneficial in preventing or minimizing the occurrence of problems. When prevention fails, however, managers must turn their attention to containing the damage that flows from unwanted events and to addressing their consequences. In this, managers are best served by aggressive, positive, and proactive efforts to identify the harmed stakeholders, to return them as much as is possible to the positions and conditions they experienced before the event, and to communicate with them openly and extensively in doing so.

REVIEW QUESTIONS

1. Define communicating, and draw a model of the basic communication process.

2. Describe both contextual and interpersonal barriers to communicating effectively in programs, and identify ways these barriers can be managed.

3. Describe the directional flows of communication within health programs, and give an example of each type of flow.

4. Describe three common types of communication networks, and give an example of each.

5. Discuss the role of informal communication in programs.

6. Identify two especially important external stakeholders for programs, and discuss communication with them.

7. Discuss the role of communication with both internal and external stakeholders when something goes wrong in a health program.

KEY TERMS AND CONCEPTS

advocacy

boundary spanners

channels

communicating

communication flows

communication networks

communication process

contextual and interpersonal barriers

decoded

encoded

feedback

grapevine

message

receivers

senders

stakeholder map

stakeholder relations

References

Berkowitz, Eric N. *Essentials of Health Care Marketing*, 3rd ed. Burlington, MA: Jones & Bartlett Learning, 2011.

BusinessDictionary. "Communication." Accessed May 20, 2014. http://www.businessdictionary.com/definition/communication.html

Chuang, You-Ta, Liane Ginsburg, and Whitney B. Berta. "Learning from Preventable Adverse Events in Health Care Organizations: Development of a Multilevel

Model of Learning and Propositions." *Health Care Management Review* 32, no. 4 (October-December 2007): 330–340.

Dunn, Rose T. *Dunn and Haimann's Healthcare Management*, 9th ed. Chicago: Health Administration Press, 2010.

Freeman, R. Edward. *Strategic Management: A Stakeholder Approach*. New York: Cambridge University Press, 2010.

Freeman, R. Edward, Jeffrey S. Harrison, Andrew C. Wicks, Bidhan L. Parmar, and Simone DeColle. *Stakeholder Theory: The State of the Art*. New York: Cambridge University Press, 2010.

Harris, Thomas E., and John C. Sherblom. *Small Group and Team Communication*, 5th ed. Boston: Pearson Education, 2011.

James, Brent C., and Lucy A. Savitz. "How Intermountain Trimmed Health Care Costs through Robust Quality Improvement Efforts." *Health Affairs* 30, no. 6 (June 2011): 1185–1191.

Kohn, Linda T., Janet M. Corrigan, and Molla S. Donaldson, eds. *To Err Is Human: Building a Safer Health System*. Washington, DC: National Academies Press, 2000.

Kovner, Anthony R., Ann Scheck McAlearney, and Duncan Neuhauser. *Health Services Management: Readings, Cases, and Commentary*, 9th ed. Chicago: Health Administration Press, 2009.

Longest, Beaufort B., Jr. *Health Policymaking in the United States*, 5th ed. Chicago: Health Administration Press, 2010.

O'Rourke, James S. *Management Communication: A Case Analysis Approach*, 5th ed. Upper Saddle River, NJ: Prentice Hall, 2012.

Pride, William M., and O. C. Ferrell. *Marketing*, 17th ed. Mason, OH: South-Western, Cengage Learning, 2014.

Rice, James A. *Leadership Insights*. La Jolla, CA: International Health Summit, 2003.

Richmond, Virginia Peck, James C. McCroskey, and Larry Powell. *Organizational Communication for Survival*, 5th ed. Upper Saddle River, NJ: Pearson, 2012.

Robbins, Stephen P., and Mary Coulter. *Management*, 12th ed. Upper Saddle River, NJ: Pearson, 2013.

Seglin, Jeffrey L. "Ethics: Good for Goodness' Sake." *CFO* 18, no. 10 (October 2002): 75–77.

Smith, Mark, Robert Sanders, Leigh Stuckhardt, and J. Michael McGinnis, eds. *Best Care at Lower Cost: The Path to Continuously Learning Health Care in America*. Washington, DC: National Academies Press, 2012.

White, Kenneth R., and John R. Griffith. *The Well-Managed Healthcare Organization*, 7th ed. Chicago: Health Administration Press, 2010.

CHAPTER 7

MANAGING QUALITY—TOTALLY

Managers of health programs typically place a high priority on effectively managing the quality of services provided. Not only is quality important to those who receive the services of a program, playing an important role in their future service-seeking decisions, but also it is important to professionals who work in programs. In spite of the importance of achieving quality, however, the United States is failing to reach its potential in regard to the quality of health services (Smith et al. 2012). It has been noted that over the past fifty years, systematic and sustained improvement in quality has been sought, although "with only limited success" (Chassin and Loeb 2011, 559).

Like decision making and communicating, discussed in the previous two chapters, *managing quality* is a facilitative activity that managers engage in as they perform their core activities of developing/strategizing, designing, and leading as well as the other facilitative activities (see Figure 1.4). Managing quality well is among the most challenging responsibilities for managers. A major study conducted in the British National Health Services suggested some of the reasons why it is so challenging, including "the inertia built into established ways of working, and the effort needed to implement new work processes" (Ham, Kipping, and McLeod 2003, 434).

The Institute of Medicine (2001) has given a great deal of attention to the issues of quality and safety in health care, as reflected in its list of ten things that patients/customers should be able to expect from providers of health services, no matter what the setting. Clearly an ideal to be pursued, these expectations, listed in Figure 7.1, suggest the difficulty of fully meeting the challenges associated with satisfying contemporary patients/customers in regard to the quality and safety of health services.

LEARNING OBJECTIVES

After reading this chapter, you should be able to:

- Define quality in the context of health services, and describe the two components of quality

- Understand structural, process, and outcome measures of quality

- Understand a total quality framework for managing quality in health programs

- Understand the application of the three components of a total quality approach: patient/customer focus, continuous improvement, and teamwork

1. **Beyond patient visits:** You will have the care you need when you need it . . . when-ever you need it. You will find help in many forms, not just in face-to-face visits. You will find help on the Internet, on the telephone, from many sources, by many routes, in the form you want it.
2. **Individualization:** You will be known and respected as an individual. Your choices and preferences will be sought and honored. The usual system of care will meet most of your needs. When your needs are special, the care will adapt to meet you on your own terms.
3. **Control:** The care system will take control only if and when you freely give permission.
4. **Information:** You can know what you wish to know, when you wish to know it. Your medical record is yours to keep, to read, and to understand. The rule is: "Nothing about you without you."
5. **Science:** You will have care based on the best available scientific knowledge. The system promises you excellence as its standard. Your care will not vary illogically from doctor to doctor or from place to place. The system will promise you all the care that can help you, and will help you avoid care that cannot help you.
6. **Safety:** Errors in care will not harm you. You will be safe in the care system.
7. **Transparency:** Your care will be confidential, but the care system will not keep secrets from you. You can know whatever you wish to know about the care that affects you and your loved ones.
8. **Anticipation:** Your care will anticipate your needs and will help you find the help you need. You will experience proactive help, not just reactions, to help you restore and maintain your health.
9. **Value:** Your care will not waste your time or money. You will benefit from constant innovations, which will increase the value of care to you.
10. **Cooperation:** Those who provide care will cooperate and coordinate their work fully with each other and with you. The walls between professions and institutions will crumble, so that your experiences will become seamless. You will never feel lost.

Figure 7.1   What Patients/Customers Should Expect of Health Services
Source: Institute of Medicine. *Crossing the Quality Chasm: A New Health System for the 21st Century.* Washington, DC: National Academies Press, 2001, 23. Reprinted with permission.

The challenge of managing quality is substantial, and there is much room for improvement in efforts to meet that challenge. Participants at the National Roundtable on Health Care Quality convened by the Institute of Medicine concluded, "At its best, health care in the United States is superb. Unfortunately, it is often not at its best. Problems in health care quality are serious and extensive; they occur in all delivery systems and financing mechanisms. Americans bear a great burden of harm because of these problems, a burden that is measured in lost lives, reduced functioning, and wasted resources" (Institute of Medicine, National Roundtable on Health Care Quality 1998, 11).

After defining quality as it applies to health services and describing its measurement, a total quality (TQ) framework for the systematic management of quality in health programs is presented. The total quality framework presented and discussed in this chapter includes three interconnected components: (1) patient/customer focus, (2) commitment to continuous improvement, and (3) teamwork. Before discussing these components, however, we should define quality in the health services context and discuss its measurement.

Quality Defined

Quality in the context of health services has been defined by the Institute of Medicine (1990, 21) as "the degree to which health services for individuals and populations increase the likelihood of desired health outcomes and are consistent with current professional knowledge." There are, of course, many other definitions of quality as it applies to health services. Most such definitions have been influenced by the seminal paradigm established by Avedis Donabedian, a physician and health services researcher who founded the study of quality in health services. Donabedian's (1966, 1980) paradigm described the dual nature of quality in terms of its technical and inter-personal components.

In an analysis that reviewed many definitions of quality, researchers confirmed Donabedian's perspective on quality by noting that most definitions reflect two components of quality: high technical quality and humane and culturally appropriate treatment of people (Brook, McGlynn, and Shekelle 2000). These authors used "high technical quality" to mean that "the patient receives only the procedures, tests, or services for which the desired health outcomes exceed the health risks by a sufficiently wide margin and . . . each of these procedures or services is performed in a technically excellent manner" (282). In defining the second component of quality, the authors argued "that all patients wish to be treated in a humane and culturally appropriate manner and be invited to participate fully in deciding about their therapy [treatment]" (282).

An individual's value system and the conditions and circumstances confronting him or her in a particular situation influence which component is more important to that person. A person with an immediate and acute concern, such as whether or not he or she is HIV positive, may be primarily interested in the technical expertise of those doing the testing. In contrast, people with chronic conditions, such as well-controlled diabetes, may be more concerned about being treated humanely and in a culturally sensitive manner over a long period of time.

James and Savitz (2011) characterized the two components of quality as (1) content quality and (2) delivery and service quality. Content quality means clinical expertise and the technical aspects of providing health services. Delivery and service quality means the interpersonal aspects of service provision, such as empathy and communication, and how well the requirements and expectations of patients/customers are being met in terms of such things as convenience and timeliness. For managers of health programs, both components of quality are relevant and must be addressed.

Studies using focus groups of patients and other research methods have shown that patients want their health services to be of high technical quality and to contain an appropriate interpersonal component (Gerteis et al. 2002; Smith et al. 2012). Inclusion of an appropriate interpersonal component requires that attention be given to the following:

- Patients/customers' values and preferences

- Patients/customers' physical comfort, including pain control

- Patients/customers' emotional and psychological comfort, including alleviation of fear and anxiety

- Patients/customers' need for information from and open communication with those who provide services

There is also an ethical dimension to quality. Ethics considerations and ethical issues routinely emerge in the provision of health services and in the overall management of health programs. Remember from our discussion of ethical program management in Chapter 1 that managers should be guided by the application of four key *ethics principles:* respect for persons, justice, beneficence, and nonmaleficence.

These principles may seem abstract, but they can be very useful in guiding those who seek to consider the ethical aspects of quality in health services. For example, the application of these principles can be seen in the Institute of Medicine's recommendations concerning desirable attributes of health services. These attributes and how they reflect the four key ethics principles can be described as follows (Institute of Medicine 2001, 39–40):

Safe—avoiding injuries to patients from the care that is intended to help them. [Reflects the principles of respect for persons and nonmaleficence]

Effective—providing services based on scientific knowledge to all who could benefit and refraining from providing services to those not likely to benefit (avoiding underuse and overuse). [Reflects the principles of respect for persons, justice, beneficence, and nonmaleficence]

Patient-centered—providing care that is respectful of and responsive to individual patient preferences, needs, and values and ensuring that patient values guide all clinical decisions. [Reflects the principles of respect for persons and beneficence]

Timely—reducing waits and sometimes harmful delays for both those who receive and those who give care. [Reflects the principles of respect for persons and nonmaleficence]

Efficient—avoiding waste, including waste of equipment, supplies, ideas, and energy. [Reflects the principles of respect for persons and nonmaleficence]

Equitable—providing care that does not vary in quality because of personal characteristics such as gender, ethnicity, geographic location, and socioeconomic status. [Reflects the principle of justice]

Measuring Quality

Measuring quality, including both its technical and interpersonal components, is essential to managing and improving the quality of the services provided in a program. Sometimes called *quality assessment,* the measurement of quality has its origins in the work of Donabedian (1966, 1980). He pointed out that the measurement of quality includes structural measures (innate characteristics of those who provide services and of the settings in which they are provided); process measures (what service providers do to patients/customers); and outcome measures (what happens to the health of patients/customers as a result of services). Donabedian's pioneering work offered the first conceptual framework for measuring health services quality, and it "has powerfully influenced all subsequent efforts to improve quality" (Chassin and Loeb 2011, 560).

Structural measures of quality in a health program are measures of available inputs or resources that can be associated with quality. These measures include such indicators as the number and credentials of staff; the presence of specialized, state-of-the-art equipment; the use of active peer review; and accreditation or approval by outside agencies. Process measures include indicators of compliance with protocols, such as the percentage of elderly patients/customers served who appropriately receive an influenza vaccine or whether children served receive the immunizations they need when they need them. Outcome measures include indicators that reflect changes in patients/customers' health status and level of satisfaction. These are "bottom-line" measures of how well the delivery of health services is going.

The National Quality Measures Clearinghouse, which is sponsored by the Agency for Healthcare Research and Quality (AHRQ), maintains a Web site (www.qualitymeasures.ahrq.gov) containing extensive information on specific, evidence-based quality measures and measure sets. Another Web site (www.guidelines.gov) maintained by AHRQ is for the National Guideline Clearinghouse (NGC); it contains a comprehensive database of evidence-based clinical practice guidelines.

Managing Quality

Achieving high levels of quality and safety in health programs cannot be separated from other management work. For example, the presence of five specific management practices is associated with a greater likelihood that a program will achieve a high level of quality and safety. These practices are (1) achieving a balance between requirements for productivity and requirements for quality and safety, (2) establishing and maintaining trust among participants, (3) managing the process of change effectively, (4) permitting high levels of involvement by participants in decision making, and (5) operating the program as a learning organization (Lukas et al. 2007; Page 2004; Smith et al. 2012).

Above all else, managing quality in a program requires a systematic approach. Over the years, there have been several different systematic approaches to managing quality in the delivery of health services. These are best viewed as steps in an evolutionary process leading to the contemporary approaches. Important aspects of this history are presented here as background information.

One early approach to managing quality was *quality assurance (QA)*, which has been described as a formal and systematic exercise of identifying problems in health services delivery, and then designing and implementing means to resolve these problems (Brook and Lohr 1985). In essence, QA is a process of eliminating defects (Kelly 2003), and as such is a negative process (Longest and Darr 2014). Supplanting the QA approach, *quality improvement (QI)* arose as a more positive and broader approach to managing quality.

The more positive QI approach builds on the work of such industrial-quality experts as Philip Crosby (1989), W. Edwards Deming (1982), and Joseph Juran (1989). QI has also been called *continuous quality improvement (CQI)* (Sollecito and Johnson 2013). James (1989, 4) suggested that the essence of the CQI approach to quality is to answer three questions: "Are we doing the right things? Are we doing things right? How can we be certain that we do things right the first time, every time?"

More recently, the concepts and activities of QI have been called quality management (Kelly 2003); *total quality management (TQM)* (McLaughlin and Kaluzny 1990); a total quality, or TQ approach (Dean and Bowen 1994); or simply improvement (Sollecito and Johnson 2013). Other approaches include Six Sigma, Lean, Plan-Do-Check-Act, and hybrid approaches (Lighter 2013).

Contemporary approaches to quality tend to be conceptually broad and often reflect a management philosophy of careful attention to quality (Chassin and Loeb 2011; Kaplan et al. 2010). Although the variety of terms and associated abbreviations can be confusing, these newer approaches to improving quality and safety are characterized by the application of similar principles, practices, and techniques. Above all else, they are characterized by their use of robust *process improvement* techniques and their systematic nature. According to Chassin and Loeb (2011, 564), the systematicness of these approaches means that they incorporate the following tasks:

- Reliably measuring the magnitude of a problem
- Identifying the root causes of the problem and determining the importance of each cause
- Finding solutions for the most important causes
- Proving the effectiveness of those solutions
- Ensuring sustained improvements over time

A Total Quality Approach to Managing Quality

In keeping with the value of taking a systematic approach to managing quality, which we are calling a *total quality (TQ)* framework, three things should guide managers in managing quality in health programs: (1) patient/customer focus, (2) commitment to continuous improvement, and (3) teamwork (Dean and Bowen 1994). Figure 7.2 illustrates the interconnected nature of the components that underpin a TQ approach.

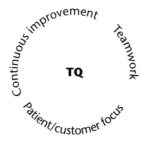

Figure 7.2   Components of a TQ Approach to Managing Quality

Patient/customer focus requires managers in pursuit of quality to identify what a program's patients/customers need and want, and then to design and deliver services that satisfy those needs and wants. Patient/customer focus, or a patient/customer-focused approach, does not mean simply agreeing with the patient/customer at all times. "Rather, it entails meaningful awareness, discussion, and engagement among patient (or customer), family, and clinician on the evidence, risks and benefits, options, and decisions in play" (Smith et al. 2012, 15).

Commitment to continuous improvement requires managers to continuously examine and refine the processes through which services are provided. Ongoing efforts to improve the performance of health services delivery in the United States has resulted in a situation that can accurately be described as one in which "pockets of excellence coexist with enormously variable performance across the delivery system" (Chassin and Loeb 2011, 562).

Finally, teamwork is an important component of a TQ approach to managing quality because achieving quality is a collective responsibility of all those involved in a program. Teams, which are collections of individuals who share interdependent tasks and responsibility for outcomes or results (LaFasto and Larson 2001; Smith and Imbrie 2013), if they work together smoothly and effectively, can contribute to a program's ability to achieve quality in the delivery of health services.

The patient/customer focus, continuous improvement, and teamwork triad of a TQ approach can be used in the smallest program or in the largest corporation. For example, General Electric (2014), one of the world's largest and most successful corporations, has said that customer, process, and employee are the three key elements of quality, and that "everything [it does] to remain a world-class quality company focuses on these three essential elements." In the health services context, Hospital Corporation of America (2014), one of the nation's largest providers of health services, has said that it "puts patients first and works to constantly improve the care [it gives] them by implementing measures that support [its] caregivers, help ensure patient safety and provide the highest possible quality."

Each of the three components of a TQ approach to managing quality—patient/customer focus, commitment to continuous improvement, and teamwork—is described in more detail in the following sections.

Patient/Customer Focus

The purpose of the ***patient/customer focus*** component of a TQ approach to managing quality (see Figure 7.2) is to make certain that services that satisfy patients/customers' wants and needs are designed and delivered. For example, Stanford Hospital & Clinics (2014) has said that it "prioritizes quality improvement initiatives based on the positive impact the plan will have for patients and their families." Patient/customer satisfaction is a vital element in the long-term success of any program.

The prominent place of patient/customer focus in the selection criteria for the Malcolm Baldrige National Quality Award Program reflects the importance in this organization's view of focusing on patients/customers in achieving overall performance excellence in health programs (National Institute of Standards and Technology 2014). The award criteria are intended to encourage managers to take an integrated approach to performance management. To compete for the award, health services organizations must have a patient/customer focus that is evidenced by how the organization engages its patients/customers through listening to them and building relationships with them.

An effective patient/customer focus requires first that patients/customers be carefully identified. As is discussed fully in Chapter 8, health programs can have many different patients/customers and other stakeholders. Although in a TQ approach managers must concern themselves with all of them, patients/customers who receive services are typically the primary focus for health programs. After all, the provision of services to patients/customers is the principal reason such programs exist.

Continuous Improvement

The second component of a TQ approach to managing quality is ***continuous improvement (CI),*** as shown in Figure 7.2. Underpinning this component is the concept that by continuously improving their processes, programs can more completely meet the needs and wants of their patients/customers. CI can be defined as "a structured organizational process for involving personnel in planning and executing a continuous flow of improvements to provide quality health care that meets or exceeds expectations" (Sollecito and Johnson 2013, 4).

Certainly, in the complex processes through which health services are provided in programs, there are many opportunities for improvement. These opportunities are inherent in the idea that a goal for health services can be achieving perfection or near perfection in their provision. For example, Chassin (1998, 578) stated such goals as follows:

• Always providing effective health services to those who could benefit from them

- Always avoiding the provision of ineffective health services

- Eliminating all preventable complications in the health services that are provided

Although realistically absolute perfection is not attainable in the provision of health services in any setting, contemporary CI efforts increasingly involve establishing goals at very high levels, including those that might encourage programs to achieve performance that approaches perfection. Three of the most popular CI approaches, widely used in health services settings, are described in the next three subsections.

Six Sigma

Sigma is a statistical term that simply refers to standard deviation, and when applied to CI it can be used to measure how much a given process deviates from perfection (Barry, Murcko, and Brubaker 2002; Inozu et al. 2012). Technically, the statistical term *six sigma*, from which the **Six Sigma** approach draws its name, means that in a process governed by a normal distribution, values more than six standard deviations away from the average will occur only 3.4 times in a million opportunities. This very small number, when practically applied to QI, means that errors in a process would occur only 3.4 times in a million opportunities. Although not perfection, this is very close to it.

The central idea behind Six Sigma is that if the number of defects or errors existing in a process can be measured, then steps can be taken to move the process as close to zero defects as possible. Six Sigma is data driven and relies on extensive use of statistical analysis. As Revere and Black (2003) noted, Six Sigma complements, embellishes, and expands CI, especially in that the goals developed in the Six Sigma approach are very aggressive. Adopters of the Six Sigma approach to CI typically follow these steps in their efforts to improve performance:

Step 1: Identify a critical process where improved performance is important.

Step 2: Quantify present performance by measurement and statistical analysis, and have present performance serve as a baseline.

Step 3: Consider possible changes to improve the process.

Step 4: Implement changes on a trial basis.

Step 5: Monitor and assess the implementation experience.

Step 6: Extend successful changes, and make them permanent.

Step 7: Monitor the new process on an ongoing basis to ensure stability.

Step 8: Identify another process to be improved, and repeat the cycle.

Toyota Production System

Another popular contemporary approach to CI is the *Toyota Production System (TPS)* (Black and Miller 2008; Kenney 2011; Liker and Franz 2011). Over many years, the Toyota Motor Manufacturing Corporation developed a set of principles that facilitate a self-reflective process involving designing, testing, and improving work so that all participants contribute at or near their full potential. According to Spear and Bowen (1999, 98), "Toyota uses a rigorous problem-solving process that requires a detailed assessment of the current state of affairs and a plan for improvement that is, in effect, an experimental test of the proposed changes." These authors also described the principles that underlie TPS, noting that this approach to CI is built on ideas about how people work, how they connect with other people in performing work, and how production processes are best set up. Above all else, in their view, the success of TPS lies in teaching all participants how to use the scientific method in pursuing improvement.

FOCUS-PDCA Model

Although Six Sigma and TPS incorporate unique features, they are based on the fundamental conceptual approach underlying all comprehensive CI efforts: the *FOCUS-PDCA model.* Figure 7.3 shows the complete FOCUS-PDCA model, which is the oldest CI model yet is still widely used (Tague 2004). The FOCUS part of the model's name derives from the following:

Find a process to improve.

Organize an improvement team and necessary resources.

Clarify current knowledge about the process.

Understand the process and sources of variation in it.

Select an improvement or intervention.

The PDCA part of the model's name is based on a model developed by Walter A. Shewhart at Bell Laboratories in the 1930s. Shewhart observed that constant evaluation of processes is essential to CI, along with the willingness of managers to adopt or reject changes in the processes based on evidence of their utility. Establishing what has come to be called the

Step 1: Find a process to improve.

↓

Step 2: Organize an improvement team and necessary resources.

↓

Step 3: Clarify current knowledge about the process.

↓

Step 4: Understand the process and sources of variation in it.

↓

Step 5: Select an improvement or intervention.

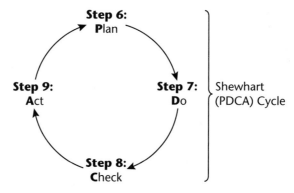

Figure 7.3   FOCUS-PDCA Model

Shewhart Cycle, he developed the Plan-Do-Check-Act (PDCA) cycle to guide managers in their efforts to make process improvements, with managers first planning an action intended to improve a process (the action having been chosen based on careful study of the process), then implementing the action on a small scale, then checking to see how results conform to the plan, and then acting on what has been learned. The Shewhart cycle has the manager proceed in improving a process by following these steps:

Plan how to implement the improvement or intervention.

Do the improvement or intervention by initiating it, often on a small scale at first.

Check the results of the early implementation of the improvement or intervention.

Act on what was learned in the "check" step. If the improvement or intervention was successful, incorporate it on a larger scale and make it permanent. If it wasn't successful, go through the cycle again with a different plan.

Applied Example of the Use of the FOCUS-PDCA Model

The work of a CI team established in a family practice program provides an example of the application of the FOCUS-PDCA model (Schwarz, Landis, and Rowe 1999). This team attempted to improve the care of people with type 2 diabetes using the model as a guide, proceeding through the steps in Figure 7.3 as follows:

Step 1: Find a process to improve. The program's CI team's efforts began as many do, with consideration of how the program's processes compared to so-called best practices. The program manager wanted to be certain that the care of patients measured up to the best practice standards in caring for patients with type 2 diabetes. In effect, one of the most basic CI tools, benchmarking, was used as a means of identifying a process to improve. Unless current performance of a process measures up to the corresponding benchmark, it is a candidate for improvement.

Benchmarking is a process whereby those pursuing CI establish operating targets that are based on leading performance standards for particular processes. Benchmarks are more than mere metrics against which to judge performance. Benchmarking reflects a philosophy that, when applied, guides CI activities toward the goal of achieving the best possible performance in processes. This goal is pursued through emulating the performance levels achieved by those performing processes in an exemplary or benchmark-worthy manner. The use of benchmarking requires managers and others involved in CI to identify whom or what to benchmark, collect information on best practice standards, and use the information to guide CI efforts.

Step 2: Organize an improvement team and necessary resources. The CI team was formed by the program manager based on each member's knowledge of the process to be improved. The members were a physician, a nurse, and a laboratory technician. A representative from the business office served as a consultant to the team. The physician member was the team leader, and another member who had been trained in facilitation served as the facilitator. (More information on teams and teamwork is provided in a subsequent section in this chapter.)

Step 3: Clarify current knowledge about the process. The CI team conducted a literature review to gather information about appropriate clinical guidelines for the care of patients with diabetes, then collected and reviewed data concerning the program's patients. In undertaking the literature review, they focused on the process through which patients with type 2 diabetes were seen in well-run programs, and they became especially interested in whether their own program's patients were receiving appropriate hemoglobin A1c (HbA1c) tests. (The HbA1c test is an excellent way to monitor blood sugar levels in patients over three-month periods.)

To establish a baseline of information in their own program, the CI team identified all patients who had the type 2 diabetes diagnosis during the past year. The team audited a random sample of these patients' charts to determine the program's rate of ordering HbA1c tests, as well as the average HbA1c value. After reviewing the results, the team decided they could improve diabetes management by increasing the number of patients who received at least two HbA1c tests per year.

Step 4: Understand the process and sources of variation in it. The processes through which health services are provided comprise operations, steps, or activities through which people, materials, or information flows. One of the best ways to understand a process is to carefully document or chart it to identify places where improvements can be made. Flow charting involves establishing the boundaries of a process; identifying the steps in the process and their sequence; and showing the flow of people, materials, or information.

Figure 7.4 is a flowchart developed by the CI team to help them understand the care process for patients with type 2 diabetes. Symbols are used in flowcharts to illustrate what happens in each step of a process: for example, a parallelogram represents the starting point, a rectangle represents a task or activity performed during the process, a diamond represents a yes-no decision point, and an oval represents the end point of the process.

Step 5: Select an improvement or intervention. Based on the previous steps, the CI team decided that a potentially useful improvement or intervention was to attach a reminder form to the first page of the medical record at every encounter with every patient who had been diagnosed with type 2 diabetes. This form provided guidelines on the frequency of tests and procedures to improve care of these patients. The form and its use constituted the team's selected improvement or intervention.

Step 6: Plan how to implement the improvement or intervention. Planning is vital to the successful implementation of any improvement or intervention. In seeking to implement the use of diabetes care reminders, the CI team found that the office, nursing, and laboratory staff, as well as physicians, needed instructions about how to use the new reminders. They also had to decide who would print out the reminders, who would ensure that they were attached to the first page of each medical record, and who would enter the laboratory values on that record. All of this required careful planning.

Step 7: Do the improvement or intervention by initiating it, often on a small scale at first. The CI team initiated the intervention by having the

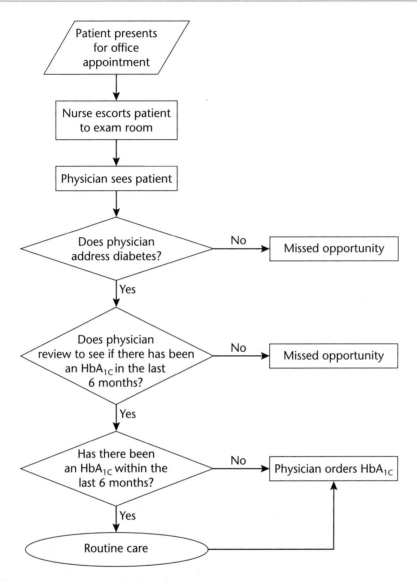

Figure 7.4   Pre-Intervention Flowchart of the Patient Care Process
Source: Reprinted with permission from "A Team Approach to Quality Improvement," April 1999, Vol 6, No. 4, *Family Practice Management.* Copyright © 1999 American Academy of Family Physicians. All rights reserved.

reminder forms attached to all medical records for all encounters with patients with the diabetes diagnosis, and by encouraging the use of the reminder forms.

Step 8: Check the results of the early implementation of the improvement or intervention. It is important that improvements or interventions be monitored to determine if they are having the desired effect. This step may trigger necessary revisions before an improvement or intervention is considered completely developed. In checking on whether their intervention was improving diabetes care, the CI team monitored changes in the frequency with which HbA1c tests were ordered.

Step 9: Act on what was learned in the "check" step. If an improvement or intervention was deemed successful, the CI team could incorporate it on a larger scale and make it permanent. If not, they could go through the cycle again with a different plan. The CI team was very pleased with the intervention and the resulting improvement in care for patients. They gave each physician in the program individualized and program-wide data on the more appropriate use of the HbA1c test, and celebrated their success with a catered lunch.

Looking to the future, the team established two goals: that 80 percent of the program's patients with type 2 diabetes would have all tests and procedures completed (and documented on the reminder form), and that 80 percent would have their most recent HbA1c values at less than 7.5 percent. To meet these goals, the CI team planned to explore additional improvements or interventions, including automatic HbA1c reminders for patients and educational support group sessions for patients.

Step 9 reflects the reality that CI is an ongoing process. Not only can successful improvements or interventions be identified and made permanent, but also successes can stimulate and encourage participants to look for additional opportunities to improve processes.

Whether an approach to CI is Six Sigma, Toyota Production System, FOCUS-PDCA, or something else, effective, systematic approaches to process improvement all share the common characteristic that they begin with diagnosing something about a process that needs to be changed and extend through to the implementation and evaluation of changes that are made to that process. The steps are similar to those routinely taken in managing changes. Longest (1998), for example, described these steps as identification, planning and preparation, implementation, and evaluation. The steps in a CI approach are also similar to those in the general approach to making good management decisions discussed in Chapter 5 (see Figure 5.2).

Tools for CI

Going beyond the benchmarking and flow charting noted previously, several additional tools are useful in conducting CI activities (Spath 2013)—especially in determining what should be changed about a process to improve it.

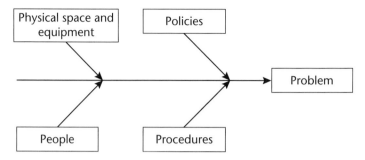

Figure 7.5   Generalized Cause-and-Effect (Fishbone) Diagram

Cause-and-Effect (Fishbone) Diagram

One of the simplest and most useful tools is a ***cause-and-effect diagram,*** also popularly known as a fishbone diagram because of its shape. The fishbone pattern is readily visible in Figure 7.5, a generalized cause-and-effect diagram. You may wish to review Figure 5.3, which is a specific example of the application of a cause-and-effect diagram.

Use of this diagram in determining the possible causes of a problem in a process and in deciding what can be done to improve that process is based on organizing the examination or study of the process. Is the problem noted in Figure 7.5 caused by something people are doing or not doing? Is it a matter of inadequate equipment or a poor layout in terms of the physical space? Perhaps the problem is caused in part by a confusing policy or an incomplete procedural protocol. A carefully constructed fishbone diagram of the potential causes of a problem often yields multiple causes or process variables that can be changed to improve the process.

Pareto Chart

Because problems may have numerous underlying causes, another useful tool in CI is a ***Pareto chart,*** which is a bar graph that can show the relative importance of elements in a process that contribute to a problem. For example, the Pareto chart depicted in Figure 5.4, which you may wish to review, shows the relative importance of process variables in causing cases of nosocomial pneumonia. In that instance, a Pareto analysis determined that relatively few variables caused most of the problem. These few variables became the focus of efforts to improve the process at hand.

Run Chart

A ***run chart,*** which is a graphic representation of data over time, can be very useful in monitoring the progress of a CI intervention and in confirming that

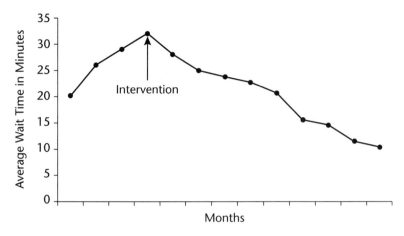

Figure 7.6   Run Chart of an Intervention to Shorten Wait Times

the intervention actually led to improvement. Figure 7.6 is a run chart of average patient wait times in a program before and after an intervention designed to shorten wait times by using better personnel scheduling practices.

This run chart shows that for several months prior to the intervention, the average patient wait time increased. Following the intervention, the average wait time declined for subsequent months, indicating that the intervention had the desired effect and improved this process.

Additional information about CI and tools to support it can be found on the Web site of the Institute for Healthcare Improvement (IHI; www.ihi.org). IHI is a nonprofit organization devoted to improving the delivery of health services. Another useful resource is the Institute for Clinical Systems Improvement (ICSI; www.icsi.org). ICSI is a collaboration of organizations also devoted to improving the delivery of health services by helping its members identify and accelerate the implementation of best clinical practices for their patients/customers.

Teamwork

The third component of a TQ approach to managing quality is *teamwork* (see Figure 7.2). Most significant improvements in processes that lead to better quality are accomplished by teams rather than by individuals. When team members work collaboratively, the knowledge, experience, and skills of individual members are combined with those of the others, usually generating more problem-solving power than any individual member possesses. The keys to achieving collaboration among team members include (1) managers' establishing an organizational culture that encourages collaboration, (2) managers' promoting and encouraging teamwork, and (3) managers' making certain that team members are responsible for working together collaboratively and cooperatively (Fallon, Begun, and Riley 2013). As noted previously, the emphasis on teamwork reflects the fact that CI is a collective responsibility of the participants in a program when a TQ approach is being taken.

Collaborative efforts in a TQ approach tend to occur in the context of what are typically called improvement teams. Such teams can be formed to address specific problems or issues, or for the more general purpose of improving performance in particular areas. In some situations, all participants in a program are thought of as a team. In other situations, smaller groups of participants form teams. In both cases, teams are collections of participants who share interdependent tasks as well as responsibility for outcomes or results.

Team Effectiveness

Managers purposefully design effective improvement teams; successful teams do not just form spontaneously. For teams to succeed at improving quality, they must be empowered. This means granting them a significant degree of control over processes, including the ability to revise processes to improve them. Managers who wish to empower improvement teams must ensure that participants have the necessary training as well as the tools and resources to bring about improvements.

Another part of empowerment is that managers must establish a climate in which participants feel comfortable participating actively in TQ efforts. A good example of this is found at University Hospitals Case Medical Center (www.uhhospitals.org/locations/case), which received the 2012 American Hospital Association–McKesson Quest for Quality Prize in recognition of its success in quality improvement efforts. In announcing the award, American Hospital Association–McKesson noted that part of the winning formula was this medical center's encouragement of employees' active roles in improving quality and their empowerment to identify and implement improvements.

Successful teams usually achieve two results that are important considerations for program managers: work is accomplished, and participants enjoy the experience. These teams are better at making process improvements, and participation in a successful team effort generally improves participants' morale and job satisfaction. Figure 7.7 summarizes the factors and the complex interactions that determine a team's effectiveness. As can

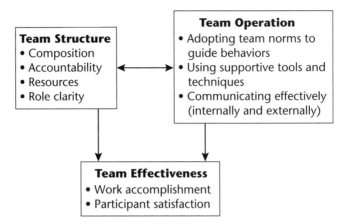

Figure 7.7   Key Determinants of Team Effectiveness

be seen in this figure, team effectiveness results from two sets of factors that a manager can influence: how teams are structured and how they operate. The following subsections address these factors.

Team Structure

In structuring and determining the composition of improvement teams, managers should consider how well potential members can work together. This consideration is secondary, however, to considerations of the knowledge or information needed and of who has or can obtain knowledge or information to accomplish improvements. Participants' difficulties in working together can usually be overcome by how a team is structured, which is discussed in this subsection, and by how a team operates, as is discussed later in the chapter. The structure of a team is a function of several variables, including composition, accountability, resources, and role clarity, as shown in Figure 7.7. Each of these structural variables in discussed in the following paragraphs.

Composition

Determination of an improvement team's composition should be guided by answers to two questions: (1) What knowledge or information is required to address a specific problem or issue or to accomplish the general objective of process improvement? (2) Who possesses or can acquire the required knowledge or information? Improvement team members typically come from within a program, but in considering team composition, managers may want to include people from outside the program. For example, a program organized to receive referrals from local hospitals may find it beneficial to include participants from those organizations as members of improvement teams or as consultants to the teams.

Accountability

A basic part of structuring an improvement team is establishing accountability for and within the team. For example, managers can appoint a team leader and imbue him or her with authority over other participants. Appointed team leaders can also be held responsible for team performance. Alternatively, managers can leave it to teams to select their own leaders or to function under a team-developed plan for rotating the role of leader. The experiences of improvement teams in many settings have shown that teams are more participative and democratic when managers assign accountability to the team and leave it to participants to negotiate the leader role as well as how the work of the team will be accomplished.

Resources

Another important structural consideration is the resources needed for a team to be effective. Resource requirements vary across situations, but all improvement teams require resources. No resource tends to be more important than appropriate training in team participation techniques and strategies for participants. Specific training in the use of the tools and techniques of CI for those who lead or facilitate improvement teams is vital to the success of the teams.

Other resource allocation decisions managers face in structuring improvement teams have to do with financial resources or budget commitments; the time allocated for participants to attend team meetings and engage in team activities; and the level of access to information needed for an improvement team to effectively address a problem or identify and make general process improvements. In regard to the last consideration, a team might, for example, need access to management reports, clinical data, regulatory requirements, and the program's strategic and operational plans.

Role Clarity

Teams also need role clarity if they are to succeed. Managers establish teams for explicit purposes. The purposes must be specified for a team, and at the outset of its work, any constraints or limits on the team must be clarified, including required timelines, budgets, or the channels the team is to use to communicate results of its work. This process of making the purpose of a team clear at the outset is sometimes called chartering a team. A team charter, which can be provided verbally but is more useful in written form, typically includes information such as the following, which is specific to a team established to address a specific process rather than to pursue more general improvements:

- A brief overview of the process to be improved

- A statement about why the process needs to be improved or considered for improvement

- A statement about how the team will demonstrate that the process has been improved

- A timeline for the team's work

- A list of resources available to the team and constraints on the team

- A description of how and to whom the team should communicate its progress and its final product

Establishing role clarity does not necessarily mean that managers impose all the norms or operational practices (which are discussed next) on a team. A team may have considerable latitude in determining for itself how it will approach resolving a problem or accomplishing an improvement. Teams formed for the general purpose of improvement, in fact, may even be free to select the problems or issues they wish to address. However, a team's freedom to establish its agenda and all aspects of a team's purpose must be clearly established as part of the team's structure.

Two specific and particularly important roles filled by team participants are those of team leader and team facilitator. It is possible, but not necessary, for these roles to be occupied by a single individual. Both roles are necessary for a team to be effective, because the work of teams has two components: task and process. The task component involves accomplishing the work for which the team has been formed—that is, making improvements in one or more processes that enhance quality or other aspects of performance. The process component of a team's work, which is essential if the task component is to be accomplished, involves how the team members work together as they interact in performing their tasks. The team's leader can focus on the task component, while its facilitator can focus on the processes of team performance. The leader keeps participants on track toward accomplishing the purposes established for or by the team, and the facilitator monitors participation and interactions, intervening as necessary to keep things working smoothly.

An improvement team whose membership composition has been carefully considered, for which accountability has been clearly established, to which necessary resources have been made available, and whose purposes have been clearly defined is more likely to be effective than a team that does not possess these advantages. But the structure of a team does not fully explain its effectiveness, either in terms of work accomplishment or participant satisfaction. To succeed, a team must also operate effectively.

Team Operation

As can be seen in Figure 7.7, team effectiveness is determined by factors associated with team structure and team operation. As with team structure, managers have a great deal to do with how teams operate, beginning with being certain that team norms are established and followed. Managers have varying levels of input into these norms, but typically they are developed within teams by members. The manager's task is to be certain that norms are developed and used.

Adopting Team Norms to Guide Behaviors

Team operation requires that teams adopt and use norms that can guide individual participant and team behaviors. A team norm is a "standard that is shared by team members and regulates member behavior" (Fried, Topping, and Edmondson 2012, 138). How teams develop norms is largely influenced by how accountability and responsibility for and within a team are established by managers. Operational norms can be imposed by managers, or managers can permit teams themselves to determine them. The latter is usually a better approach.

Norms that support an improvement team's operation include the following examples: being committed to continuous improvement, attending and participating in team meetings regularly, valuing achievement of consensus in decision making, giving full attention to tasks, respecting diverse opinions and views, and accepting responsibility for the team's success. The most important operational norm for improvement teams is commitment to continuous improvement. This commitment by team members can be buttressed in part by the program manager's commitment to improvement.

Using Supportive Tools and Techniques

A second team operation variable that influences effectiveness is a team's use of supportive CI tools and techniques. Several of these tools and techniques have been described previously, including benchmarking, flow charting, cause-and-effect (fishbone) diagrams, Pareto charts, and run charts. Also useful to improvement teams are strategies to accomplish

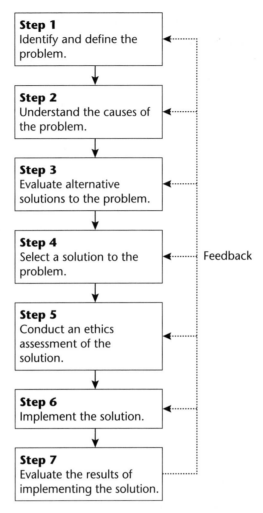

Figure 7.8   Model of the Problem-Solving Process for Improvement Teams

such group processes as conflict resolution and negotiation (LaFasto and Larson 2001; Runde and Flanagan 2010).

Improvement teams often benefit from considering themselves problem-solving groups and using a basic problem-solving process model as an integral technique in their work. Figure 7.8 is one such model. Please note that this problem-solving process model bears a close resemblance to the basic decision-making process model shown in Figure 5.2.

Communicating Effectively (Internally and Externally)

A final team operation variable that is crucial to team effectiveness is how well a team communicates, both internally and externally. As defined in Chapter 6, communicating effectively means creating or exchanging understanding between senders and receivers. Managers must ensure that communication occurs both within a team and between that team and others. A model of the technical process of communicating is shown in Figure 6.3, which depicts the contextual and interpersonal barriers that hinder effective communication. You may wish to review this figure and the corresponding material in Chapter 6, paying close attention to the discussion of how the barriers to communication can be overcome. This information about overcoming such barriers is highly relevant to effective communication within improvement teams, as well as to any communication about a team's work that occurs between the team and people not directly involved with the team (for example, the team might describe its results or offer its recommendations to non-members).

In many situations, the most important communication in a CI effort occurs at the first meeting of the improvement team. This is when the tone and pattern are set for subsequent work, when the team's purposes are clarified and to whom the team is accountable is specified, and when information is provided about how the team will operate. The initial meeting of an improvement team should be carefully planned. Those who do this planning should be the manager who is chartering or establishing the team; the team leader, if the person is appointed rather than selected later by the team; and the team facilitator. A typical agenda for a first meeting of an improvement team includes the following items:

1. Introduce participants (as needed), clarify team leader and facilitator roles, and explain what other team members can contribute to the improvement effort.

2. Discuss the team's charter, if there is one, or discuss the purposes for which the team has been established.

3. Discuss the development of norms (which can be added to later) that will guide the team.

4. Discuss the approach the team will take, such as by applying the FOCUS-PDCA model, or by using some other CI tool or technique.

5. Develop a schedule for the team's work, focusing on the next meeting by deciding who will do what and by when.

6. Evaluate the meeting by discussing what went well and what did not. This step permits the team to improve as it goes and brings closure to the meeting.

Subsequent meetings can be structured by following steps 3 through 9 of the FOCUS-PDCA model of improvement (see Figure 7.3). These meetings will be more productive if the team leader and team facilitator establish objectives for each meeting and develop and distribute an agenda, including the time allocated for each agenda item, prior to every meeting.

Summary

This chapter emphasizes that quality is important not only to those who receive services from health programs but also to the participants who work in them. The importance of quality both to those who receive and to those who provide a program's services is relevant to its manager. Patients/customers want health services to be of high technical quality, with appropriate attention paid to their values, their physical and psychological comfort, and their need for open communication with those who provide the services. The importance of quality for participants derives from the fact that those who work in a program that strives to continuously improve quality typically enjoy higher levels of satisfaction from their work.

Quality, as it applies to health services, is defined as "the degree to which health services for individuals and populations increase the likelihood of desired health outcomes and are consistent with current professional knowledge" (Institute of Medicine 1990, 21). Quality is described as having two important components: (1) a content component, which is the clinical expertise and the technical aspects of providing health services; and (2) a delivery and service component, which is the interpersonal aspects of providing health services. Interpersonal aspects include empathy, communication, and being able to meet patients/customers' requirements and expectations in regard to convenience, timeliness, and the like. The relationship between ethics and quality is also considered.

Measurement of quality is described in terms developed by Donabedian (1980), who noted that the measurement of quality rests on structural measures (innate characteristics of those who provide services and of the settings in which they are provided); process measures (what service providers do to patients/customers); and outcome measures (what happens to the health of patients/customers as a result of services).

Following a brief review of the evolution of various approaches to managing quality, a systematic total quality approach is described in detail. Such an approach to managing quality in programs has three interrelated components: (1) patient/customer focus, (2) commitment to continuous improvement, and (3) teamwork. Figure 7.2 illustrates the interconnected nature of these components.

Patient/customer focus requires that a health program manager identify what the program's patients/customers need and want, and then design and deliver services that satisfy those needs and wants. Continuous improvement means a manager commits to ongoing efforts to examine the processes through which services are provided in search of better ways to provide those services. Teamwork is emphasized because TQ efforts are a collective responsibility of all those involved in a program.

The FOCUS-PDCA model (Tague 2004), the oldest continuous improvement model and one that is still widely used, is described in detail and shown in Figure 7.3.

Application of the FOCUS-PDCA model is exemplified in the chapter by a description of how a continuous improvement team, established in a family practice program to improve the care of people with type 2 diabetes, followed the steps in the model in undertaking a successful CI effort.

A number of tools useful in support of CI are described, including benchmarking, flow charting, cause-and-effect (fishbone) diagrams, Pareto charts, and run charts. A comprehensive model (see Figure 7.7) of the determinants of successful improvement teams is presented, showing that a team's effectiveness results from several aspects of how it is structured and how it operates.

REVIEW QUESTIONS

1. Define quality as it applies to health programs. Distinguish between content quality and delivery and service quality.

2. Discuss the importance of managing quality in a health program.

3. Discuss Donabedian's approach to measuring quality.

4. List and briefly describe the three components of a total quality approach to managing quality in health programs.

5. Discuss the role of continuous improvement in managing quality.

6. Draw the FOCUS-PDCA model of CI.

7. List and briefly describe several tools and techniques that are useful in CI.

8. Draw a model of the determinants of improvement team effectiveness.

9. Describe the role of team leader and the role of team facilitator in a successful CI team.

10. Write an agenda for a first meeting of a newly formed CI team, and describe briefly why each agenda item is important.

KEY TERMS AND CONCEPTS

cause-and-effect diagram

continuous improvement (CI)

continuous quality improvement (CQI)

ethics principles

FOCUS-PDCA model

managing quality

measuring quality

Pareto chart

patient/customer focus

process improvement

quality

quality assessment

quality assurance (QA)

quality improvement (QI)

run chart

Six Sigma

teamwork

total quality (TQ)

total quality management (TQM)

Toyota Production System (TPS)

References

Barry, Robert, Amy C. Murcko, and Clifford E. Brubaker. *The Six Sigma Book for Healthcare*. Chicago: Health Administration Press, 2002.

Black, John, and David Miller. *The Toyota Way to Healthcare Excellence: Increase Efficiency and Improve Quality with Lean.* Chicago: Health Administration Press, 2008.

Brook, Robert H., and Kathleen N. Lohr. "Efficacy, Effectiveness, Variations and Quality: Boundary-Crossing Research." *Medical Care* 23, no. 5 (1985): 710–722.

Brook, Robert H., Elizabeth A. McGlynn, and Paul G. Shekelle. "Defining and Measuring Quality of Care: A Perspective from U.S. Researchers." *International Journal for Quality in Health Care* 12, no. 4 (2000): 281–295.

Chassin, Mark R. "Is Health Care Ready for Six Sigma Quality?" *Milbank Quarterly* 76, no. 4 (December 1998): 565–591.

Chassin, Mark R., and Jerod M. Loeb. "The Ongoing Quality Improvement Journey: Next Stop, High Reliability." *Health Affairs* 30, no. 4 (April 2011): 559–568.

Crosby, Philip B. *Let's Talk Quality.* New York: McGraw-Hill, 1989.

Dean, James W., Jr., and David E. Bowen. "Management Theory and Total Quality: Improving Research and Practice through Theory Development." *Academy of Management Review* 19, no. 3 (July 1994): 392–418.

Deming, W. Edwards. *Quality, Productivity, and Competitive Position.* Boston: MIT Press, 1982.

Donabedian, Avedis. "Evaluating the Quality of Medical Care." *Milbank Memorial Fund Quarterly* 44, no. 3 (July 1966): 166–206.

Donabedian, Avedis. Explorations in Quality Assessment and Monitoring. Vol. 1, *The Definition of Quality and Approaches to Its Assessment.* Chicago: Health Administration Press, 1980.

Fallon, L. Fleming, Jr., James W. Begun, and William Riley. *Managing Health Organizations for Quality and Performance.* Burlington, MA: Jones & Bartlett Learning, 2013.

Fried, Bruce J., Sharon Topping, and Amy C. Edmondson. "Teams and Team Effectiveness in Health Services Organizations." In *Shortell and Kaluzny's Health Care Management: Organization Design and Behavior,* edited by Lawton Robert Burns, Elizabeth H. Bradley, and Bryan J. Weiner, 6th ed., 121–162. Clifton Park, NY: Delmar, Cengage Learning, 2012.

General Electric. "Key Elements of Quality." Accessed May 21, 2014. http://www.ge.com/sixsigma/keyelements.html.

Gerteis, Margaret, Susan Edgman-Levitan, Jennifer Daley, and Thomas L. Delbanco, eds. *Through the Patient's Eyes: Understanding and Promoting Patient-Centered Care.* San Francisco: Jossey-Bass, 2002.

Ham, Chris, Ruth Kipping, and Hugh McLeod. "Redesigning Work Processes in Health Care: Lessons from the National Health Service." *Milbank Quarterly* 81, no. 3 (September 2003): 415–439.

Hospital Corporation of America. "About Our Company." Accessed May 21, 2014. http://hcahealthcare.com/about/.

Inozu, Bahadir, Dan Chauncey, Vickie Kamataris, and Charles Mount. *Performance Improvement for Healthcare: Leading Change with Lean, Six Sigma, and Constraints Management.* New York: McGraw-Hill, 2012.

Institute of Medicine. *Medicare: A Strategy for Quality Assurance.* Vol. 1. Washington, DC: National Academies Press, 1990.

Institute of Medicine. *Crossing the Quality Chasm: A New Health System for the 21st Century.* Washington, DC: National Academies Press, 2001.

Institute of Medicine, National Roundtable on Health Care Quality. *Statement on Quality of Care.* Washington, DC: Institute of Medicine, 1998.

James, Brent C. *Quality Management for Health Care Delivery.* Chicago: Health Research and Educational Trust of the American Hospital Association, 1989.

James, Brent C., and Lucy A. Savitz. "How Intermountain Trimmed Health Care Costs through Robust Quality Improvement Efforts." *Health Affairs* 30, no. 6 (June 2011): 1185–1191.

Juran, Joseph M. *Juran on Leadership for Quality: An Executive Handbook.* New York: Free Press, 1989.

Kaplan, Heather C., Patrick W. Brady, Michele C. Dritz, David K. Hooper, W. Matthew Linam, Craig M. Froehle, and Peter Margolis. "The Influence of Context on Quality Improvement Success in Health Care: A Systematic Review of the Literature." *Milbank Quarterly* 88, no. 4 (December 2010): 500–559.

Kelly, Diane L. *Applying Quality Management in Healthcare.* Chicago: Health Administration Press, 2003.

Kenney, Charles. *Transforming Health Care: Virginia Mason Medical Center's Pursuit of the Perfect Patient Experience*. New York: Productivity Press, 2011.

LaFasto, Frank, and Carl Larson. *When Teams Work Best*. Thousand Oaks, CA: Sage, 2001.

Lighter, Donald E. *Basics of Health Care Performance Improvement: A Lean Six Sigma Approach*. Burlington, MA: Jones & Bartlett Learning, 2013.

Liker, Jeffrey K., and James K. Franz. *The Toyota Way to Continuous Improvement: Linking Strategy and Operational Excellence to Achieve Superior Performance*. New York: McGraw-Hill, 2011.

Longest, Beaufort B., Jr. "Organizational Change and Innovation." In *Handbook of Health Care Management*, edited by W. Jack Duncan, Peter M. Ginter, and Linda E. Swayne, 369–398. Malden, MA: Blackwell, 1998.

Longest, Beaufort B., Jr., and Kurt Darr. *Managing Health Services Organizations and Systems*, 6th ed. Baltimore: Health Professions Press, 2014.

Lukas, Carol VanDeusen, Sally K. Holmes, Alan B. Cohen, Joseph Restuccia, Irene E. Cramer, Michael Schwartz, and Martin P. Charns. "Transformational Change in Health Care Systems: An Organizational Model." *Health Care Management Review* 32, no. 4 (October-December 2007): 309–320.

McLaughlin, Curtis P., and Arnold D. Kaluzny. "Total Quality Management in Health: Making It Work." *Health Care Management Review* 15, no. 3 (Summer 1990): 7–14.

National Institute of Standards and Technology. *Health Care Criteria for Performance Excellence*. Washington, DC: National Institute for Standards and Technology, 2014.

Page, Ann. *Keeping Patients Safe: Transforming the Work Environment of Nurses*. Washington, DC: National Academies Press, 2004.

Revere, Lee, and Ken Black. "Integrating Six Sigma with Total Quality Management: A Case Example for Measuring Medication Errors." *Journal of Healthcare Management* 48, no. 6 (November-December 2003): 377–391.

Runde, Craig E., and Tim A. Flanagan. *Developing Your Conflict Competence: A Hands-On Guide for Leaders, Managers, Facilitators, and Teams*. San Francisco: Jossey-Bass, 2010.

Schwarz, Miriam, Suzanne E. Landis, and John E. Rowe. "A Team Approach to Quality Improvement." *Family Practice Management* 6, no. 4 (April 1999): 25–33.

Smith, Karl A., and P. K. Imbrie. *Teamwork and Project Management*, 4th ed. New York: McGraw-Hill Higher Education, 2013.

Smith, Mark, Robert Sanders, Leigh Stuckhardt, and J. Michael McGinnis, eds. *Best Care at Lower Cost: The Path to Continuously Learning Health Care in America*. Washington, DC: National Academies Press, 2012.

Sollecito, William A., and Julie K. Johnson. *McLaughlin and Kaluzny's Continuous Quality Improvement in Health Care*, 4th ed. Burlington, MA: Jones & Bartlett Learning, 2013.

Spath, Patrice L. *Introduction to Healthcare Quality Management*, 2nd ed. Chicago: Health Administration Press, 2013.

Spear, Steven, and H. Kent Bowen. "Decoding the DNA of the Toyota Production System." *Harvard Business Review* 77 (September-October 1999): 96–106.

Stanford Hospital & Clinics. "Key Quality Initiatives." Accessed May 21, 2014. http://www.stanfordhospital.org/quality/whatisquality/initiatives.

Tague, Nancy R. *The Quality Toolbox*, 2nd ed. Milwaukee, WI: ASQ Quality Press, 2004.

CHAPTER 8

COMMERCIAL AND SOCIAL MARKETING

Managers of health programs use two important forms of marketing as they perform their work, both of which are discussed in this chapter. The financial or commercial success of many programs is affected by the use of commercial marketing. In addition, especially in programs focused on health promotion and education, social marketing is used as a mechanism in the provision of services. Like decision making, communicating, managing quality, and evaluating, marketing is a facilitative activity that managers engage in as they perform their core activities of developing/strategizing, designing, and leading (see Figure 1.4).

Marketing is increasingly pervasive in health services. For example, marketing occurs when a group practice of physicians advertises to attract new patients; when a hospital establishes a comprehensive cancer center to meet an unmet need for more cancer care in a community; when a health plan improves benefits to attract new subscribers; when a pharmaceutical manufacturer hires more sales representatives to increase sales of its products; when Health Canada sponsors a campaign to motivate more Canadians to stop smoking; and when the Centers for Disease Control and Prevention (CDC) mounts a campaign to encourage people to get flu shots.

To succeed, health services organizations from the largest medical centers to the smallest programs rely on marketing. As we will see in this chapter, marketing is the activity through which program managers exchange things of value with a program's patients/customers and with other stakeholders. At the simplest level, services are exchanged for payment.

To properly use marketing in a program, managers must understand how both commercial and social marketing take place. We will discuss strategies for both forms of

LEARNING OBJECTIVES

After reading this chapter, you should be able to:

- Define commercial marketing, and understand the basic elements in a commercial marketing strategy for health programs, including the five Ps of commercial marketing

- Define social marketing, and understand the basic elements of using social marketing in health programs

- Understand the use of the epidemiological planning model in marketing

marketing. As background, however, definitions of both forms are provided in the following sections.

Commercial Marketing

The American Marketing Association (2014) has defined commercial marketing as "the activity, set of institutions, and processes for creating, communicating, delivering, and exchanging offerings that have value for customers, clients, partners, and society at large." Adapting this and other widely cited definitions of commercial marketing (Berkowitz 2011; Keller and Kotler 2011; Pride and Ferrell 2014), this chapter defines *commercial marketing* in a health program as the process of planning, implementing, and evaluating activities designed to bring about satisfying exchange relationships with patients/customers and other stakeholders in the program's dynamic environment.

Commercial marketing focuses on facilitating exchanges between a program and its target markets, including identifying and quantifying the target markets. These exchanges involve things of value to the parties. Obvious target markets of a health program include the existing patients/customers who directly use its services; potential new patients/customers who may use its services; as well as others who can influence existing or potential patients/customers, such as referring physicians and health plans that may permit or limit use of the services by their subscribers or members. Other important target markets are a program's potential participants, donors, and volunteers, and the organization in which the program is embedded.

Social Marketing

The American Marketing Association (2014) has defined social marketing as "marketing designed to influence the behavior of a target audience in which the benefits of the behavior are intended by the marketer to accrue primarily to the audience or to the society in general and not to the marketer." *Social marketing* involves the use of marketing knowledge, concepts, and techniques to enhance social ends. Stated another way, social marketing is "a process for influencing human behavior on a large scale, using (commercial) marketing principles for the purpose of societal benefit rather than commercial profit" (Smith 2000, 11).

An example of social marketing is the efforts of the American Cancer Society to influence people to stop smoking. Adapting the definition provided by the American Marketing Association and other widely cited definitions of social marketing (Andreasen 2005; French et al. 2010; Lee and Kotler 2011; Weinreich 2011), this chapter defines social marketing in health programs as the application of commercial marketing technologies to planning, implementing, and evaluating services that are designed to influence the voluntary behavior of people in target markets to improve their personal welfare and that of society.

With the distinguishing definitions of commercial and social marketing in mind, we are ready to consider how both forms of marketing can success-fully take place in health programs. Each form of marketing is an important facilitative program management activity. We begin by considering com-mercial marketing in the next section.

Commercial Marketing in Health Programs

Often the success and longevity of a program may depend on its manager's at least moderate success in marketing the program commercially. This is the case because the central concept of commercial marketing is the establishment and facilitation of voluntary and mutually beneficial exchanges between parties.

The most obvious examples of commercial marketing exchanges involve those between buyers and sellers. The services provided through a program (for example, a well-baby care or eldercare program) may be perceived to have value by certain people who will then buy the services either directly or through insurance coverage. When the services are seen as valuable and purchased to a sufficient extent, the program can be a commercial success. And there are also many other types of exchanges that are important to programs. Other exchanges occur because

- It is essential to attract participants (and volunteers in some situations) to fill the positions in a program's organization design.
- Many programs rely on donors or grant makers for financial support.
- It may be necessary to satisfy public and private payers, such as Medicaid programs or insurance plans, to cover the services provided.
- Success may depend on convincing physicians or other health services providers to refer patients to a program.
- Finally, it is important for a program to convince its host organization of the value of the program to sustain its continuation and perhaps its expansion.

All of these, and other, parties to potential exchanges with a program can be reached through commercial marketing efforts. In effect, the individuals, organizations, and groups with which exchanges are needed are the focus of a program manager's marketing efforts. They are the target markets. Identifying and understanding their wants and needs is central to effective marketing and is discussed in the next subsection.

The Concept of Target Markets

The broad range of parties to potential exchanges with a program in effect represents the individuals, organizations, and groups making up the *target markets* for the program. The purposes of commercial marketing can be summarized as building and maintaining *exchange relationships* with people in various target markets to optimize the achievement of the program's mission and objectives. It is important to emphasize at the outset of this discussion that target markets are made up of people, including those who are or may become patients/customers as well as those who lead or participate in other organizations or groups with which exchange relationships are established. It is also important to note that the foci of social marketing initiatives are typically called *target audiences*. They will be discussed more fully in a later section, where the focus is on social marketing in health programs.

Regardless of which target market, or segment or subgroup within a target market, is the focus of a given commercial marketing effort, the key to marketing a program successfully is knowledge of the wants and needs of the people in the target market and its segments, coupled with the ability to satisfy some of those wants and needs.

Even though establishing and facilitating voluntary and mutually beneficial exchanges between a program and the people in its target markets presumes knowledge of the needs and wants of those people, identifying their needs and wants is not always simple or straightforward. In part, the determination of the needs and wants of patients/customers, donors, participants, or others with whom exchanges may be necessary or desirable is complicated by the fact that people have various types of needs and wants.

The Needs and Wants of People in Target Markets

As a starting point, people have perceived needs—that is, what they think they need. Perceived needs become wants, and people often feel very strongly about what they want. For example, certain patients/customers, perhaps influenced by ubiquitous pharmaceutical marketing efforts, may be convinced that they need a specific new drug to address their health problem. The nature of perceived needs varies across individuals. For example, one donor making a significant financial gift to a program may want anonymity, whereas other donors may seek widespread publicity concerning their generosity. Because these donors have different needs, they must be dealt with in different ways if successful exchanges are to occur.

People sometimes demonstrate or express their needs through their decisions and actions. Without knowing what the people who enroll in a program actually perceive their needs to be, one might infer merely from a high level of enrollment that the services of the program are needed and wanted. Thus, a second type of needs is expressed needs. This type of need is typically revealed in the numbers of people using particular services.

Especially in regard to sophisticated health services, it may be difficult or impossible for people either to perceive their own needs or to exhibit an expressed need for the services. They simply do not know of the services or of the benefits they might derive from receiving them. It may therefore be necessary to determine levels of needs and wants existing in a target market by assessing these levels in some way (Hoffman and Bateson 2011).

The use of guidelines or norms established by experts is a frequently employed means of assessing levels of needs and wants in a target market. For example, determination of what are called normative needs in regard to health services is routinely based on the opinions of experts about the appropriate (needed) levels of health services for individuals and populations. A panel of public health experts may decide what they believe to be the appropriate levels of certain services to meet the need for these services in populations of people. On a smaller scale, the manager of a specific program may be able to normatively determine the need for services among its target markets by applying incidence rates that are often available from such sources as the CDC or state and local public health agencies.

A thorough understanding of the needs of people in a program's target markets is the basis for building effective exchange relationships with them. These needs are best understood if perceived, expressed, and normative needs are all taken into account. It is important to determine the different needs and wants of people in each of a program's target markets, whether patients/customers, potential participants, donors, health professionals who might refer patients/customers, or others. For programs that are established to provide services, however, the potential patients/customers who might use the services are a critical target market and are likely to be the focus of significant commercial marketing efforts.

Identification and quantification of vital patient/customer target markets are described in general in the next subsection. After that, a specific target market is used in an example of how to develop a commercial marketing strategy to facilitate exchanges with people in a target market.

Although the specific example used is for a patient/customer target market, the processes of identifying and quantifying target markets and of designing and implementing marketing strategies to facilitate exchanges with them are similar for all types of target markets.

Identifying and Quantifying Patient/Customer Target Markets

Managers seek to identify and quantify target markets, as well as to understand the needs and wants of people in these markets, so that they can tailor effective marketing strategies accordingly. To facilitate commercial marketing focused on a patient/customer target market, it may be useful to segment the market along any number of dimensions. Examples of patient/customer *market segments* (or subgroups) are listed in Table 8.1.

Of course, the identification and quantification of target markets and segments within them are only the beginning of understanding the potential of the target markets and segments to produce actual demand for the services of a program. Making such a determination requires additional analysis, which can be aided by use of a technique called the epidemiological planning model (White and Griffith 2010). An example of the application of this model follows.

Epidemiological Planning Model

Healthy Start is a national initiative of the Health Resources and Services Administration of the U.S. Department of Health and Human Services; it has programs in thirty-nine states, the District of Columbia, and Puerto Rico (U.S. Department of Health and Human Services 2014). One of these

Table 8.1 Examples of Patient/Customer Market Segments

Type of Market Segment	Shared Group Characteristics
Demographic segment	Measurable statistics, such as age, gender, race, income, occupation, or health insurance coverage
Psychographic segment	Lifestyle preferences, such as a preference for urban, suburban, or rural life; a preference for alternative medicine; or a willingness to use new products or services
Use-based segment	Frequency of usage, for example in regard to the use of medical and dental services, health clubs, or fitness centers
Benefit segment	Desire to obtain certain product or service benefits, such as luxury, cost-effectiveness, scheduling convenience, or ease of access
Geographic segment	Location, such as a zip code, community, region, or state

programs is based in Pittsburgh, Pennsylvania (Healthy Start 2014). This program is designed to reduce the rate of infant mortality and improve perinatal outcomes through grants for interventions in areas with high annual rates of infant mortality.

Several of the services provided by Healthy Start Pittsburgh are designed for teenage mothers, whose babies are twice as likely to die before their first birthday as are babies born to women in their twenties. The teenage mothers make up an important target market for this program, which represents a typical situation in which the level of demand for a service can be estimated using the ***epidemiological planning model (EPM)*** (White and Griffith 2010).

The EPM is an equation, in the following general form, through which an estimate of the demand for a particular service can be made:

$$\left\{\begin{array}{c}\text{Demand for}\\\text{a service}\end{array}\right\}=\left\{\begin{array}{c}\text{Population}\\\text{at risk}\end{array}\right\}\times\left\{\begin{array}{c}\text{Incidence}\\\text{rate}\end{array}\right\}\times\left\{\begin{array}{c}\text{Average use}\\\text{per incident}\end{array}\right\}\times\left\{\begin{array}{c}\text{Market}\\\text{share}\end{array}\right\}$$

For programs like Healthy Start, the EPM has many marketing and planning uses. For example, managers in such programs may be interested in estimating the demand for counseling services for teenage mothers. An estimate of demand for these services will help ensure that a given program can provide appropriate services in an effective and timely manner. Successful commercial marketing strategies require that the needs and wants—which translate into demand for services—of the people in target markets are known, and that a program can effectively satisfy the demands.

The estimate of the demand for counseling services for teenage mothers would be based on current information for terms in the EPM equation, or on projections if a manager was interested in projecting demand in future years. In this example, where the service area is Pittsburgh and its surrounding county, the demand calculation for counseling for teenage mothers is made as follows:

• The population at risk is determined from information on the county's population. There are about 82,000 female teenagers in the county.

• The incidence rate is determined by using national data on birth rates for teenagers. Assume in this example that the overall birth rate is approximately 35 births per 1,000 female teenagers annually. This means there are about 2,870 births to teenage mothers in the county annually ($35 \times 82 = 2{,}870$).

• Average use of counseling sessions per incident is determined by the number of counseling sessions that the program manager plans to provide for each client; assume three sessions per client.

- Market share in this situation is based on the fraction of the population at risk that the manager thinks the program will serve; this number can be guided by actual experience in an ongoing program. In this instance, assume that 50 percent of the population at risk will be served.

Thus, demand for Healthy Start's counseling services can be *estimated* by the following calculation at 4,305 counseling sessions per year:

$$
\begin{Bmatrix} \text{Demand for} \\ \text{counseling} \\ \text{sessions} \end{Bmatrix} = \begin{Bmatrix} \text{Population at} \\ \text{risk =} \\ 82{,}000 \end{Bmatrix} \times \begin{Bmatrix} \text{Incidence} \\ \text{rate =} \\ 35/1{,}000 \end{Bmatrix} \times \begin{Bmatrix} \text{Average use} \\ \text{per incident =} \\ 3 \end{Bmatrix} \times \begin{Bmatrix} \text{Market} \\ \text{share =} \\ 50\% \end{Bmatrix}
$$

When target markets and segments within them are clearly identified and quantified, managers are better able to develop effective commercial marketing strategies to achieve productive exchanges with the people in the target markets and segments. Such commercial marketing strategies are developed around several interrelated elements, which are discussed in the next section. To provide a concrete example, these elements are applied to Healthy Start's efforts to establish effective exchanges with teenage mothers as part of the discussion.

The Five Ps of Commercial Marketing

The development of a commercial marketing strategy traditionally was discussed in terms of the four Ps of the strategy: **p**roduct or service, **p**rice, **p**lace, and **p**romotion (Berkowitz 2011). Contemporary thought adds a fifth P for **p**eople in target markets. Successful commercial marketing strategies in any context involve these five essential elements—the *five Ps of commercial marketing*. The first four elements of a *commercial marketing strategy* (that is, product or service, price, place, and promotion) require concurrent and interactive decisions if desired exchanges with the fifth element of the strategy (that is, people in target markets) are to be accomplished. Figure 8.1 illustrates these relationships.

Product or service, price, place, and promotion each affect the appeal of a program's services. The manner in which these four elements are packaged in an overall marketing strategy will directly affect the likelihood that the people in the program's target markets will enter into the desired exchanges with the program. These five elements of a commercial marketing strategy, which are also sometimes referred to as a *marketing mix*, are discussed in the following subsections.

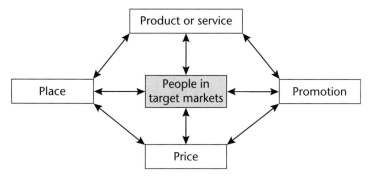

Figure 8.1   Elements of a Commercial Marketing Strategy

Product or Service

In the context of health programs, outputs are far more often services than products. Whether a program produces services or products, however, they are critical to successful commercial marketing. From a commercial marketing perspective, a successful service is one that satisfies the needs and wants of people in target markets in such a way that those individuals select the service over alternatives provided by competitors, or over the alternative of not using any service. The challenge for program managers is to make the services provided through a program so attractive and convenient for people in target markets that these services are selected over others that might be available, or in lieu of not using any services. In the example of counseling services for teenage mothers provided by Healthy Start, the services must appeal to people in this specific target market—that is, the appeal must be specific to teenage mothers.

The Difficulty of Marketing Services

Services are typically more difficult to successfully market than products for a variety of reasons, including their having such characteristics as intangibility, inseparability, perishability, and variability (Ginter, Duncan, and Swayne 2013). Products, such as clothing or computers, are tangible. Products can be picked up, put in a bag, taken home after purchase, and used by the consumer. Services, in contrast, are intangible. They are an experience. Production and consumption of services occur simultaneously; consumption is inseparable from provision. Provision of health services typically involves repeated episodes in which service providers directly interact with patients/customers. The fact that production and consumption occur simultaneously means that services cannot be produced in advance and stored for later delivery. The services are in effect perishable.

Thus, a key ingredient in successfully marketing service-based programs is a careful matching of the provision of services with the demand for them. It does not matter that services are readily available on weekdays if people want them on weekends, or that they are available between the hours of 8:00 a.m. and 4:00 p.m. if people prefer them in the evening.

Many variables enter into each service episode: specific program participants who provide services vary in terms of ability and attitude; patients/customers vary in terms of needs and expectations; and conditions vary in terms of, for example, how busy a program is on a particular day or the availability of support, such as computer systems. These factors lead, typically, to greater variability in the provision of services compared to the provision of tangible products. Services provided through programs are difficult to standardize, in other words, and this complicates efforts to commercially market them. However, there are a number of steps that a manager can take to successfully market services.

Overcoming the Challenges of Marketing Services

The most important thing that program managers can do to ensure that services are commercially successful is to make certain that they are of high quality. This means providing services with high content quality and high delivery and service quality as discussed in Chapter 7. An important part of delivery and service quality is making services attractive and appealing to patients/customers. The best way to accomplish this is to base the services on input from current and potential patients/customers in the target markets identified for the services. This information can be gathered in a variety of ways, such as by using questionnaires, surveys, or focus groups.

Although developed outside the health care context and certainly not perfect, the SERVQUAL (from "service quality") model of ensuring service quality can be useful in guiding efforts to provide services in a manner that satisfies a given health program's patients/customers (Zeithaml, Parasuraman, and Berry 1990). This model identifies five dimensions of service that are important to patients/customers:

- *Reliability*—providing services dependably and accurately
- *Assurance*—demonstrating knowledge and courtesy when providing services, and also conveying trust and confidence
- *Responsiveness*—demonstrating willingness to assist patients/customers and to provide services promptly
- *Empathy*—providing patients/customers with services in a caring and individualized manner

- *Tangibles*—maintaining the appearance and amenities of the physical facilities and the appearance and attitudes of those who work in the program

In addition to determining what aspects of services will be attractive and appealing to patients/customers, managers can do several other things to overcome the challenges inherent in marketing services. They can, for example,

- Select and train staff carefully, including training them in interacting with patients/customers in culturally appropriate ways.
- Pay attention to the physical aspects of service episodes. Décor, ambience, and amenities are important to most people and have a significant bearing on how they view their experience with a program.
- Pay attention to the entire process through which interactions occur with patients/customers. Even if people receive excellent health services that fully address their health issues, they will be concerned about all aspects of their interactions with a program. Were they received courteously when they arrived for their appointment? Were they treated with respect, and were their dignity and privacy honored? Did they have to wait past the appointment time? Did they receive a correct bill, or was the insurance paperwork properly handled?
- Routinely ask probing questions of themselves and other program participants about how program services are actually experienced. This requires empathy.

Patients/customers' levels of satisfaction with the interactions through which they receive services are determined both by clinical and service aspects of those interactions. It is not enough to provide services that are clinically excellent, although this must be done if patients/customers are to be satisfied with services. A broader approach to patient/customer satisfaction acknowledges both clinical and nonclinical aspects of the services a health program provides.

A suitably broad approach to patient/customer satisfaction takes into account accessibility and convenience, the availability of resources, continuity of care, the efficacy and outcomes of care, financial considerations, humaneness, how information is gathered, how information is provided, the pleasantness of surroundings, and the quality and competence of health service providers (Berkowitz, Pol, and Thomas 1995). All of these variables are relevant in the service element of a commercial marketing strategy. No matter how effectively services are designed to satisfy the needs and wants of patients/customers, however, successful commercial marketing strategies require consideration of additional elements.

Price

Another of the five Ps of a commercial marketing strategy is price (see Figure 8.1). Even if the services of a program respond to the needs and wants of patients/customers, successful exchanges with them may depend in part on the price of the services. The most obvious aspect of the price of health services is the dollar amount patients/customers are expected to pay in exchange for them. But there is more to price than monetary value. Using services may have other costs, such as inconvenience, loss of time, loss of a sense of well-being, or even feelings of indignity.

In regard to many health services, the financial price is not paid directly by patients/customers—or at least not fully and exclusively paid by them. This is the case, for example, with the counseling services available to teenage mothers through Healthy Start, which are free to them. In other situations, services are covered by insurance plans. In these cases, price, except when there are deductibles or co-payment provisions in the coverage, may be of little importance to the direct consumer. In contrast, in other instances where services are not covered by public or private insurance, price may be very important to patients/customers, although its importance in their decision making may vary with their personal financial circumstances.

The existence of private and public insurance frequently affects the role of price in marketing health services, shifting concerns about price from patients/customers to those who pay on their behalf. For example, if services are covered by commercial insurance plans, then the prices charged to the plans for their subscribers who receive the services are more important to the plans than to the subscribers. Similarly, the prices charged to public payers such as Medicare and Medicaid for services provided to beneficiaries of these programs are important to the government agencies responsible for reimbursing providers for these services.

Price considerations in the decisions people make about consuming services are often weighed in association with quality and utility or usefulness considerations. Many people seek services they think are of high quality, useful to them, and offered at a fair price. In effect they are seeking value.

In the case of the counseling services provided by Healthy Start, the teenage mothers considering using the services will take it into account that the services are available free of charge to them, but they will also weigh such costs as time and inconvenience against their assessment of the benefits they will derive from participating in the counseling sessions. They will also consider the quality of the counseling and its usefulness to them. If they do not value the sessions, it will not matter that they are offered for free.

Teenage mothers, then, will take a number of considerations into account as they make decisions about using the counseling services of Healthy Start. The program must factor all of these considerations into the design of an effective commercial marketing strategy. Even if a program has carefully designed its services to meet the needs of patients/customers and has made certain that financial price is not a barrier, other elements must also be considered. For example, the physical location, or place, of a program and the associated convenience or inconvenience for potential patients/ customers can play an important role in the program's commercial success, and are discussed next.

Place

The place (see Figure 8.1) where a program is physically located can support or hinder its overall success. The teenage mothers to whom Healthy Start wants to offer counseling services will make their decisions about using the services in part based on where they will receive the services. Invariably, a program's accessibility to the people in its target markets influences their decisions about using the program's services.

Accessibility is about more than physical location. It encompasses days and hours of operation. Further, the availability of parking and ease of access for people with disabilities are part of the place consideration. Programs that extend weekday hours and remain open on weekends enhance accessibility for many of those who may wish to use their services. Similarly, opening new locations or operating satellite units can improve access to a program's services.

Beyond the importance of physical location, attention must also be given to various other aspects of how patients/customers are treated and made to feel. For example, comfortable, attractive, well-lit reception areas can make them feel welcome. A courteous, respectful, and culturally sensitive reception is an important aspect in terms of the place element in a commercial marketing strategy for any program.

Luallin and Sullivan (1998) have emphasized the importance of how a program responds to the expectations of those it attracts and serves. The first step in ensuring that a program is responsive to its patients/customers is for the manager to routinely assess responsiveness in several areas. This can be done by answering such questions as the following:

Accessibility	Are office hours convenient for employed patients/customers?
	Are exterior and interior signs attractive and legible?
	Is parking adequate, and are provisions made for elderly people and people with disabilities?
	Are all public areas clean and attractive?
Patient/Customer Flow	Are patients/customers greeted quickly and courteously on arrival?
	Are those who have contact with patients/customers and other visitors professional, helpful, and friendly?
	Are waiting areas comfortable?
	Are waiting patients/customers kept informed of their situation and seen as quickly as possible?
Patient/Customer Communication	Are all patients/customers treated as valued clients in all communication with them?
	Do service providers explain procedures before starting?
	Are educational and informational materials of high quality and readily available?
	Is there an effective way to obtain patient/customer feedback?
	Are patient/customer confidentiality and privacy ensured?

Another step in ensuring that a program responds effectively to actual and potential patients/customers it seeks to serve is to select high-potential participants and train them properly. This step ensures that program participants—including direct service providers and those who support them in their work—contribute positively to the place element of the overall commercial marketing strategy. Recall from the discussion in Chapter 3 that staffing is the process of filling the individual positions established in an organization design for a program with appropriate participants.

To be suited for work in a program, an individual must possess relevant technical proficiency in the work, hold the required credentials and certifications, and have relevant experience. In addition, from a commercial marketing strategy perspective, appropriate participants include those who can relate to patients/customers in a culturally and linguistically sensitive manner. They must be able to work with people in highly stressful conditions and respond to their needs under such circumstances.

Program managers should establish performance standards and expectations that go beyond the procedural aspects of work and extend to the service aspects. Luallin and Sullivan (1998) recommended the use of patient/customer-centered performance standards in the following areas:

- *Communication procedures*—making clear that patients/customers are entitled to prompt, courteous communication, and requiring such actions as (1) answering the phone promptly and speaking in a friendly, helpful tone of voice; (2) when putting callers on hold, asking, "Will you hold, please?"; and then (3) thanking them for holding when returning to the line.

- *Patient/customer handling*—making clear that patients/customers are to be greeted and treated with respect and dignity, and requiring such actions as (1) greeting patients/customers and other visitors promptly and establishing eye contact with them; (2) looking for ways to reassure anxious patients/customers; and (3) concluding every patient/customer encounter by thanking the patient/customer for the opportunity to provide services.

- *Communicating with patients/customers*—making clear that they are to receive prompt, courteous, and accurate responses to their questions and concerns, and requiring such actions as (1) making certain that the information given to patients/customers is accurate; (2) explaining procedures carefully and asking if there are questions before proceeding; (3) participants' telling patients/customers what they plan to do and not making promises that cannot be kept; (4) following through on all promises made to patients/customers; and (5) addressing patient/customers' problems as responsively as possible.

- *Professional standards*—making clear that patients/customers will be assured of high-quality care and services that are delivered professionally, and requiring such actions as (1) following dress codes and wearing name badges correctly; and (2) being courteous to patients/customers and other program participants.

The standards and actions just listed must be tailored to specific circumstances and settings, but they provide a template for adding a service focus to what is expected of participants who work in any program. For the standards to have their full impact, it is necessary for managers to recognize performance that meets the standards, including offering merit pay increases that reflect service performance as well as the technical competence displayed in work.

As Healthy Start's manager considers a commercial marketing strategy to encourage and facilitate mutually beneficial exchanges with teenage mothers, in addition to giving careful attention to designing services to meet teenage mothers' needs and making the place where services will be received appealing and convenient, the manager must also address another element in the overall commercial marketing strategy: promotion.

Promotion

Through promotion (see Figure 8.1), a program's manager seeks to establish and maintain the program's reputation or image, as well as to inform patients/customers and their intermediaries about the types and quality of services offered and how to access the services.

A program with multiple target markets is likely to have a different image with each of them. For example, patients/customers may see a program as a convenient source of health services of a particular type. Present and potential participants may see it as a good place to work. Referring physicians may see it as a good place to send patients, because of the high quality of the services. Insurance plans may see it as a program with better quality and outcomes than those of competitors. The general public may have an image of the program as a potential source of particular services, should they ever need them.

Health programs typically seek to establish familiarity and positive images with target markets through such promotional activities as issuing annual reports; using social media and other online platforms, such as blogs, Wikipedia, YouTube, Facebook, LinkedIn, and Second Life; maintaining informative Web sites; publishing newsletters and brochures; and having managers and other participants give public lectures on topics related to the program. At the extreme, promotion may include purchased media exposure, support or sponsorship of local athletic or social events, and distribution of such items as coffee mugs or T-shirts bearing the name and logo of the program.

Internet and Social Media

Increasingly, people rely on the ***Internet*** for all sorts of information, including health-related information. Based on a recent national survey (Fox and Duggan 2013), 85 percent of adults in the United States use the Internet. Ninety-one percent of adults own a cell phone, and 56 percent own a smartphone. Fifty-nine percent of adults reported looking on the Internet for health information in the past year. The vast majority begin their searches using a search engine, such as Google, Bing, or Yahoo. A small percentage begin their search at a ***social media*** site, such as Facebook.

The term *social media* refers to a large and expanding group of Internet-based applications that foster the creation and exchange of user-generated content (Kaplan and Haenlein 2010). Effective promotion of health programs increasingly relies on the Internet and social media. In using social media, managers must make careful choices. There are too many applications for managers to participate in all of them, and whatever social media applications are used must be integrated with more traditional media.

Kaplan and Haenlein (2010) advised that use of social media for marketing purposes, such as program promotion, requires that the users be active, interesting, humble, honest, and "unprofessional." By being unprofessional, they mean not being too professional or flashy in producing content. It works best when social media content blends in with the content generated by other users.

Program Brochures

Well-designed brochures can be among a program manager's best tools for promotion. They are sometimes called identity and capabilities brochures, which denotes their basic uses: providing enough information about a program for readers to identify it, and providing descriptions that inform readers about the program's capabilities and services. In some instances, a brochure may also contain information that supports access to and use of the services provided. For example, a section of a brochure may contain a map and parking information, contact information, and information about referral arrangements as well as payment and billing practices.

Although brochures tend to be idiosyncratic, depending on the nature of the program, effective ones include the following types of information:

- *Welcome and introduction.* This section should reflect the program's appreciation for being selected as a service provider, and should include a statement of desire to warrant and maintain the trust of patients/customers.

- *Mission statement.* This section, in addition to containing the program's mission statement, might also include a brief history of the program and its important affiliations.

- *Services and capabilities.* This section describes in easily understood terminology the specific services available through the program, as well as special capabilities. For example, if the program provides counseling services, these may be described, along with special capabilities in regard to communicating in various languages. (In fact, depending on the target market demographics, it might be necessary to provide brochures in more than one language.)

- *Operating policies and practices.* This section, which is optional but often needed, contains practical information, such as how to schedule an appointment, billing and payment options, and how insurance forms are processed.

- *Staff.* This section contains information about the program's key professional participants. Depending on the number of people involved, this might be in the form of a list with a note about how to obtain additional information from a Web site or directory. If space permits, brief biographies of key professional participants can be included in the brochure.

Media Opportunities for Promotion

Print and electronic media provide several opportunities to promote programs. The following activities are useful means through which managers can use the media in efforts to promote a program:

- Developing and distributing press kits to local media that contain detailed information about the program, including awards and measures of performance, along with photographs and information about specific services. The kits can include contact information for satisfied patients/customers who might be interviewed, if this has been cleared with them beforehand.

- Issuing press releases to alert the press to major events, such as receiving prizes or awards, large grants, or accreditation. Including information that explains who, what, where, why, and when—and perhaps photographs and quotations—helps reporters do their job and improves the likelihood that they will develop the material into a story.

- Producing public service announcements to reach target markets through television and radio stations. In many communities, radio stations and some television stations provide public service announcements free of charge for nonprofit programs. The production costs must of course be covered, but sometimes assistance with this can be obtained on a pro bono basis from production companies.

- Writing informative articles for local newspapers and magazines reflecting technical expertise about health issues, and describing what a program is doing to address the issues. This promotes the author as well as the program with which he or she is affiliated.

- Writing editorials and letters to the editor for local newspapers and magazines, especially if these brief documents present a balanced viewpoint in about three hundred to nine hundred words.

Working with Others

Some programs benefit from the assistance of others in their promotional efforts. For example, the Healthy Start program in Pittsburgh benefits from the fact that similar programs established in communities across the United States have formed an association, the National Healthy Start Association (www.healthystartassoc.org). The mission of this association is to promote the national Healthy Start program and its community-based programs, such as the one in Pittsburgh, through a wide range of activities and efforts. The association's efforts are rooted in the communities with Healthy Start programs, and the promotional efforts actively focus on the local programs' target markets.

In some instances, as is the case with Healthy Start, image building reaches the level of branding. In addition to programs that are associated with widespread initiatives, such as Healthy Start, other programs may benefit from the promotional efforts of the organization in which they are embedded when the host organization undertakes branding efforts. For example, the Osteoporosis and Bone Health Program of Magee–Womens Hospital of the University of Pittsburgh Medical Center (www.upmc.com/locations/hospitals/Magee/for-women/bone-health/Pages/default.aspx) benefits from its association with the hospital's branding efforts to establish itself as the premier place in Pittsburgh for women's health services. Furthermore, the hospital is part of a large, integrated health system, and both the program and the hospital also benefit from the system's branding efforts.

We can conclude our discussion of commercial marketing by noting that when the people in a program's target markets or segments are accurately identified, and when their demographics are quantified; when the needs and wants (translated into demand) of the people in the target markets or segments are understood; and when a commercial marketing strategy is appropriately developed and implemented by integrating the product or service, price, promotion, and place aspects of a marketing strategy, then commercial marketing can provide a program with great value.

A successful commercial marketing strategy will help encourage and facilitate mutually beneficial exchanges between a program and its patients/customers. This marketing strategy can also encourage and facilitate mutually beneficial exchanges with participants, donors, and volunteers. Further, the strategy can help strengthen the support of the organization in which the program is embedded, and can improve relationships with regulatory agencies, grant makers, and other stakeholders.

As noted at the beginning of this chapter, two types of marketing are important to health programs. In addition to commercial marketing, some programs also use social marketing as a key tool in providing their services. Managers use commercial marketing to convince patients/customers to purchase a product or service. They use social marketing to influence the behavior of certain target markets, or as they are frequently called when they are targets of social marketing, target audiences. This type of marketing is discussed in the next sections.

Social Marketing in Health Programs

Social marketing was defined earlier in this chapter as the application of commercial marketing technologies to planning, implementing, and evaluating services that are designed to influence the voluntary behavior of target audiences to improve their personal welfare and that of society. Remember, target markets are the focus of commercial marketing, but social marketing focuses on target audiences. This distinction is largely one of terminology, not concept. Social marketing has been used widely in such areas as energy conservation and recycling, and especially in addressing such health issues as smoking prevention and cessation, safety, drug abuse, drinking and driving, HIV and AIDS, nutrition, physical activity, immunization, breast cancer screening, mental health, family planning, and many others (Grier and Bryant 2005). Appendix C at the end of this chapter provides a comprehensive example of social marketing in a health program.

Around the world, many national governments are increasingly using social marketing as a means of keeping their respective populations healthy. Canada has led the way in this by making significant use of social marketing in seeking to improve the health of Canadians through widespread social marketing campaigns sponsored by Health Canada (www.hc-sc.gc.ca/index-eng.php), which is the federal department responsible for helping Canadians maintain and improve their health. In late 2013 the first Global Health Conference on Social Marketing and Franchising was held in India (www.smfconference.com/).

In the United States, where health services are primarily provided by the states through their respective health departments and even more so by numerous private-sector health programs, the role of the federal government in health-related social marketing centers on providing funding and other resources and encouraging the states and programs to use social marketing as a means of improving health. A good example of this facilitation activity by the federal government is an excellent online course,

Social Marketing for Nutrition and Physical Activity (www.cdc.gov/nccdphp/ dnpa/socialmarketing/training/index.htm), provided by the CDC's Division of Nutrition, Physical Activity, and Obesity. This division also provides other resources on social marketing and encourages use of these resources on its Web site (www.cdc.gov/nccdphp/dnpao/socialmarketing/index.html).

The following section outlines how program managers can use social marketing to accomplish missions and objectives that involve helping people in target audiences (which, as with the target markets of commercial marketing, can be individuals, organizations, and groups) improve their personal welfare and that of society by changing behaviors.

Conducting Social Marketing Initiatives in Health Programs

Managers can enhance the likelihood of success in their social marketing initiatives by taking a systematic approach to developing and implementing social marketing strategies. One of the most widely used systematic frameworks for the use of social marketing in health programs is the *Social Marketing Assessment and Response Tool (SMART)* (Thackeray and Neiger 2003), which contains the interactive phases of activities shown in Figure 8.2.

Another framework for using social marketing in health programs is described in the CDC's (2014) Social Marketing for Nutrition and Physical Activity online course. Using this framework, managers planning social marketing initiatives concern themselves primarily with four components of the plan at hand: the problem/health issue, the target audience, behavior to be changed, and strategies for bringing about the change (CDC 2014). These components, along with the basic questions that must be asked and answered in the planning process, are shown in Figure 8.3.

To fully answer the questions posed about each of the components in Figure 8.3, a number of specific and detailed questions will need to be asked and answered. Examples of these questions, adapted from the CDC's (2014, 39) Social Marketing for Nutrition and Physical Activity online course, are as follows:

I. Problem/Health Issue

1. What is the problem?
2. What factors contribute to the problem? What causes or contributes to those factors?

Phase I   Preliminary Planning for Social Marketing Intervention
              • Identify the health issue or problem of focus
              • Develop goals for interventions
              • Outline preliminary plans for evaluation of interventions

Phase II   Patient/Customer Analysis
              • Identify target markets and segment them
              • Determine patient/customer needs and wants
              • Develop preliminary ideas for interventions

Phase III   Social Marketing Strategy
              • Establish plans for 4 Ps (product/service, price, place, and promotion)
              • Identify partners, competitors, and allies
              • Identify individual and societal exchange goods, benefits, values

Phase IV   Develop Interventions
              • Design interventions based on patient/customer analysis and
                social marketing strategy
              • Communicate with partners and clarify roles
              • Pretest and refine the interventions

Phase V   Implement Social Marketing Strategy
              • Activate the interventions
              • Document the process and compare to goals and plans
              • Continually refine the interventions

Phase VI   Evaluate Social Marketing Strategy
              • Assess the degree to which target markets are receiving
                the interventions
              • Ensure that interventions are consistent with plans and protocols; refine
                interventions as necessary
              • Analyze changes in the target markets

Figure 8.2   Phases of the Social Marketing Assessment and Response Tool
Source: Adapted from Thackeray, Rosemary, and Brad L. Neiger, "Use of Social Marketing to Develop Culturally Innovative Diabetes Interventions." *Diabetes Spectrum* 16, no. 1 (January 2003): 15–20. Copyright © 2003 American Diabetes Association. Adapted with permission from the American Diabetes Association.

3. Who is affected by the problem?

4. Who is most likely to change?

5. Who is able to change?

6. What evidence demonstrates there is a health problem? Do you have evidence to show the burden of the health problem in your community?

Plan Component	Questions to Ask and Answer
I. Problem/health issue	What is the problem we need to address?
II. Target audience	Who is affected by the problem and how can they be reached?
III. Behavior	What do we want the audience to do?
IV. Strategies for change	How can we get the target audience to adopt the desired behavior(s)?

Figure 8.3   Main Components of a Social Marketing Plan
Source: Adapted from Centers for Disease Control and Prevention. *Social Marketing: Nutrition and Physical Activity*. Atlanta: Centers for Disease Control and Prevention, Division of Nutrition, Physical Activity, and Obesity, 38. Accessed May 26, 2014. http://www.cdc.gov/nccdphp/dnpa/socialmarketing/training/index.htm.

II. Target Audience

Identifying People in Appropriate Target Audiences

1. Who is the most appropriate audience for your intervention?

2. What are some meaningful ways to distinguish one group from another?

3. Which audiences do your partners and stakeholders most care about? Which audiences are your partners and stakeholders interested in reaching?

4. Which audiences do you or your partners have access to?

5. Which audiences fit in with your organization's priorities?

Segmenting the Target Audience

6. What are the segments in your target audience? How do they differ from each other with regards to their behavior?

7. Which audience segments are most affected by the problem? Or, who has the ability to change the environment of those affected by the problem?

8. Which audience segments are most likely and most willing to change their behavior?

III. Behavior

Selecting a Behavior

1. What is the current behavior of your target audience?

2. What specific behavior are you going to address with your intervention?

3. What is the most realistic behavior change for the target audience to adopt?

4. What behavior can you feasibly try to change?

5. Will a change in this behavior actually affect the problem?

6. Should you select one behavior or a series of behaviors?

Understanding the Behavior in Your Target Audience

7. What will the audience like about the new behavior? What are the consequences of change?

8. What might keep the audience from adopting the new behavior?

9. Are there environmental factors that play a role? What are they?

10. Are there policies or standards (for example, government laws or corporate policies) that either help or hinder the behavior change?

11. What recommendations or guidelines (i.e., *HealthyPeople 2020* objectives, clinical guidelines) exist related to your behavior?

12. What makes the audience's current behavior easy? What makes the target behavior difficult?

13. Is it a measurable behavior? Is it observable? How would you measure it?

14. What happens on days where your audience is successful at doing the behavior? What's different about those days? What made it easier to do it on those days?

15. What about days when they don't do the behavior? What happens on those days? What is different?

IV. Strategies for Change

1. What strategies were used in interventions that have similar goals? Who was the target audience of those other interventions? How are the audiences similar to or different from your target audience?

2. Which strategies are promising?

3. Which strategies have not worked in the past?

4. Are there strategies that have been fully evaluated or draw on a base of evidence?

In addition to questions about people in target audiences noted earlier, other specific planning questions can be asked about the product or service, price, place, and promotion aspects of possible strategies for change as follows (adapted from CDC 2014, 39):

Product or Service

1. What does your target audience like about the behavior? (answers help you identify benefits)

2. What is appealing about it? (benefits)

3. What benefits can you reasonably offer to your audience?

4. What new behavior will be easiest for them to adopt?

5. What could they fit into their lives?

6. What kinds of things do they value in their life?

7. What does your audience believe about the behavior? Do they believe it will provide them with a certain benefit? What do they think, and how do they feel about that benefit?

8. Does the audience believe they can do the behavior?

9. What social supports exist to help your audience adopt the behavior?

Price

10. What does your audience not like about the behavior? (barriers/costs)

11. What is unappealing about it? (barriers/costs)

12. What things keep them from doing the behavior? (barriers/costs)

13. What barriers/costs do you have the ability to modify or reduce?

14. What will the audience need to give up to adopt the desired behavior?

Place

15. Where does the audience do the desired behavior (or its competition)? Where are they thinking about the behavior? Where do they have the opportunity to try the desired behavior?

16. Where does the audience get information about the target behavior?

17. Where does the audience spend time?

Promotion

18. What does your audience value in their lives? What are their hopes and dreams? What do they want out of life?

19. Who influences/could influence your audience to do the behavior? To start it? To maintain it?

20. Whom do they listen to about this behavior? Who is a credible source of information? Who is most motivating?

21. Who would be a credible source of information to the audience about the health topic or about the behavior?

Answers to these questions will serve as a base of information for the program manager who wants to undertake an effective social marketing initiative. In addition, however, there are other steps a manager can take to improve the likelihood of success. These steps are listed in the next section.

Ensuring the Success of Social Marketing Initiatives

Social marketing initiatives work best when those who are designing and implementing them do the following (adapted from Lagarde, 1998):

- Adopt a patient/customer-centered orientation, rather than simply focusing on the message to be conveyed. Conducting formative research, which may be as simple as making sure that the people in the target audiences can read and understand the message, supports this orientation. This orientation requires that representatives of target audiences be actively involved as the social marketing initiative is initially developed so that it fits their needs, wants, perceptions, life-styles, media habits, and other attributes. The use of focus groups made up of representatives of target audiences can be especially useful in ensuring patient/customer focus.

- Carefully segment target audiences. Segmentation based on pre-disposition, motives, values, and lifestyle is essential when designing social marketing strategies. For example, social marketing pertaining to exercise will be different for teenagers and for the elderly.

- Take into account real and perceived barriers (things that prevent people from adopting a new behavior) facing target audiences. Taking barriers into account means being willing to modify interventions to surmount the barriers, including taking action to address the systems or structures that create them. For example, part of an antismoking initiative might involve taking steps to ensure that antismoking regulations that are intended to inhibit smoking in public places are vigorously rather than laxly enforced.

- Demonstrate the benefits of the desired change for people in the target audiences by showing how their needs and interests are served. This requires recognizing that the needs and wants of people in target audiences may differ from those ascribed to them by public health professionals and other program participants, and therefore can only be determined by analysis of the target audiences.

- Use a variety of means or channels to reach target audiences through the media, face-to-face communication, and planned and structured events. The methods selected should be based on analysis of the target audiences.

- Pretest interventions and monitor and evaluate them as an initiative is implemented. Modify the interventions as necessary based on the results of ongoing evaluation (see the discussion of evaluation in Chapter 9).

- Form partnerships that enhance credibility with and facilitate access to target audiences. Partnerships also may help mobilize the human and financial resources necessary to implement a social marketing initiative.

- Create synergy and complementarity with other approaches to social change. Social marketing strategies alone are rarely sufficient to bring about and sustain change. These strategies sometimes work best when related public policies are enacted. For example, laws requiring the use of seat belts, or helmets for motorcyclists, strengthen efforts to encourage their use in target audiences through social marketing strategies.

- Make a long-term commitment to the initiative at hand. The types of changes that most social marketing strategies are aimed at creating take years and decades rather than weeks or months to accomplish. Commitment also often entails sustained financial support for the initiative.

Ethics Considerations in Commercial and Social Marketing Strategies

Ethics considerations and ethical issues routinely emerge in the provision of health services and in the overall management of health programs, including in the development and implementation of both commercial and social marketing strategies (Andreasen 2001). Remember from our discussion of ethical program management in Chapter 1 that managers should be guided by the application of four key ethics principles: respect for persons, justice, beneficence, and nonmaleficence.

Kass (2001) suggested a framework for considering the ethical aspects of health interventions, which readily applies to health services that use social marketing. She indicated that conducting a careful *ethics analysis* increases the likelihood that those who are planning interventions will be meticulous in their reasoning and will design interventions that are based on science and facts and not merely on beliefs. Using the example of a health education–based cardiac risk reduction intervention, the steps in conducting an ethics analysis are outlined as follows:

Step 1: Determine the objectives of the intervention. Establishing objectives is the starting point in an ethics analysis of a health intervention. The objectives may already have been established by someone else planning the intervention. If they do not already exist, however, objectives must be established and used in conducting the analysis. These objectives might typically be expressed in terms of health improvements, such as reduction of morbidity or mortality. Using the cardiac risk reduction intervention as an example, those who are planning this health education intervention for a target audience would be likely to establish an objective of reducing the number of heart attacks among individuals in the target audience. Other objectives could include producing certain educational information about cardiac risk and distributing it to people in the target audience, and having individuals in the target audience learn relevant facts about cardiac risk and change their risk-related behavior.

Step 2: Assess the potential effectiveness of the planned intervention in relation to achieving the established objectives. In this step, those planning the intervention would consider the question of how the intervention will achieve the desired results. All interventions have a hypothesis embedded in them, even if the hypothesis is only implicit. Those planning an intervention hypothesize that if they do a, b, and c, then the result will be x, y, and z. For example, the hypothesis on which the cardiac risk reduction intervention rests is that if individuals in the target audience are exposed to risk-reduction information, then they will change their behavior (for example, stop smoking, modify their diet, increase exercise) in ways suggested by the information provided—and that the changes in behavior will result in fewer heart attacks for those in the target audience. The planners of this intervention should challenge the assumptions in their hypothesis by examining existing data and evidence about the effectiveness of such interventions. Only if a planned intervention is reasonably likely to achieve the objectives established for it should the intervention be implemented.

Step 3: Determine and minimize the known or potential burdens of the planned intervention. Interventions can impose a variety of potential burdens or harms, ranging from physical harm to issues of privacy and confidentiality. Among the various types of interventions, health education interventions tend to impose relatively few burdens. Education-based interventions are voluntary and seek to empower people in the target audience with information that equips them to make their own choices and decisions concerning their health. Even though the potential burdens and harms in the planned health education–based cardiac risk reduction intervention may be relatively minor, however, the known and potential burdens must be determined so that they can be minimized.

Once identified, the known and potential burdens of the intervention must be reduced to the lowest possible level. For example, health education interventions are potentially paternalistic when they emphasize changes in behavior. Paternalism is inconsistent with the ethics principle of respect for persons in terms of treating people as autonomous beings. Similarly, health education–based interventions can stereotype people in a target audience if care is not exercised. For example, decisions about who is pictured in educational materials should be carefully considered. If only obese people are pictured, it may convey the incorrect message that obesity is the only relevant risk factor related to the health education–based cardiac risk reduction intervention.

Step 4: Ensure that the intervention is implemented fairly. This step is based on the principle of justice, which requires that the benefits and the burdens of an intervention be distributed fairly among those affected. For example, unless the cardiac risk reduction intervention is being planned for a specific segment within the target audience (such as women, the elderly, or African American males), perhaps because they have been identified as being at particularly high risk, the intervention should be designed to benefit all members of the target audience. Similarly, the intervention should be readily and conveniently available to the entire target audience.

Summary

Overall, this chapter presents a picture of how both *commercial marketing* strategies and *social marketing* interventions or initiatives play a role in the success of health programs. Commercial marketing, which is important to all health programs, is defined as the process of planning, implementing, and evaluating activities designed to bring about satisfying exchange relationships with patients/customers and other stakeholders in a program's dynamic environment. Social marketing, which is useful in many health programs, is defined as the application of commercial marketing technologies to planning, implementing, and evaluating services that are designed to influence the voluntary behavior of target audiences to improve their personal welfare and that of society.

Effective commercial marketing strategies help managers identify, quantify, and understand the needs and wants of people in their target markets, whether patients/customers or other stakeholders who can contribute to the success of a program. When effectively packaged with product or service, price, place, and promotion elements, a complete commercial marketing strategy can emerge (see Figure 8.1). The purpose of a commercial marketing strategy is to facilitate mutually beneficial exchanges with people in a program's target markets.

This chapter's discussion includes how managers identify and quantify target markets, and how they seek to understand the needs and wants of people in these markets. The importance of understanding the perceived, expressed, and normative needs of people in target markets and market segments is emphasized.

The epidemiological planning model, which is useful in estimating the size and scope of markets for the services provided by many programs, is described, along with an applied example. It is noted, however, that even after people in target markets and in segments within the markets are identified, quantified, and understood, managers must develop commercial marketing strategies to facilitate exchanges with them.

When effectively managed, commercial marketing strategies will help attract patients/customers directly and through referrals, and they can help attract participants, donors, and volunteers, as well as gain the support of the organization in which a program is embedded. Commercial marketing strategies can also improve relationships with regulatory agencies and grant makers.

Many programs also find social marketing initiatives useful in achieving their respective missions and objectives. This is especially so when the program's work involves health promotion and education as part of efforts intended to change the behavior of individuals and groups. Social marketing has been used to address such health issues as smoking cessation, safety, drug abuse, drinking and driving, HIV and AIDS, nutrition, physical activity, immunization, breast cancer screening, mental health, family planning, and numerous others.

Two widely used systematic frameworks for the use of social marketing in health programs are presented in the chapter. The Social Marketing Assessment and Response Tool (Thackeray and Neiger 2003) is described in terms of the interactive phases of activities shown in Figure 8.2. Another framework for using social marketing in health programs described in the chapter is the CDC's (2014) Social Marketing for Nutrition and Physical Activity online course. The four components of this framework, along with the basic questions that must be asked and answered in the planning process, are shown in Figure 8.3.

It is noted that ethics considerations routinely arise in the development and implementation of both commercial and social marketing strategies and initiatives, and that managers must pay attention to how these issues are addressed. Managers can be guided in these efforts by the application of four key ethics principles: respect for persons, justice, beneficence, and nonmaleficence.

REVIEW QUESTIONS

1. Define commercial marketing and social marketing as they apply to health programs. Why are both important to health programs?

2. Discuss the importance of identifying target markets and segments as a basis for developing effective commercial marketing strategies.

3. Discuss the usefulness of the epidemiological planning model in developing effective commercial marketing strategies.

4. Briefly describe the five Ps of a commercial marketing strategy.

5. List and describe the five dimensions of service that are important to patients/customers in the SERVQUAL model of ensuring service quality.

6. Write an outline of the topics that should be covered in an identity and capabilities brochure for a program.

7. Describe ways that a program can use the media in promotional efforts.

8. Discuss the key components of an effective social marketing strategy.

9. Discuss how managers can avoid ethics problems in developing and implementing commercial and social marketing strategies.

KEY TERMS AND CONCEPTS

commercial marketing

commercial marketing strategy

epidemiological planning model (EPM)

ethics analysis

exchange relationships

five Ps of commercial marketing

Internet

marketing mix

market segments

social marketing

Social Marketing Assessment and Response Tool (SMART)

social media

target audiences

target markets

References

American Marketing Association. "Marketing." Accessed May 24, 2014. http://www.marketingpower.com/_layouts/dictionary.aspx?dLetter=M

Andreasen, Alan R. *Ethics in Social Marketing*. Washington, DC: Georgetown University, 2001.

Andreasen, Alan R. *Social Marketing in the 21st Century*. Thousand Oaks, CA: Sage, 2005.

Berkowitz, Eric N. *Essentials of Health Care Marketing*, 3rd ed. Burlington, MA: Jones & Bartlett Learning, 2011.

Berkowitz, Eric N., Louis G. Pol, and Richard K. Thomas. *Healthcare Market Research: Tools and Techniques for Analyzing and Understanding Today's Healthcare Environment*. New York: McGraw-Hill, 1995.

Centers for Disease Control and Prevention. *Social Marketing: Nutrition and Physical Activity*. Atlanta: Centers for Disease Control and Prevention, Division of Nutrition, Physical Activity, and Obesity. Accessed May 26, 2014. http://www.cdc.gov/nccdphp/dnpa/socialmarketing/training/index.htm

Fox, Susannah, and Maeve Duggan. *Health Online 2013*. Washington, DC: Pew Research Center's Internet & American Life Project, January 15, 2013. http://www.pewinternet.org/2013/01/15/health-online-2013/

French, Jeff, Clive Blair-Stevens, Dominic McVey, and Rowena Merritt. *Social Marketing and Public Health: Theory and Practice*. New York: Oxford University Press, 2010.

Ginter, Peter M., W. Jack Duncan, and Linda E. Swayne. *Strategic Management of Health Care Organizations*, 7th ed. San Francisco: Jossey-Bass, 2013.

Grier, Sonya, and Carol A. Bryant. "Social Marketing in Public Health." *Annual Review of Public Health* 26 (2005): 319–339.

Healthy Start. "Welcome to Healthy Start." Accessed January 24, 2014. http://www.healthystartpittsburgh.org/index.php?cID=1

Hoffman, K. Douglas, and John E. G. Bateson. *Essentials of Services Marketing: Concepts, Strategies, and Cases*, 4th ed. Mason, OH: South-Western, Cengage Learning, 2011.

Kaplan, Andreas M., and Michael Haenlein. "Users of the World, United! Challenges and Opportunities of Social Media." *Business Horizons* 53, no. 1 (January 2010): 59–68.

Kass, Nancy E. "An Ethics Framework for Public Health." *American Journal of Public Health* 91, no. 11 (November 2001): 1776–1783.

Keller, Kevin, and Philip Kotler. *Framework for Marketing Management*, 5th ed. Upper Saddle River, NJ: Prentice Hall, 2011.

Lagarde, François. "Best Practices and Prospects for Social Marketing in Public Health." Speech given at the 89th Annual Conference of the Canadian Public Health Association on Best Practices in Public Health, Montreal, Quebec, June 8, 1998.

Lee, Nancy R., and Philip Kotler. *Social Marketing: Influencing Behaviors for Good*, 4th ed. Thousand Oaks, CA: Sage, 2011.

Luallin, Meryl D., and Kevin W. Sullivan. "Marketing in a Changing Environment." In *Ambulatory Care Management*, edited by Austin Ross, Stephen J. Williams, and Ernest J. Pavlock, 3rd ed., 287–307. Clifton Park, NY: Delmar, 1998.

Pride, William M., and O. C. Ferrell. *Marketing*, 17th ed. Mason, OH: South-Western, Cengage Learning, 2014.

Smith, William A. "Social Marketing: An Evolving Definition." *American Journal of Health Behavior* 24, no. 1 (January-February 2000): 11–17.

Thackeray, Rosemary, and Brad L. Neiger. "Use of Social Marketing to Develop Culturally Innovative Diabetes Interventions." *Diabetes Spectrum* 16, no. 1 (January 2003): 15–20.

U.S. Department of Health and Human Services. "Healthy Start." Accessed January 24, 2014. http://mchb.hrsa.gov/programs/healthystart/index.html.

Weinreich, Nedra K. *Hands-On Social Marketing: A Step-by-Step Guide to Designing Change for Good*. Thousand Oaks, CA: Sage, 2011.

White, Kenneth R., and John R. Griffith. *The Well-Managed Healthcare Organization*, 7th ed. Chicago: Health Administration Press, 2010.

Zeithaml, Valarie A., A. Parasuraman, and Leonard L. Berry. *Delivering Quality Service: Balancing Customer Perceptions and Expectations*. New York: Free Press, 1990.

A Step-by-Step Social Marketing Process

The Georgia Division of Public Health worked closely with the Fulton County Health Department in Atlanta to develop a nutrition and physical activity intervention targeted to tweens (children 9–12 years old) to address obesity. They chose to follow the social marketing process to influence tween behavior regarding nutrition and physical activity. State and county representatives, along with their partners, formed a work group and began discussing this intervention in January. They followed a process, including: (1) describing the problem, (2) choosing a target audience, (3) conducting formative research with that audience, and (4) developing an intervention strategy based on social marketing.

The social marketing process began with a "Social Marketing 101" training class for all work group members in February. This training highlighted the differences between social marketing and other planning processes. It also emphasized the need to take time to plan and learn about the target audience before choosing intervention strategies.

Describing the Problem

A local graduate student worked with the work group to describe the obesity problem in Georgia. She gathered information comparing Georgia's obesity prevalence to national levels and used it to write the problem description for a social marketing plan.

This appendix is a case study that has been adapted from Centers for Disease Control and Prevention. *Georgia Uses Step-by-Step Social Marketing Process.* Atlanta: Centers for Disease Control and Prevention, Nutrition and Physical Activity Communication Team, September 2006. http://www.cdc.gov/nccdphp/DNPAO/socialmarketing/pdf/Georgia_0906.pdf.

The problem description had several components. It identified the populations with the greatest need and those most likely to change their behavior. A second part was a list of behavioral factors that could potentially contribute to obesity. Some examples were low fruit and vegetable intake, frequent television viewing, and consumption of sweetened beverages. A third part was a description of behavior-change models that could apply to this problem. These models were revisited as the team formed its intervention strategy. Another part of the problem description identified potential behavioral theories that might aid in developing the intervention. The concepts of "self-efficacy" and "influence of the environment" from social cognitive theory were particularly useful in planning. Finally, the problem description included best practices and lessons learned from other programs that had addressed overweight in children.

Choosing a Target Audience

The work group identified two potential audiences: preschoolers (2–5 years old) and tweens (9–12 years old). It was difficult to decide which audience to target, because they felt like they could make a case for either age group. However, they chose tweens for several reasons. The group felt that it would be easier to intervene with tweens because they could be targeted directly, instead of through their parents. Tweens are at a stage of life where they are beginning to make some of their own decisions. Finally, Georgia already provides a variety of services to younger children, so the group wanted to offer something to older children as well.

Georgia had data on tween overweight prevalence as well as information about their current behavior. Some data came from the Georgia Student Health Survey (Youth Risk Behavior Survey [YRBS]), including self-reported heights and weights, physical activity levels, and TV viewing habits. The YRBS collects data on middle school children aged 11–14 and high school children aged 14–18. Georgia used the middle school data as an estimate for tweens. Other data sources included the Continuing Survey of Food Intakes by Individuals (CSFII) and a tween audience analysis from the Health Communications Unit in Toronto, Canada.

The choice of "tweens" was still a broad target audience. A specific segment of this target audience was chosen after the work group conducted formative research with the target audience. The work group also discussed possible secondary target audiences—parents or caregivers, school cafeteria workers, physical educators, after-school programs, and tween peers. Final decisions about secondary audiences were also saved until the work group had conducted its formative research.

The work group began to learn more about the broad target audience and to make some initial decisions about behavioral objectives and the intervention setting. The problem description contained information from the literature on best practices and lessons learned about obesity prevention. These resources helped the group choose the main behaviors to target for change. The group chose increasing physical activity and increasing healthy snack and beverage choices. These behaviors were refined in June as the team met with school representatives, teachers, and community organizations. In this meeting, the group identified the existing strengths, weaknesses, opportunities, and threats (a SWOT analysis) to working with tweens. The participants felt that gaining access to the target audience would be easier in the community instead of through the school system. Therefore, they decided to conduct the intervention in a community setting. This meeting also provided an opportunity for Georgia to gain input from the "experts"—people who were currently working with tweens and could give some insight into their behaviors and motivations.

Some of these early decisions were difficult for the team, and some members of the work group wanted to revisit them in future meetings. To keep progressing, the leaders decided to add two items to their standing agenda: "decisions made" and "action steps," so that the decisions were clear and the group could move on to the next steps. This was done only after getting agreement from all of the work group members.

Conducting Formative Research

The work group decided to use focus groups to understand more about tweens. The focus groups served two purposes: to help the work group understand its audience better, and to find out what strategies could be effective at reaching tweens. A series of focus groups for tweens and their parents were conducted.

A literature review led to the first draft of focus group questions. The questions addressed barriers and enablers to performing the desired behaviors, and ways to reach the audience. Next, the team refined the questions by using some examples from VERB™ (a campaign that also targets tweens) and the Lexington Tweens Nutrition and Fitness Coalition in Kentucky. The team also looked at other focus groups that had been done in Georgia to learn from those experiences. They gave the questions to the Nutrition and Physical Activity Communication Team (NuPAC) at the Centers for Disease Control and Prevention (CDC) for review. Lastly, the team informally pretested the questions by asking for feedback from team members who had access to tweens or their parents.

The work group recruited participants for the focus groups from the Atlanta Public School System. One of the work group members who worked with the school district gave the team contact information for eight schools with after-school programs. Institutional review board committees from the Atlanta Public School System and Georgia's Department of Human Resources granted approval.

Principals from all eight schools were contacted, and two agreed to participate. The work group then worked with the after-school coordinators to recruit participants; they posted flyers and offered food and gift certificates to a local grocery store as incentives. Parents who had a child in the 4th or 5th grade were eligible to participate.

Overall, four focus groups were conducted—two with parents and two with their tweens. Groups for the tweens and parents were held at the same time but in separate rooms. All focus groups were held in the schools and were moderated either by work group members or a consultant with another local health department. Because they were not allowed to audiotape the tween focus groups, the team also had note-takers present.

Following the focus groups, the work group collaborated with a local university to analyze the data from the tween groups and a local health promotion organization to analyze the data from parent groups. These two groups then met with work group members to review responses given by the parents and tweens.

Creating the Social Marketing Strategy

Continuing to follow the social marketing process, the Georgia Division of Public Health and the Fulton County Health Department took the fourth step in the process: developing an intervention strategy based on social marketing. This step involved several components as follows.

Segmenting the Target Audience

Once the focus groups were conducted and the results had been analyzed, the work group met to brainstorm about potential audience segments. Their desire was to segment tweens by their current behaviors, instead of just demographics. In August, the work group met for a two-part series of meetings to make final decisions about primary and secondary target audiences.

During these meetings, the team narrowed the target audience's age range even further, to 9–11 years old. Other target audience characteristics included: being African American, living in Southeast Atlanta in Fulton County, and attending public schools. Even though these children attend public schools, the intervention will focus on their out-of-school time. The team further specified the target audience by describing a particular segment they called "Your Regular Kid." These children have the following characteristics: they are somewhat active, they are healthy, they participate in after-school programs, and they come from single-parent families. The work group eliminated school personnel as a potential secondary audience and chose to focus on parents/caregivers and peers instead.

Refining Behavioral Objectives

At the same meetings, the work group revised its broad behavioral objectives to make them more specific. For example, the group took the broad goal of "increase levels of physical activity" and revised this to "increase active play outside of school time, with your peers, for 60 minutes per day." This will be revised further to include a baseline (the percentage of students who are already doing this) and a target goal for improvement.

Developing the Strategy

During its two-part series of meetings, the team combined the findings from its literature review, expert advice, and focus group results. All of this formative research allowed it to identify its audience's benefits from and barriers to participating in the desired behaviors. For example, tweens valued energy, strength, and active play as benefits of physical activity. Some barriers were lack of time for physical activity and embarrassment over lack of skill. The team also identified activities that may compete with the target behavior, such as shopping and spending time with friends. Finally, they identified other factors that may be important (e.g., the tweens know about healthy eating and physical activity but are also confused about what is healthy) and possible channels to reach the target audience (e.g., TV, malls near public transportation). All of these components will be used to determine strategies and activities to design the final intervention. The work group also spent time prioritizing the factors that related specifically to their chosen audience segment.

Next Steps

Georgia plans to hire a project coordinator to lead this intervention. They are currently working on developing a job description for this person and hope to hire someone soon. They will continue to refine their strategy and intervention components, create specific behavioral objectives, identify and recruit more community partners, and identify a specific geographic location or neighborhood in which to place the intervention.

CHAPTER 9

EVALUATING

Managers of health programs engage extensively in evaluation. Evaluation plays a key role in everyday program management, yielding feedback on both program design and execution. These activities are akin to other management activities, such as routinely monitoring and controlling performance, especially as these tasks relate to progress toward accomplishing a program's mission and objectives. However, program evaluation tends to be more structured and formalized than routine monitoring of performance (McDavid, Huse, and Hawthorn 2013). Evaluations can be designed to answer a range of questions about programs to assist program managers with decision making. They may be conducted to assess an entire program, or they may focus on a specific aspect or component of a program, such as a particular service provided by the program or a particular activity within the overall program, such as marketing.

Program evaluations may be conducted internally by program managers or other participants, including experts from the host organization. Alternatively, program evaluations may be conducted by others external to a program, such as when an independent assessment of a program's strengths and weaknesses is needed. Independent assessments are typically conducted at critical decision points—for example, when a decision must be made about whether to continue or discontinue a program, or whether to make major adjustments in its funding. Independent program evaluations are generally in the hands of professional evaluators and are not the focus of this chapter. Instead, we will examine how program managers can use evaluation to make better decisions about developing/strategizing, designing, and leading in their programs.

LEARNING OBJECTIVES
After reading this chapter, you should be able to:

- Define program evaluation, and understand what program managers evaluate
- Understand the roles of program theory and logic models in program evaluation
- Distinguish among different types of evaluations and understand their appropriate uses
- Understand the Centers for Disease Control and Prevention's six-step framework for designing program evaluations
- Outline a written report of a program evaluation

Like decision making, communicating, managing quality, and marketing, *evaluating* is a facilitative activity that managers engage in as they perform their core activities of developing/strategizing, designing, and leading as well as their other facilitative activities (see Figure 1.4).

In Chapter 1, programs were defined as organizational units intended to accomplish one or more objectives through a plan of action that describes what work is to be done, by whom, when, and how, as well as what resources will be used. In this chapter, we bring things full circle by exploring what program managers do to evaluate or assess whether a program's mission and objectives have been or are being achieved. This exploration begins with a definition of program evaluation.

Program Evaluation Defined

At its most basic level, evaluating something means determining "its merit, worth, value, or significance" (Patton 2012, 2). When managers evaluate a program or some component of a program, they are interested in determining its value, among other things. Such a determination of value is made by seeking answers to such practical questions as the following: How effective is our program, or some component of it? Have the mission and objectives of our program been achieved, or have the objectives of some component of our program been achieved? What are the strengths and weaknesses of our program or a component part of it? To what extent do the benefits of our program or a component part of it justify its costs? Does our program or a component part of it deserve continued funding? Increased funding? And so on. There are many ways to answer these and other similar questions. In distinguishing evaluation from other forms of inquiry, Fournier (2005, 139–140) said that evaluation "is an applied inquiry process for collecting and synthesizing evidence that culminates in conclusions about the state of affairs, value, merit, worth, significance, or quality of a program, product, person, policy, proposal or plan. Conclusions made in evaluations encompass both an empirical aspect (that something is the case) and a normative aspect (judgment about the value of something). It is the value feature that distinguishes evaluation from other types of inquiry, such as basic science research, clinical epidemiology, investigative journalism, or public polling."

As we will see, there are various types of program evaluations that managers can use, although they have much in common. McNamara (2014) identified at least thirty-five different types of program evaluations. Even with all these different types, however, *program evaluation* can be defined generically as "carefully collecting information about a program or some aspect of a program in order to make necessary decisions about the program" (McNamara 2014). This definition has the advantage of being consistent with our view that program evaluation is one of the facilitative activities of program managers in performing their management work.

Another good definition of program evaluation is given by the U.S. Government Accountability Office (GAO; 2012, 3): "Program evaluation is a systematic study using research methods to collect and analyze data to assess how well a program (or a component part of a program) is working and why. Evaluations answer specific questions about program performance and may focus on assessing program operations or results. Evaluation results may be used to assess a program's effectiveness, identify how to improve performance, or guide resource allocation."

Yet another, similar definition of program evaluation is that it is "a systematic method for collecting, analyzing, and using information to answer basic questions about a program—and to ensure that those answers are supported by evidence" (Office of Planning, Research and Evaluation 2010, 6). In a classic and widely cited definition, program evaluation is described as "the systematic assessment of the operation and/or outcomes of a program, compared to a set of standards, in order to improve the program" (Weiss 1998, 4). What is clear from these definitions is that program evaluation is an activity that program managers engage in as they seek to manage their programs in ways that improve both operations and results.

What Do Program Managers Evaluate?

At the most general level, program evaluation requires that managers pay attention to "documenting and measuring the implementation of the program and its success in achieving intended outcomes, and using such information to be accountable to key stakeholders" (Centers for Disease Control and Prevention [CDC] 2011, 1). In effect, program evaluation requires attention to three distinct aspects of a program or a component part, such as a specific intervention conducted by the program: its implementation, its effectiveness, and its accountability to key stakeholders (CDC 2011; Fallon, Begun, and Riley 2013). These three aspects are described here:

- *Program implementation.* Often a first evaluation activity involves judging whether a program or component of a program was implemented as planned. Examining the operations of a program—including answering questions, for example, about what activities took place, who conducted the activities, and whether target markets were reached by the activities—can lead to identification of the program's strengths and weaknesses, which can then lead to improvements in the program's content and operations.

- *Program effectiveness.* Programs and their components ultimately are evaluated on whether they achieve the purposes for which they were established. Programs have a mission and objectives, and can be judged on the extent to which these are accomplished.

- *Program accountability.* Evaluation is a tool with which to demonstrate program accountability to an array of stakeholders (individuals, organizations, and groups, inside or outside the program, with significant interests in it). A typical program's stakeholders include its host organization, funders and payers, patients/customers and those with the potential to become patients/customers, program participants, regulators and policymakers, and many others. The results of program evaluation can demonstrate accountability in a number of ways. For example, accountability to patients/customers is demonstrated when evaluation reveals that they experienced health improvements because of a program's intervention. Similarly, when evaluation shows that a program performed as expected and fulfilled its objectives, accountability to its funders and payers is demonstrated.

No matter what aspect of a program or a component part of it is being evaluated, a complete understanding of the program is helpful as a precursor to the evaluation. Two useful tools in understanding any program are the underlying program theory of how the program is supposed to work and the associated logic model of the program. Remember, the concepts of program theory and logic models were introduced in Chapter 2 (see Figure 2.1, which is a logic model in schematic form), and were applied to the core management activity of designing in Chapter 3. As noted there, logic models are useful in designing programs. They are also very useful in evaluating programs, especially in concert with the associated theory of how a program is intended to work. The important roles of logic models and program theory in evaluation are discussed in the next section.

Program Theory and Logic Models

Logic models, such as the one in Figure 2.1, describe schematically the relationships among the resources available to a program, the activities or work processes planned and undertaken with the resources, and the effects or results intended to be achieved through operating the program (Frechtling 2007; Funnell and Rogers 2011; W. K. Kellogg Foundation 2004). The ***logic model*** for a program is based on a ***program theory.*** Thus, to understand a logic model, one must first understand the underlying program theory on which it is based. In fact, the term logic model is used because implicit in the theory on which a program can be built is an underlying logic or rationale (Renger and Titcomb 2002).

As discussed in Chapter 2, any program can be conceptualized using a theory as the basis for how the program is intended to work. Of course, there are instances in which no one has bothered to use a program theory as a basis for a program. When a program theory is present, as is the case with most well-managed programs, the underlying theory can be expressed as follows: if inputs or resources a, b, and c are assembled and processed by doing m, n, and o with them, then the results will be x, y, and z. The important point here is that any program, if its underlying program theory is used as a guideline, can be described in terms of the relationships among the resources available for it to use, the work processes it undertakes with the resources, and the results it achieves by processing the resources. Fully understanding these elements of a program and their interrelationships will serve program managers well in their evaluation activity.

Evaluations with and without a Program Theory

A program may or may not be based on an underlying theory. Evaluations in these two circumstances are very different. It is instructive to contrast conducting a program evaluation for a program that is not based on an underlying theory with evaluating a program that is theory based. For example, imagine a program called Walk a Mile for Health, which encourages sedentary people to begin walking to improve their health. Figure 9.1 shows a representation of this program without an underlying theory, simply depicting the program followed by the intended outcome of better health. In an evaluation of this program, which would be termed a "black box evaluation" (Funnell and Rogers 2011, 4) because there is no theory of an explanatory relationship between the program and outcome available, only inputs and an outcome would be considered, without attention to the processes occurring in between.

It is very difficult, if not impossible, to interpret results from an evaluation of a program with no underlying program theory. Such an

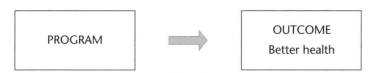

Figure 9.1   Evaluating Walk a Mile for Health without a Program Theory

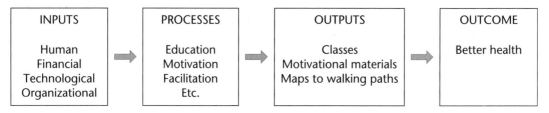

Figure 9.2   Evaluating Walk a Mile for Health with a Program Theory

evaluation would yield very little information that could be used to manage and improve the program. In contrast, if this same program were based on a program theory that reflected the causal processes that occur between encouraging sedentary people to walk and improved health, an evaluation of it could provide the program manager with much more useful information. Figure 9.2 shows a representation of this program with an underlying theory, depicting the program in terms of inputs, processes, outputs, and an outcome. The theory is that the program will use certain processes— such as educating sedentary people about the health effects of walking, motivating them to walk more, facilitating their walking with information about good locations and facilities for walking, and so on—to accomplish the desired outcome of better health for patients/customers. The program theory incorporates the well-established relationship between walking (or other forms of exercise) and improved health.

Uses of Program Theory and Logic Models in Program Evaluation

Program managers may be involved in multiple evaluations, and may engage in this activity in regard to several program components simultaneously. Correspondingly, there are multiple possible uses of program theory and logic models in evaluation, and use will vary depending on circumstances. For example, when an evaluation is undertaken as a program manager is initially developing/strategizing a program and designing how it will be structured and how it will operate, the program manager or others who are conducting the evaluation can use program theory to help do the following (Funnell and Rogers 2011, 442–443):

•   Ensure that key stakeholders have a clear and reasonably cohesive idea about what the program is all about and that there is sufficient buy-in to the program for it to be successfully implemented

•   Evaluate the likely future effectiveness of the program by ensuring that the situation and its causes have been adequately identified and incorporated in the program theory

- Make sure the objectives are achievable and important and the design is appropriate to the situation and feasible to implement

- Develop a monitoring, evaluation, and reporting framework for use during program implementation

Program managers will find different ways to use program theory once a program has begun to be implemented. In this circumstance, program theory can be used to do the following (Funnell and Rogers 2011, 443):

- Identify the critical aspects to monitor with respect to inputs, processes, outputs, immediate outcomes, and any other key factors that might affect outcomes to ensure that the program is on track and performing as well as possible, especially if this has not been done during the [initial developing/strategizing and designing activities]

- Identify key evaluation questions

- Conduct an assessment of a program's readiness for measuring and evaluating outcomes at various points in the logic model

- Conduct a formative or process evaluation concerning program implementation

When a program manager is conducting an evaluation of a mature, operational program for which a decision must be made as to whether continuation or adaptation is appropriate, program theory can be useful in yet other ways. In this circumstance, program theory can be used to decide what information needs to be collected for purposes such as these (Funnell and Rogers 2011, 443):

- Demonstrate effectiveness in achieving desired outcomes and addressing needs (additional to any that might already have been included in a routine performance monitoring system)

- Demonstrate that outcomes are attributable to the program

- Ensure that the design continues to be appropriate

- Determine what changes, if any, are needed to improve effectiveness and efficiency

In another circumstance, when a program manager is conducting a summative evaluation of a program's performance, program theory can be used in assessing accountability by identifying information needed to determine the following (Funnell and Rogers 2011, 443–444):

- What outcomes were achieved and how well did they address program objectives

- The extent to which outcomes were attributable to the program

- Lessons learned for the future about, for example, factors that affect success or unintended outcomes

Indeed, the underlying theory of a program can be used in many ways as its manager engages in the evaluating activity. In the next section, we will consider the variety of types of program evaluations with which managers should be familiar.

Types of Program Evaluations

As noted earlier, there are numerous types of program evaluations. Among the most widely used are process and outcome evaluations, formative and summative evaluations, and cost-benefit and cost-effectiveness evaluations. Each of these types has specific characteristics as follows (adapted from Office of Planning, Research and Evaluation 2010, 96–101):

- *Process evaluation*—an evaluation that examines the extent to which a program or component part of it is operating as intended by assessing ongoing operations and whether the target population (market or audience) is being served. A process evaluation involves collecting data that describes operations in detail, including the types and levels of services provided, the location of service delivery, staffing, socio-demographic characteristics of participants, the community in which services are provided, and the linkages with collaborating agencies. A process evaluation—also called a formative or implementation evaluation—helps program staff identify needed interventions, change program components to improve service delivery, or both.

- *Outcome evaluation*—an evaluation that is designed to assess the extent to which a program or a component of it has affected those targeted according to specific variables or data elements. These results are expected to be caused by program activities and tested by comparing results across sample groups in the target population. This type of evaluation is also known as an impact or summative evaluation.

- *Formative evaluation*—a type of process evaluation of a new program or a component of it that focuses on collecting data on operations so that needed changes or modifications can be made to the program or component in its early stages. Formative evaluations are used to provide program managers and staff with feedback about the program components that are working and those that need to be changed.

- *Summative evaluation*—a type of outcome evaluation that assesses the results or outcomes of a program or component. This type of evaluation is concerned with the overall effectiveness of a program or component. Summative evaluations often occur at the conclusion of a program to estimate the program's effectiveness. Evaluations conducted after a program has concluded have their uses, but evaluations that occur while a program is ongoing can result in a steady stream of improvements for the program or component, and tend to be more beneficial. Summative evaluations can be usefully conducted on an annual or biannual basis for ongoing programs.

- *Cost-benefit evaluation*—a type of evaluation that involves comparing the relative costs of operating a program or component (expenses, staff salaries, and so on) with the benefits (gains to individuals or society) it generates. For example, a cost-benefit evaluation of an intervention to reduce cigarette smoking would focus on the difference between the dollars expended for converting smokers into nonsmokers and the dollar savings from reduced medical care for smoking-related disease, days lost from work, and the like.

- *Cost-effectiveness evaluation*—a type of evaluation that involves comparing the relative costs of operating a program or component with the extent to which the program or component met its objectives. For example, an evaluation of an intervention to reduce cigarette smoking would involve estimating the dollars that had to be expended to convert each smoker into a nonsmoker.

Program managers typically use multiple types of evaluations in carrying out the evaluating activity. Over the life of a program, its manager might use any or all of the types just listed, and perhaps other types as well, depending on the purpose of any particular evaluation. For example, as we discussed in Chapter 8, knowing how commercial or social marketing strategies have worked in reaching and influencing target markets and target audiences is an important step in using marketing effectively and in improving future marketing efforts. Managers must answer such questions as, Did our message reach the intended target markets or audiences? Did they believe and accept our message? Ultimately, did they respond as we had hoped they would? Answering such questions requires that marketing strategies be evaluated (Russ-Eft and Preskill 2009).

A program manager interested in evaluating a commercial marketing strategy for a program or in evaluating a social marketing intervention might use several types of evaluations. A formative evaluation could be undertaken to help those responsible for developing a marketing strategy determine how people in the target markets or audiences will react to messages and materials as the messages and materials are being developed. This evaluation would entail testing the messages and means of distributing them to ensure that target markets or audiences will understand the information communicated through the marketing effort.

A second type of evaluation, process evaluation, could be used to track how effectively the message is reaching the target markets or audiences. It would involve tracking when, where, and how often messages are delivered, as well as how often those in the target markets or audiences actually see or hear the messages. A third type of evaluation, outcome evaluation, would focus on what happened with people in the target markets or audiences as a result of the marketing effort.

No matter what type of evaluation is being contemplated or undertaken, managers should put it into the context of an overarching evaluation framework. One very useful framework has been developed by the CDC (1999, 2011, 2014) and is discussed next. This extended discussion provides the structure for much of the remainder of this chapter.

The CDC Framework for Conducting Program Evaluations

Evaluations of programs or components of programs can range from simple to complex. Even simple evaluations, however, benefit from a framework that outlines the essential elements of an evaluation and illustrates how to organize and conduct a program evaluation. Using a comprehensive evaluation framework to design and conduct an evaluation accomplishes two purposes: (1) it enhances the evaluation's quality, credibility, and usefulness, and (2) it allows program managers to make effective use of the time and resources devoted to the evaluating activity.

The CDC (1999, 2011, 2014) has developed and encourages use of a framework, consisting of six steps and four sets of standards, for conducting evaluations of health programs or components of them, as shown in Figure 9.3. *The CDC framework for program evaluation* can assist program managers as they plan, design, implement, and use the results of program evaluations.

It should be noted at the outset of this discussion of a framework for conducting program evaluations that the CDC evaluation framework is not the only one. For example, another very useful framework for conducting program evaluations has been developed by the W. K. Kellogg Foundation (2004). Interested readers might wish to compare the CDC and W. K.

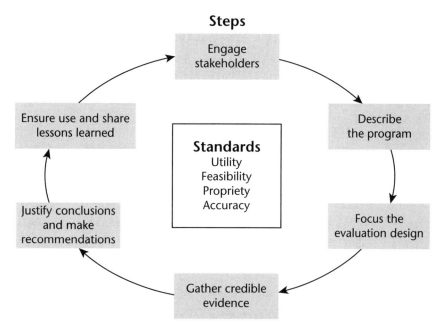

Figure 9.3   CDC Framework for Program Evaluation

Source: Adapted from Centers for Disease Control and Prevention. "Framework for Program Evaluation in Public Health." *Morbidity and Mortality Weekly Report* 48, no. RR-11 (September 17, 1999), 4. The original figure is also available at Centers for Disease Control and Prevention. "A Framework for Program Evaluation." Accessed May 27, 2014. http://www.cdc.gov/eval/framework/index.htm.

Kellogg frameworks. This discussion, however, is based on the CDC framework exclusively.

As we begin an extensive discussion of the CDC evaluation framework in this chapter, we will start by examining the standards, because they are what the quality of almost all program evaluations is judged against. In fact, the CDC based its standards on core attributes of evaluation quality developed with oversight by the Joint Committee on Standards for Educational Evaluation (www.jcsee.org), a coalition of respected professional associations concerned with the quality of evaluation (Yarbrough, Shulha, Hopson, and Caruthers 2011).

Standards in the CDC Evaluation Framework

There are thirty standards in total, although they are organized into four sets as follows (CDC 2014; see the section on evaluation standards):

- *Utility standards* ensure that an evaluation will serve the information needs of intended users.

- *Feasibility standards* ensure that an evaluation will be realistic, prudent, diplomatic, and frugal.

- *Propriety standards* ensure that an evaluation will be conducted legally, ethically, and with due regard for the welfare of those involved in the evaluation, as well as those affected by its results.

- *Accuracy standards* ensure that an evaluation will reveal and convey technically adequate information about the features that determine worth or merit of the program being evaluated.

It is important to note that the **CDC framework standards** do not tell program managers how to conduct evaluations; instead, they serve to guide managers in choosing from among many options available to them at each step in the framework. For example, in the step of engaging stakeholders shown in Figure 9.3, the standards can help a manager decide which stakeholders should be engaged and how by suggesting these questions:

- *Utility*—Who will use the results of the evaluation?
- *Feasibility*—How much time and effort can a manager devote to stakeholder engagement?
- *Propriety*—To be ethical, which stakeholders should a manager consult (for example, only those served by the program, or members of the larger community in which it operates)?
- *Accuracy*—How much information does a manager need to provide to give stakeholders a complete and accurate picture of the program?

Although the standards are important in making certain that evaluations are conducted in a high-quality manner, the framework's greater value to managers conducting program evaluations lies in the carefully sequenced steps in the framework. Following these steps can guide a manager through the intricacies of program evaluation.

Steps in the CDC Evaluation Framework

The CDC evaluation framework depicted in Figure 9.3 includes six interconnected steps that form a pathway for tailoring an evaluation. In general, the earlier **CDC framework steps** provide the foundation for subsequent steps. The steps are as follows (CDC 2014; see the section on evaluation steps):

1. *Engage stakeholders*, including those involved in program operations; those served or affected by the program; and primary users of the evaluation.

2. *Describe the program*, including the need, expected effects, activities, resources, stage, context, and logic model.

3. *Focus the evaluation design* to assess the issues of greatest concern to stakeholders while using time and resources as efficiently as possible. Consider the purpose, users, uses, questions, methods, and agreements.

4. *Gather credible evidence* to strengthen evaluation judgments and the recommendations that follow. These aspects of evidence gathering typically affect perceptions of credibility: indicators, sources, quality, quantity, and logistics.

5. *Justify conclusions* by linking them to the evidence gathered and judging them against agreed-upon values or standards set by the stakeholders. Justify conclusions on the basis of evidence using these five elements: standards, analysis/synthesis, interpretation, judgment, and recommendations. [As shown in Figure 9.3, *making recommendations* is an essential component of this step.]

6. *Ensure use and share lessons learned* with these steps: design, preparation, feedback, follow-up, and dissemination.

    Each of these steps is discussed in more detail in the following sections.

Engaging Stakeholders

The first step in conducting an effective evaluation is to engage stakeholders, especially the people, organizations, and groups that have an investment in what will be learned through the evaluation and what will be done with the knowledge (see the first step in Figure 9.3). "Stakeholders can help (or hinder) an evaluation *before* it is conducted, *while* it is being conducted, and *after* the results are collected and ready for use" (CDC 2011, 13). Engaging stakeholders means seeking their input and fostering their participation. Engaging a program's internal stakeholders is especially important because doing so successfully increases the likelihood that the evaluation's results will be used. Engaging these stakeholders also can help increase the evaluation's credibility among program participants, clarify their roles and responsibilities in the evaluation, and avoid real or perceived conflicts among participants.

In regard to conducting evaluations, according to the CDC (2011, 14), often particular stakeholders are given more attention by program managers because the stakeholders

- Can increase the *credibility* of . . . [the] evaluation.

- Are responsible for day-to-day *implementation* of the activities that are part of the program.

- Will *advocate* for or *authorize changes* to the program that the evaluation may recommend.

- Will *fund* or *authorize the continuation or expansion* of the program.

Stakeholders play important roles throughout a program evaluation. Their perspectives can influence every step in the CDC evaluation framework. For example:

> Stakeholder input in "describing the program" ensures a clear and consensual understanding of the program's activities and outcomes. This is an important backdrop for even more valuable stakeholder input in "focusing the evaluation design" to ensure that the key questions of most importance will be included. Stakeholders may also have insights or preferences on the most effective and appropriate ways to collect data from target respondents. In "justifying conclusions," the perspectives and values that stakeholders bring to the evaluation are explicitly acknowledged and honored in making judgments about evidence gathered. Finally, the considerable time and effort spent in engaging and building consensus among stakeholders pays off in the last step, "ensuring use," because stakeholder engagement has created a market for the evaluation results. (CDC 2011, 16–17)

Describing the Program

A comprehensive program description conveys the mission and objectives of the program being evaluated and a great deal more (see the second step in Figure 9.3). It covers all the components of a program, including its intended effects or results (CDC 2011, 2014). The description sets the frame of reference for all subsequent decisions in an evaluation. A useful way to organize the program description is to include the following sections:

- *Need.* This section describes the problem or opportunity that the program is intended to address. It presents a rationale for the existence of the program. The more thoroughly and accurately the need for the program is described, the better. This section should leave no doubt that the program exists to respond to a real and significant problem or an important opportunity.

- *Expected effects or desired results.* This section describes what the program is expected to accomplish. It is where the program's mission and objectives are stated. Expected effects or desired results may also be described in terms of outputs and impact. For most programs, effects or results unfold over time, and this progression should be addressed in this section. For example, expected short-, middle-, and long-term effects or desired results can be described.

- *Activities.* This section describes what the program does to accomplish expected effects or desired results. Activities, which may also be called processes, reflect the actions undertaken to accomplish the program's mission and objectives.

- *Resources.* This section describes the people, technology, money, equipment and space, and other assets required to conduct program activities and accomplish expected effects or desired results. It is important to include resources, which may also be called inputs, in a comprehensive program description, because accountability for the use of resources is often the focus of evaluations. In addition, any sort of financial or economic evaluation is based on an understanding of a program's inputs and costs. It is axiomatic that when a program's intended effects are not occurring, or when its activities are not going as intended, inadequate resources may well be the root cause.

- *Stage of development.* This section describes where the program is located along a continuum of development at the time of the evaluation. All programs go through identifiable stages of development, akin to the life cycle of an organization, as they mature and change over time. In general, stages of development for programs include planning, implementation, and maintenance. In addition, a fourth stage, conclusion or termination, is applicable in some cases. A program in the planning stage will focus and conduct evaluations differently than will a more mature one in the maintenance stage; the evaluations are likely to have different purposes. The purpose when a program is in the planning stage may be to refine plans. The purpose when a program is in the maintenance stage is likely to be to determine both the degree to which expected effects or desired results are being realized and the factors facilitating or hindering the achievement of these effects or results.

- *Context.* This section describes the larger environment in which the program exists. Because the most important contextual variable is often the host organization in which the program is embedded, the description should include information about the host organization and the program's relationship to it. In addition, numerous other environmental or contextual variables are relevant. These include public policies relevant to the program, such as those having to do with Medicare or Medicaid, as well as general social and economic conditions that might affect the program, demographics of the program's service area, target markets and target audiences, the public- and private-sector funding environment of the program, what competitor programs are doing or planning, and perhaps relevant aspects of the history of the program.

- *Logic model.* This section describes schematically and discusses the relationships among the resources available to the program, the activities or work processes planned and undertaken with the resources, and the effects or results intended to be achieved through operating the program (Frechtling 2007). A logic model and its associated program theory are key components of a comprehensive description of the program.

Focusing the Evaluation Design

The third step in the CDC framework (see Figure 9.3) for conducting program evaluations is focusing the evaluation so that the most important evaluation questions are asked, and the most appropriate design for the evaluation is determined and selected (CDC 1999, 2011, 2014). Essentially, a good evaluation design reflects the best ways to provide credible evidence (that is, information) pertaining to the evaluation questions within the time frame and given the resources available. No matter what the specific design chosen, all evaluation designs should include the following basic components (GAO 2012, 18):

- the evaluation questions, objectives, and scope;

- information sources and measures, or what information is needed;

- data collection methods, including any sampling procedures, or how information or evidence will be obtained;

- an analysis plan, including evaluative criteria or comparisons, or how or on what basis program performance will be judged or evaluated;

- an assessment of study limitations

It is important to remember in this step that evaluations are studies designed to answer specific questions about how a program or some component of a program is working, or about how it did work in the case of summative evaluations. Thus, establishing an evaluation design should begin with developing the right questions to ask. Depending on what is being evaluated, there may be few or many questions. It may be possible for all questions to be answered within one overall evaluation design, although it is more likely that some questions will require specific designs. For example, a program manager conducting an evaluation of overall program performance may have an interest in the level of patient/customer satisfaction being achieved. Assessing satisfaction levels would require a design tailored to answer questions about satisfaction, whereas performance in other areas, such as financial performance or clinical performance, could be measured using the program's standard operating information. Once the program manager decides what questions the evaluation will attempt to answer, the rest of the process of designing an evaluation follows three specific steps (adapted from GAO 2012, 7):

1. Select an appropriate evaluation approach or design for each evaluation question.

2. Identify data sources and collection procedures to obtain relevant, credible information.

3. Develop plans to analyze the data in ways that allow valid conclusions to be drawn from the information obtained.

Adhering to the CDC framework's standards noted earlier, the manager will want an evaluation design that has utility, is feasible to conduct, and will meet standards of propriety and accuracy. This requires careful attention to the design, beginning with framing evaluation questions that are understandable and can be answered quantitatively or qualitatively as appropriate.

Different Purposes, Leading to Different Designs

Evaluations are conducted for various purposes. Different purposes lead to different evaluation questions, and thus to different designs. For example, a program evaluation may be conducted to do any of the following (adapted from GAO 2012, 13):

• Assess the extent of the program's effectiveness in achieving desired results

• Identify effective practices for achieving desired results

• Identify opportunities to improve program performance

• Ascertain the success of corrective actions

• Guide resource allocation within the program

• Support program budget requests

If the purpose of a program evaluation is to guide resource allocation, for example, then the evaluation questions might be tailored to identify which patients/customers are in greatest need of services, or which of the program's activities are most effective in achieving the desired results. If the purpose is to identify opportunities to improve program performance, then the questions should be about how various activities have been implemented or the adequacy of available resources.

Categories of Evaluation Designs

With the evaluation questions formulated, it is possible to determine the appropriate evaluation design. There are three categories of designs available: experimental, quasi-experimental, and observational. Typical program evaluations, especially those conducted by program managers or other program participants, are of the third type. Experimental and quasi-experimental designs are generally the domain of professional evaluators and researchers, and are not covered here. There are excellent books on experimental and quasi-experimental designs, such as those by Rossi, Lipsey, and Freeman (2004) and Wholey, Hatry, and Newcomer (2010).

Observational designs are commonly used in evaluating performance, whether of an entire program or of a component of a program, and include time-series analyses, cross-sectional surveys, and case studies. Goal-based evaluation designs are also popular in conducting program evaluations. Typically, the predetermined mission and objectives serve as the standards against which performance is evaluated. In a situation in which a logic model has been developed for a program being evaluated, desired results expressed as a mission and objectives can straightforwardly be used as the standards against which performance is evaluated.

Strong Designs

Well-designed evaluations "employ methods of analysis that are appropriate" to the question or questions on which the evaluation is focused (GAO 2012, 28). Such evaluations "support the answer with sufficient and appropriate evidence; document the assumptions, procedures, and modes of analysis; and rule out competing explanations" (28). Further, a strong design should do all of the following (adapted from GAO 2012, 28–29):

- *Be appropriate for the evaluation questions and context.* The design should address all key questions, clearly state any limitations in scope, and be appropriate to the nature and significance of the program or issue. For example, evaluations should not attempt to measure outcomes before a program has been in place long enough to be able to produce them.

- *Fully address the evaluation questions.* The strength of the design should match the precision, completeness, and conclusiveness of the information needed to answer the questions. Criteria and measures should be narrowly tailored, and comparisons should be selected to support valid conclusions and rule out alternative explanations.

- *Fit available time and resources.* Time and cost are constraints that shape the scope of the evaluation questions and the range of activities that can help answer them. Producing timely information enhances its usefulness. This aspect of a good evaluation design is especially important in the conduct of many health program evaluations, where available resources are constrained. Health programs typically do not allocate a large share of their financial resources to evaluating activities. Useful evaluations can be conducted, however, even when resources are constrained. For example, Table 9.1 illustrates how different types of evaluations typically used in evaluating programs' marketing activities can be undertaken with varying levels of resources, including levels that are minimal or modest.

- *Rely on sufficient, credible data.* No data collection process is free of error, but the data should be sufficiently free of bias or other significant errors that could lead to inaccurate conclusions. This attribute of a strong design is discussed in more depth in the next section. Whatever the design selected, it will influence the timing of data collection, how the data is analyzed, and the types of conclusions that can be drawn from the analyses.

Gathering Credible Evidence

In conducting a program evaluation, it is important for the manager to collect data and information that convey a well-rounded picture of the program, if the evaluation is to be seen as credible by its users. It is important to remember the definitions of data and information given in Chapter 2. Although related, data and information differ, and both are important in conducting evaluations. Data is "information in raw or unorganized form (such as alphabets, numbers, or symbols) that refer[s] to, or represent[s], conditions, ideas, or objects" (BusinessDictionary 2014a). Information is "data that is (1) accurate and timely, (2) specific and organized for a purpose, (3) presented within a context that gives it meaning and relevance, and (4) [possibly leading] to an increase in understanding and decrease in uncertainty" (BusinessDictionary 2014b).

Continuing to follow the CDC evaluation framework (CDC 1999, 2011, 2014; see the fourth step in Figure 9.3), the aspects of evidence (or data and information) that typically affect the evidence's credibility include the indicators selected, sources of data and information and collection methods,

Table 9.1   Options for Evaluating Commercial or Social Marketing Activities in Programs

Type of Evaluation	Minimal Resources	Modest Resources	Substantial Resources
Formative	• Focus groups to determine the service location and scheduling preferences (commercial) • A readability test of educational material (social)	• A limited survey to determine the program's name recognition (commercial) • Intercept interviews to determine target audience attitudes about health behaviors (social)	• Extensive market research designed to segment target markets (commercial) • Extensive assessment of the need for services among people in target audiences (social)
Process	• Record keeping to track how messages are delivered and received by target markets or audiences (commercial and social)	• A checklist review of implementation milestones (commercial and social)	• A complete management audit of implementation, including a review by external experts (commercial or social)
Outcome, short term	• Tracking changes in the use of services, such as in the number of visits or screenings (commercial) • Tracking people in target audiences' adherence to, attendance at, or compliance with an intervention (social)	• Analyzing changes in referral patterns (commercial) • Monitoring the percentage of people in target audiences who are aware of or participating in an intervention (social)	• Calculating changes in target market share (commercial) • Assessing people in target audiences for changes in knowledge through pre- and posttests (social)
Outcome, long term	• Monitoring trends in media coverage (commercial) • Monitoring trends in grant support for an intervention (social)	• Conducting public surveys to determine opinions about the program (commercial) • Conducting telephone surveys of target audiences to determine changes in health behaviors (social)	• Conducting a complete review of program performance after five-years, including audited financial performance (commercial) • Conducting formal studies of health status changes in people in target audiences (social)

as well as the quality and quantity of data and information and the logistics and protocols that guide its creation.

Indicators Selected

Indicators are specific, observable, and measurable pieces of data and information that help define exactly what is being sought as evidence or relevant data and information in a program evaluation. Indicators can pertain to program activities (process indicators), outcomes or effects (outcome indicators), or both. Examples of process indicators include levels of patient/customer satisfaction and efficiency of resource use. Examples of outcome indicators include changes in behavior, health status, or quality of life among patients/customers.

Sources of Data and Information and Collection Methods

After managers or other evaluators have decided what program activities or processes to measure or what results or outcomes to measure, the sources of data and information and methods of collecting them can be considered. The initial determination here is often whether there are existing data and information that can be collected from secondary sources or whether new data and information will have to be collected from primary sources.

A number of secondary data and information sources have direct relevance to many health programs, including

- The Current Population Survey and other U.S. Census files
- The Behavioral Risk Factor Surveillance System (BRFSS)
- The Youth Risk Behavior Survey (YRBS)
- The Pregnancy Risk Assessment Monitoring System (PRAMS)
- Cancer registries
- State vital statistics
- Various surveillance databases
- The National Health Interview Survey (NHIS)

When primary data and information are required in conducting a program evaluation, common sources include the following (CDC 2011, 59):

- Surveys, including personal interviews, telephone interviews, and instruments completed by respondent, received through the mail or e-mail
- Group discussions/focus groups
- Observation [of program activities]
- Document review, such as medical records, diaries, logs, minutes of meetings, etc.

Quality of Data and Information

The quality of data and information used in a program evaluation certainly affects the credibility of the evaluation. Quality in this context refers to the appropriateness and integrity of the data and information used. High-quality data and information are reliable, valid, and informative for their intended use. The following factors influence quality (CDC 2011):

- Design of the evidence (data and information) collection instruments and the wording of questions
- Evidence collection procedures

- Training of evidence collectors
- Selection of sources of evidence
- How the pieces of data are coded
- Data and information management
- Routine error checking as part of quality control

Quantity of Data and Information

Quantity in this context refers to the amount of data and information (evidence) gathered in an evaluation. The amount of evidence required can usually be estimated in advance, and end points indicating when to stop collecting data and information can be established. Determination of a sample size may require the services of a statistician. Arriving at the appropriate quantity of evidence to collect is important because it affects the potential confidence level or precision of the evaluation's conclusions. The quantity of evidence also partly determines whether the evaluation will have sufficient power to detect effects. From the manager's perspective, the appropriate quantity of data and information to collect is the amount that will ensure credibility of the evaluation, but no more. One of the manager's obligations in conducting a program evaluation is to minimize the burden placed on those providing needed data and information. This duty is balanced against the need for enough evidence to draw valid conclusions through the evaluation.

Logistics and Protocols

The final aspect of evidence collected in a program evaluation that affects the evaluation's credibility is the technical details of the methods, timing, and physical infrastructure for gathering and handling the data and information— that is, the logistics. An overriding logistical concern is, Do data and information collection procedures protect confidentiality? Other concerns include the following (adapted from CDC 2011, 67):

- When and at what intervals will data and information be collected?
- Will data and information be collected from all patients/customers, or from a sample?
- Who will collect the data and information?
- How will the security and confidentiality of the data and information be ensured?
- Will institutional review board (IRB) approval be needed before data and information are collected?

✓ Identify indicators (specific, observable, and measurable pieces of data and information) for activities and outcomes.

✓ Determine whether existing indicators will suffice, or whether new ones must be developed.

✓ Consider data and information sources, and choose the most appropriate ones.

✓ Consider data and information collection methods, and select those best suited for the evaluation.

✓ Pilot test new instruments as needed.

✓ Consider a mixed-method approach to data and information collection

✓ Consider quality and quantity issues in data and information collection.

✓ Develop a detailed protocol for data and information collection.

Figure 9.4   Checklist for Gathering Credible Evidence
Source: Adapted from Centers for Disease Control and Prevention. *Introduction to Program Evaluation for Public Health Programs: A Self-Study Guide.* Atlanta: Centers for Disease Control and Prevention, Office of Strategy and Innovation, 2011, 69.

Figure 9.4 presents a checklist for gathering credible evidence in conducting a program evaluation.

Justifying Conclusions and Making Recommendations

Once evidence—data and information—is gathered, it must be analyzed so that justifiable conclusions can be drawn and can serve as the basis for useful recommendations (see the fifth step in Figure 9.3). This is the overarching feature of program evaluations. According to the CDC (2011, 2014), conclusions are justified when the *findings* in the evaluation (the evidence) are *analyzed* and *synthesized*; then *interpreted* through the prism of *standards*; and then *judged* accordingly, with judgments serving as the basis for *recommendations.* These relationships are shown in Figure 9.5.

Justification of conclusions is important in conducting a program evaluation because it increases the chances that stakeholders will use the

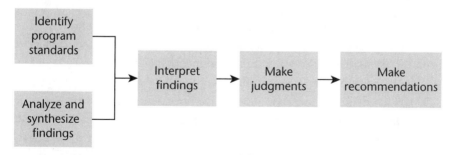

Figure 9.5   Justifying Conclusions and Making Recommendations in a Program Evaluation
Source: Adapted from Centers for Disease Control and Prevention. *Introduction to Program Evaluation for Public Health Programs: A Self-Study Guide.* Atlanta: Centers for Disease Control and Prevention, Office of Strategy and Innovation, 2011, 74.

recommendations resulting from the evaluation as a basis for working to improve or otherwise support the program. Each component of the process of justifying conclusions and making recommendations shown in Figure 9.5 is discussed in the following subsections.

Identify Program Standards

Standards are the benchmarks used to judge performance in an evaluation, whether evaluating activities or outcomes. Standards constitute the basis on which to judge that a program or a component of a program is successful, adequate, or unsuccessful. Sources of standards are numerous (CDC 2011; Phillips 2011), including

- The needs of patients/customers and other program participants
- Community values, expectations, and norms
- A program's mission and objectives
- The mission and objectives of a program's host organization
- Program protocols and procedures
- Performance by similar programs
- Performance by a control or comparison group
- Societal norms dictating that scarce resources be used wisely and efficiently
- Mandates, policies, regulations, and laws
- Judgments of participants, experts, and funders
- Societal norms for ethical behavior, social equity, and human rights

Analyze and Synthesize Findings

The "analyze and synthesize findings" box in Figure 9.5 represents the analytical processes undertaken using the evidence that has been collected for the evaluation. This work begins with organizing and classifying the evidence, perhaps in a database when the collected evidence is in the form of data. Such data can then be tabulated to provide useful information. For example, it can be stratified by various demographic variables of interest, such as race, gender, age, or income level. This data can then be presented in various ways, such as using bar graphs, pie charts, line graphs, and maps. "In evaluations that use multiple methods, evidence patterns are detected by isolating important findings (analysis) and combining different sources of information to reach a larger understanding (synthesis)" (CDC 2011, 75).

Interpret Findings

The "interpret findings" box in Figure 9.5 represents the efforts of the program manager or others conducting an evaluation to figure out what the findings mean. Evidence pertaining to the performance of a program or component is not sufficient to draw evaluation conclusions or make useful recommendations. The findings from an evaluation must be interpreted to determine their practical significance and implications. There are a number of things program managers can do to improve their interpretations of the findings from program evaluations, including the following:

- Involve others in interpreting findings (for example, stakeholders, consultants, or colleagues)

- Consider alternative explanations for findings

- Consider limitations of the findings, including validity and reliability limitations

- Compare findings with those from evaluations of similar programs

- Consider underlying theories that may support findings

- Assess patterns of findings using different data collection methods

- Consider whether findings are consistent with what was expected

Make Judgments

The "make judgments" box in Figure 9.5 represents the efforts of the program manager or others conducting an evaluation to judge the merit, worth, or significance of the program or a component of it being evaluated. These judgments are made by comparing against standards the findings and interpretations resulting from the evaluation.

It is certainly possible for stakeholders to make different—even conflicting—judgments, with discrepancies often reflecting the use of different standards. For example, a program manager using a standard of improved performance over time might judge a 10 percent increase in year-over-year enrollment very positively, whereas community members, using a social equity standard, might judge a 10 percent increase negatively, concluding that despite improvements, a minimum threshold of access to services was not reached. In the context of a program evaluation, such disagreement can catalyze discussion to clarify standards and reach consensus on which standards will be used in making judgments about the program. It is far better, however, if standards acceptable to all stakeholders have been established early in the conduct of an evaluation. This is why the first step in the CDC framework for conducting effective program evaluations is to engage stakeholders (see Figure 9.3). You may wish to go back to the discussion earlier in this chapter in the "Focusing the Evaluation Design" subsection.

Make Recommendations

The final step after justifying conclusions, as depicted in Figure 9.5, is to make recommendations (CDC 2011, 2014). The recommendations resulting from a program evaluation are unique to the particular evaluation. Typical recommendations, however, include those to continue, modify or redesign, curtail, expand, or terminate a program or some component of the program. Forming recommendations about such possible decisions and actions is a distinct element of program evaluation and goes beyond the previous step of making judgments. It is one thing to make a judgment that a program reduces risky sexual behavior, for example, but another thing to make a recommendation to continue or expand the program.

    In making recommendations, it is especially important that managers take into account the organizational context within which a program exists. Such variables in the host organization as the hierarchical structure and associated reporting relationships, leader styles, communication preferences, the degree of participation in decision making permitted, and many others should be considered in drafting recommendations. Program managers should realize that recommendations that are not based on sufficient evidence or that are not aligned with stakeholders' values and perspectives may damage an evaluation's credibility. Conversely, program managers who anticipate how recommendations will be received by stakeholders and highlight recommendations over which stakeholders can have some control improve the likelihood that their recommendations will be followed (Patton 2012). One thing a program manager can do to increase the chances that recommendations will be followed is to share the recommendations in draft form and solicit reactions and feedback from stakeholders before finalizing them. Another useful step, often appropriate, is to present recommendations as options rather than as directive statements or advice (CDC 2011, 2014).

Ensuring Use and Sharing Lessons Learned

The sixth and concluding step in the CDC (1999, 2011, 2014) framework for conducting program evaluations (see Figure 9.3) is to ensure that evaluation findings and lessons learned are disseminated and used appropriately. This requires deliberate effort by the program manager, who should remember that the primary purpose of most program evaluations is to produce information that will be used to improve the program being evaluated. Other specific uses include the following (adapted from CDC 2011, 82):

- To demonstrate accountability to stakeholders by showing them that resources are well spent and that the program is effective
- To aid in forming budgets, and to justify the allocation of resources
- To compare outcomes with those of previous years
- To compare actual outcomes with intended outcomes
- To suggest realistic intended outcomes
- To support developing/strategizing activity
- To focus attention on issues important to the program
- To promote the program
- To identify partners for collaborations
- To enhance the image of the program
- To retain or increase funding
- To provide program participants with direction
- To identify training and technical assistance needs

Program managers can increase the likelihood that the results of an evaluation will be used by giving attention to and planning for eventual users and uses of the results in the earliest design decisions about how the evaluation will be conducted (see the third step in Figure 9.3). This requires managers to plan how evaluation results will be used, with whom they will share results, and how communication about and dissemination of the results will be handled. Managers, in thinking broadly about how results will be communicated, will have to consider the audiences for those results and tailor messages and channels accordingly. (You may wish to review the discussion of communication in Chapter 6.)

A formal, written report is the primary means of communicating the results of most program evaluations. Figure 9.6 contains an outline for a typical **program evaluation report**. Various authors' tips on how to improve written evaluation reports can be summarized as follows (Fitzpatrick, Sanders, and Worthen 2010; Mertens and Wilson 2012; Royse, Thyer, and Padgett 2010):

- Include an executive summary, and consider that many in the audience will only read that part of the report.
- Provide intended users with the report in time for it to be used.

- **Executive Summary**
- **Background and Purpose**
  - Program background
  - Evaluation rationale
  - Stakeholder identification and engagement
  - Program description
  - Key evaluation questions and focus
- **Evaluation Methods**
  - Design
  - Sampling procedures
  - Measures or indicators
  - Data collection procedures
  - Data processing procedures
  - Analysis
  - Limitations
- **Results**
- **Discussion and Recommendations**
- **Technical Appendices**

Figure 9.6   Outline of a Program Evaluation Report
Source: Centers for Disease Control and Prevention. *Introduction to Program Evaluation for Public Health Programs: A Self-Study Guide.* Atlanta: Centers for Disease Control and Prevention, Office of Strategy and Innovation, 2011, 86.

- Tailor the report's content, format, and style for the intended audience.
- Summarize the description of the stakeholders and how they were engaged.
- Describe essential features of the program, including the program's logic model.
- Explain the focus of the evaluation and its limitations.
- Include a descriptive summary of the evaluation plan and procedures.
- Specify the standards for evaluation judgments.
- Explain the evaluation judgments and how they are supported by the evidence collected.
- Identify and list both strengths and weaknesses of the evaluation.
- Discuss recommendations for decisions and actions, with their advantages, disadvantages, and resource implications.
- Ensure confidentiality for the program's patients/customers and other stakeholders.

- Anticipate how people, organizations, or groups might be affected by the findings.

- Present minority opinions or rejoinders where appropriate.

- Verify that the report is accurate and unbiased.

- Organize the report logically, and include appropriate details.

- Avoid or remove technical jargon.

- Use examples, illustrations, graphics, and stories generously.

- Provide all necessary technical information in appendices when appropriate.

The CDC framework (1999, 2011, 2014) for conducting program evaluations described in this section is purposely general; it is intended as a guide for designing and conducting a wide variety of evaluations. Following the steps in conducting evaluations of health programs shown in Figure 9.3 can be of great assistance to program managers as they perform the facilitative management activity of evaluating.

Summary

This chapter addresses program managers' facilitative activity of evaluating—in particular, evaluating entire programs or component parts of programs. It is noted that at its most basic level, evaluating anything means determining "its merit, worth, value, or significance" (Patton 2012, 2). Program evaluation is defined generically as "carefully collecting information about a program or some aspect of a program to make necessary decisions about the program" (McNamara 2014). Program managers evaluate three distinct aspects of their programs or component parts of them: their implementation, their effectiveness, and their accountability to key stakeholders.

It is noted that evaluations of entire programs or component parts of programs benefit from a thorough understanding of the program as a starting point. Two useful tools in understanding any program are the underlying program theory of how the program is supposed to work, and the associated schematic logic model of the program. The logic model for a program is based on the program's theory.

Among numerous types of program evaluations, the widely used process and outcome evaluations, formative and summative evaluations, and cost-benefit and cost-effectiveness evaluations are defined and described.

Much of the chapter is organized around a comprehensive framework for use in designing and conducting evaluations. The framework, developed by the Centers for Disease Control and Prevention (1999, 2011, 2014), is shown in Figure 9.3 and includes six steps and four sets of standards for conducting evaluations of health programs or components of them. The standards, which guide managers in choosing from among many options available to them at each step in the framework, are in the areas of utility, feasibility, propriety, and accuracy (CDC 2014). The six interconnected steps in the CDC framework shown in Figure 9.3 are as follows:

1. Engage stakeholders.
2. Describe the program.
3. Focus the evaluation design.
4. Gather credible evidence.
5. Justify conclusions and make recommendations.
6. Ensure use and share lessons learned.

A formal, written report is the primary means of communicating the results of most program evaluations. Figure 9.6 contains an outline for a typical evaluation report, and a number of tips on how to improve written evaluation reports are provided.

REVIEW QUESTIONS

1. Define program evaluation, and discuss it as a facilitative management activity.
2. What do program managers evaluate?
3. Define program theory and logic models. Discuss the relationship between them.
4. Discuss the uses of program theory and logic models in program evaluation.
5. List and describe six of the most widely used types of program evaluations.
6. Draw a schematic diagram of the CDC framework for conducting program evaluations. Include the steps and standards in the framework.
7. Discuss how program managers can use the standards in the CDC framework to design and conduct a program evaluation.
8. Describe what program managers do in focusing an evaluation design.
9. Discuss what program managers do when justifying conclusions and making recommendations in a program evaluation. Draw a schematic diagram of this process.
10. Make an outline for a typical evaluation report.

KEY TERMS AND CONCEPTS

CDC framework for program evaluation

CDC framework standards

CDC framework steps

cost-benefit evaluation

cost-effectiveness evaluation

evaluating

formative evaluation

logic model

outcome evaluation

process evaluation

program evaluation

program evaluation report

program theory

summative evaluation

References

BusinessDictionary. "Data." Accessed May 30, 2014a. http://www.businessdictionary .com/definition/data.html

BusinessDictionary. "Information." Accessed May 30, 2014b. http://www.business-dictionary.com/definition/information.html

Centers for Disease Control and Prevention. "Framework for Program Evaluation in Public Health." *Morbidity and Mortality Weekly Report* 48, no. RR-11 (September 17, 1999): 1–40.

Centers for Disease Control and Prevention. *Introduction to Program Evaluation for Public Health Programs: A Self-Study Guide.* Atlanta: Centers for Disease Control and Prevention, Office of Strategy and Innovation, 2011.

Centers for Disease Control and Prevention. "A Framework for Program Evaluation." Accessed May 27, 2014. http://www.cdc.gov/eval/framework/index.htm

Fallon, L. Fleming, Jr., James W. Begun, and William Riley. *Managing Health Organizations for Quality and Performance.* Burlington, MA: Jones & Bartlett Learning, 2013.

Fitzpatrick, Jody L., James R. Sanders, and Blaine R. Worthen. *Program Evaluation: Alternative Approaches and Practical Guidelines*, 4th ed. Upper Saddle River, NJ: Pearson, 2010.

Fournier, Deborah M. "Evaluation Defined." In *Encyclopedia of Evaluation*, edited by Sandra Mathison, 139–140. Thousand Oaks, CA: Sage, 2005.

Frechtling, Joy A. *Logic Modeling Methods in Program Evaluation.* San Francisco: Jossey-Bass, 2007.

Funnell, Sue C., and Patricia J. Rogers. *Purposeful Program Theory: Effective Use of Theories of Change and Logic Models.* San Francisco: Jossey-Bass, 2011.

McDavid, James C., Irene Huse, and Laura R. L. Hawthorn. *Program Evaluation and Performance Measurement: An Introduction to Practice*, 2nd ed. Thousand Oaks, CA: Sage, 2013.

McNamara, Carter."Basic Guide to Program Evaluation." Accessed May 26, 2014. http://managementhelp.org/evaluation/program-evaluation-guide.htm

Mertens, Donna M., and Amy T. Wilson. *Program Evaluation Theory and Practice: A Comprehensive Guide.* New York: Guilford Press, 2012.

Office of Planning, Research and Evaluation. *The Program Manager's Guide to Evaluation*, 2nd ed. Washington, DC: U.S. Department of Health and Human Services, Administration for Children and Families, Office of Planning, Research and Evaluation, 2010.

Patton, Michael A. *Essentials of Utilization-Focused Evaluation.* Thousand Oaks, CA: Sage, 2012.

Phillips, Jack J. *Return on Investment in Training and Performance Improvement Programs*, 2nd ed. New York: Routledge, 2011.

Renger, Ralph, and Allison Titcomb. "A Three-Step Approach to Teaching Logic Models." *American Journal of Evaluation* 23, no. 4 (2002): 493–503.

Rossi, Peter H., Mark W. Lipsey, and Howard E. Freeman. *Evaluation: A Systematic Approach*, 7th ed. Thousand Oaks, CA: Sage, 2004.

Royse, David, Bruce A. Thyer, and Deborah K. Padgett. *Program Evaluation: An Introduction*, 5th ed. Belmont, CA: Wadsworth, Cengage Learning, 2010.

Russ-Eft, Darlene, and Hallie Preskill. *Evaluation in Organizations: A Systematic Approach to Enhancing Learning, Performance, and Change.* New York: Basic Books, 2009.

U.S. Government Accountability Office. *Designing Evaluations.* GAO-12-208G. Washington, DC: U.S. Government Accountability Office, January 2012.

Weiss, Carol H. *Evaluation: Methods for Studying Programs and Policies*, 2nd ed. Upper Saddle River, NJ: Prentice Hall, 1998.

Wholey, Joseph S., Harry P. Hatry, and Kathryn E. Newcomer. *Handbook of Practical Program Evaluation*, 3rd ed. San Francisco: Jossey-Bass, 2010.

W. K. Kellogg Foundation. *Evaluation Handbook.* Battle Creek, MI: W. K. Kellogg Foundation, 2004.

Yarbrough, Donald B., Lyn M. Shulha, Rodney K. Hopson, and Flora A. Caruthers. *The Program Evaluation Standards: A Guide for Evaluators and Evaluation Users*, 3rd ed. Thousand Oaks, CA: Sage, 2011.

Continuous improvement (CI): (*Continued*)
health care quality, 245–254; Pareto chart
for, 253; run chart for, 253–254, 254*fig*; Six
Sigma approach, 246–247; tools for,
252–254; TPS, 247; TQ and, 15
Continuous quality improvement (CQI),
228–229, 242
Control techniques, 9–10
Controlling performance: adjusting and
correcting, 61–62; budget control, 62–66;
in developing/strategizing activity, 59–66,
76; in HIV screening program, 60*fig*;
monitoring and comparing, 60–61
Cooperating, 43, 123, 195
Coordination (or integration), 11, 114;
effective, 93–94; interdependence and,
93–94
Coordination mechanisms: categorization of,
95–98; menu of, 98–99; overview, 94;
teams, 98
Cost-benefit analysis, 183–184, 200
Cost-benefit evaluation, 317
Cost-effectiveness evaluation, 317
Counseling, 218
CQI. *See* Continuous quality improvement
Creative process, 175–177
Credibility, 321
Crosby, Philip, 242
Cross-training, 85, 177
CSFII. *See* Continuing Survey of Food Intakes
by Individuals
Current Population Survey, 329
Customs, 97–98

Daft, Richard L., 6
Data, 61; HEDIS, 71; information as raw data,
188; information quality and, 328–329;
information quantity and, 330; sources, 328
Decision grid, 178–179, 179*fig*, 200
Decision making: autocratic, 163–164, 165*fig*;
characteristics of management decisions,

166–168; consultative, 163–164, 165*fig*;
defined, 162–163, 199; management work
facilitative activities, 13, 13*fig*; with other
program participants, 163–166; overview,
161–162; summary, 199–200; Vroom's
decision making model, 163–164, 165*fig*
Decision making alternatives: assessing,
178–190; brainstorming, 176–177;
choosing alternative, 190–192; cost-benefit
analysis, 183–184, 200; creative process,
175–177; decision grid, 178–179, 179*fig*,
200; decision tree, 181, 182*fig*, 183, 200;
developing, 174–178; DSS, 188–190,
189*fig*; no-action, 190; nominal group
technique, 176–177; payoff table, 179–181,
180*fig*; PERT, 184–185, 186*fig*, 187–188;
stimulating and supporting creativity,
177–178; three questions to ask, 191–192
Decision making implementation: actual
implementation, 196–198; general
approach to, 193; Lewin's decision
implementation model, 196–198, 197*fig*;
planning for implementation, 192–196;
situational diagnosis in, 192; support for
and reducing resistance to decisions,
193–196; trial basis, 198
Decision making process, 169*fig*; assessing
alternatives, 178–190; authority and, 123,
146; awareness of problem, 168–170;
choosing alternative, 190–192; defining
problem or opportunity, 170–174;
developing relevant alternatives, 174–178;
evaluating decision, 198–199; fishbone
diagram, 171, 172*fig*, 173–174, 173*fig*;
implementing the decision, 192–198;
incubation period, 176; Pareto chart for,
171; seven-step process, 199; verification
in, 176
Decision support system (DSS), 188–190,
189*fig*
Decision tree, 181, 182*fig*, 183, 200